FRACTURES OF THE PELVIS AND ACETABULUM

FRACTURES OF THE PELVIS AND ACETABULUM

Edited by
Wade R Smith
Denver Health Medical Center
University of Colorado School of Medicine
Denver, Colorado, USA
Bruce H Ziran
St. Elizabeth Health Center
Northeastern Ohio Universities College of Medicine
Youngstown, Ohio, USA
Steven J Morgan
Denver Health Medical Center
University of Colorado School of Medicine
Denver, Colorado, USA

informa
healthcare

New York London

Informa Healthcare USA, Inc.
52 Vanderbilt Avenue, 7th Floor
New York, NY 10017

Printed in the United States of America on acid-free paper
10 9 8 7 6 5 4 3 2 1

International Standard Book Number-10: 0-8247-2846-7 (Hardcover)
International Standard Book Number-13: 978-0-8247-2846-5 (Hardcover)

Library of Congress Cataloging-in-Publication Data

Fractures of the pelvis and acetabulum / edited by Wade R. Smith, Bruce H. Ziran, Steven J Morgan.
p. ; cm.
Includes bibliographical references and index.
ISBN-13: 978-0-8247-2846-5 (hb : alk. paper)
ISBN-10: 0-8247-2846-7 (hb : alk. paper)
1. Pelvic bones–Fractures. 2. Acetabulum (Anatomy)–Fractures. I. Smith, Wade R. II. Ziran, Bruce H. III. Morgan, Steven J. IV. Title.
[DNLM: 1. Pelvic Bones–injuries. 2. Fractures, Bone–surgery. 3. Pelvic Bones–surgery. 4. Reconstructive Surgical Procedure. WE 750 S663f 2007]
RD549.S59 2007
617.5′5044–dc22 2007008980

Visit the Informa web site at
www.informa.com

and the Informa Healthcare Web site at
www.informahealthcare.com

Preface

Fractures of the pelvis and acetabulum are among the most challenging injuries to treat in orthopaedic surgery. Pelvic injuries continue to have a high acute mortality and cause severe long-term disability. Tremendous improvements in prehospital resuscitation and transfer of injured patients have brought many patients to the hospital who previously would have died in the field. The trauma team is challenged to maintain blood pressure in these patients by stopping pelvic hemorrhage and limiting systemic damage. If resuscitation of these patients is successful, the next challenge is to reconstruct high energy injuries often with concomitant nerve and articular damage. The overall severity of pelvis fractures undergoing reconstruction is likely to increase given that highly comminuted fracture patients are surviving. It may be said that the pelvis that used to die now needs "fixing," and our standard techniques may not be suitable for these highly complex injuries.

Once reconstruction occurs, the next challenge is rehabilitation of the injured patient. Surgeons have become increasingly aware that outcome is not simply an x-ray finding, or even a score on a validated scale. Outcome for the patient with pelvic and acetabular injuries is a complex analysis that comes down to the basics of life for many patients. Posttraumatic arthrosis, chronic pain, nerve damage, and bowel, bladder, and sexual dysfunction, intertwined with psychological distress are the real challenges to the patient. No matter how heroic the initial work and salvage of the patient's life, ultimately the quality of life becomes the sine qua non of a "good" result. While many centers are working diligently to improve the acute outcome of pelvic fracture patients and fixation techniques for the pelvis and acetabulum, the time has come to apply the same energy toward improvements in post-injury rehabilitation. The interface of the patient, the surgeon, the rehabilitation specialist, and society may be the next frontier in the management of pelvic and acetabular injuries.

In consideration of the preceding surmises, this book aims to cover the basics of pelvic and acetabular injuries, but also expose the reader to the detailed, practical experience of surgeons who are dealing with these complex injuries every day. The variety of authors is intentional to provide wide exposure to the gamut of philosophies and techniques. No matter the continent or the country, there are good surgeons working hard to obtain the best results possible for their patients. Our hope is that you, the reader, will find within these pages some measure of information or, better yet, inspiration to help you in your efforts.

Wade R. Smith
Bruce H. Ziran
Steven J Morgan

Contents

Contributors

Scott A. Adams Department of Orthopaedics, Denver Health Medical Center, University of Colorado School of Medicine, Denver, Colorado, U.S.A.

Deniz W. Baysal Department of Orthopaedic Surgery, University of Texas Southwestern Medical Center, Dallas, Texas, U.S.A.

Johannes K. M. Fakler Department of Trauma and Reconstructive Surgery, Charité—University Medical School Berlin, Berlin, Germany

Axel P. Gänsslen Department of Trauma, Hannover Medical School, Hannover, Germany

David J. Hak Department of Orthopaedics, Denver Health Medical Center, University of Colorado School of Medicine, Denver, Colorado, U.S.A.

Robert M. Harris Department of Orthopaedic Trauma, Atlanta Medical Center, Atlanta, Georgia, U.S.A.

Dolfi Herscovici Department of Orthopaedic Traumatology, University of South Florida, Tampa, Florida, U.S.A.

Thomas F. Higgins University of Utah, Department of Orthopaedics, Salt Lake City, Utah, U.S.A.

Daniel S. Horwitz University of Utah, Department of Orthopaedics, Salt Lake City, Utah, U.S.A.

Kyle J. Jeray Department of Orthopaedic Surgery, Greenville Hospital System, Greenville, South Carolina, U.S.A.

Enes M. Kanlic Department of Orthopaedic Surgery and Rehabilitation, Texas Tech University Health Sciences Center, El Paso, Texas, U.S.A.

Christian Krettek Department of Trauma, Hannover Medical School, Hannover, Germany

Douglas W. Lundy Orthopaedic Trauma Surgery, Resurgens Orthopaedics, Atlanta, Georgia, U.S.A.

Stefan Machtens Department of Urology, Hannover Medical School, Hannover, Germany

Steven J Morgan Department of Orthopaedics, Denver Health Medical Center, University of Colorado School of Medicine, Denver, Colorado, U.S.A.

Steven A. Olson Division of Orthopaedic Surgery, Duke University Medical Center, Durham, North Carolina, U.S.A.

Patrick M. Osborn Department of Orthopaedics, Denver Health Medical Center, University of Colorado School of Medicine, Denver, Colorado, U.S.A.

Hector O. Pacheco Department of Orthopaedic Surgery and Rehabilitation, Texas Tech University Health Sciences Center, El Paso, Texas, U.S.A.

Ian Pallister Department of Trauma and Orthopaedics, Morriston Hosptial, University of Wales Swansea, Morriston, Swansea, U.K.

Hans-Christoph Pape Department of Orthopaedic Surgery, University of Pittsburgh Medical School, Pittsburgh, Pennsylvania, U.S.A.

Rodrigo Pesantez Departamento de Ortopedia y Traumatología, Fundación Santa Fe de Bogotá, Bogotá, Colombia

Miguel Pirela-Cruz Department of Orthopaedic Surgery and Rehabilitation, Texas Tech University Health Sciences Center, El Paso, Texas, U.S.A.

Daniel R. Schlatterer Department of Orthopaedic Trauma, Atlanta Medical Center, Atlanta, Georgia, U.S.A.

Wade R. Smith Department of Orthopaedics, Denver Health Medical Center, University of Colorado School of Medicine, Denver, Colorado, U.S.A.

Philip F. Stahel Department of Orthopaedics, Denver Health Medical Center, University of Colorado School of Medicine, Denver, Colorado, U.S.A.

Adam J. Starr Department of Orthopaedic Surgery, University of Texas Southwestern Medical Center, Dallas, Texas, U.S.A.

Allison E. Williams Department of Orthopaedics, Denver Health Medical Center, University of Colorado School of Medicine, Denver, Colorado, U.S.A.

Bruce H. Ziran Department of Orthopaedic Trauma, St. Elizabeth Health Center and Department of Orthopaedic Surgery, Northeastern Ohio Universities College of Medicine, Youngstown, Ohio, U.S.A.

1
Anatomy of the Pelvis

Rodrigo Pesantez
Departamento de Ortopedia y Traumatología, Fundación Santa Fe de Bogotá, Bogotá, Colombia

Bruce H. Ziran
Department of Orthopaedic Trauma, St. Elizabeth Health Center and Department of Orthopaedic Surgery, Northeastern Ohio Universities College of Medicine, Youngstown, Ohio, U.S.A.

INTRODUCTION

Familiarity with pelvic anatomy is essential for the treatment of pelvic fractures. With an increase in minimally invasive approaches in fixation methods, knowledge of pelvic anatomy is vital to safe reduction and fixation of displaced fractures. The purpose of this chapter is to review the salient features of the anatomy of the pelvis pertinent to the treatment of traumatic conditions.

Pelvis is the Latin term for basin. The pelvic basin is divided by the pelvic rim into the true pelvis (deep) and the false pelvis (superficial). The false pelvis consists of the sacral wing and iliac fossa covered by iliacus muscle. The pelvic brim continues anteriorly to contain the pectineal eminence and becomes confluent with the superior pubic ramus. The deep pelvis is bordered by the quadrilateral surfaces, obturator membrane, rami, and sacrum. The deep pelvis contains the extra peritoneal visceral structures such as the bladder, vagina, terminal colon, rectum, and perineal and pelvic floor suspensory structures. The floor of the pelvis or pelvic diaphragm is made up of the levator and coccygeus muscles and is pierced by the urethra, the rectum, and the vagina (Fig. 1).

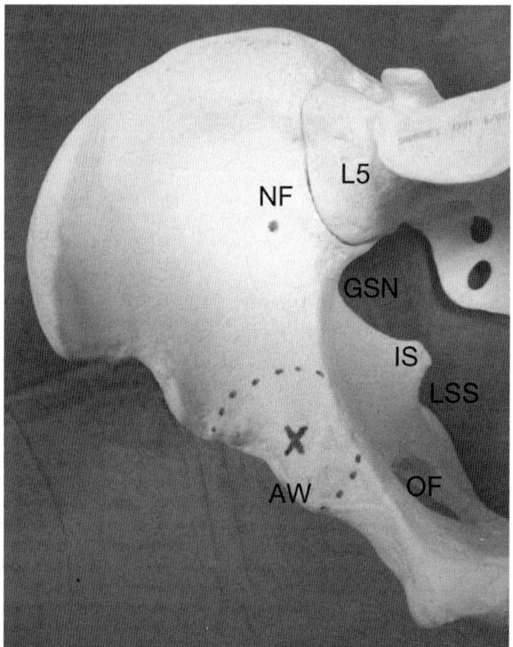

Figure 1 A model of the pelvis seen from an inlet view. The false or superficial pelvis is delineated by the area above the iliopubic ridge. The true or deep pelvis is the volume within. The *dashed lines* represent the area of the anterior wall with femoral head underneath. This region is dangerous for screw placement. The X represents the iliopectineal eminence. NF usually found in front of the sacro-iliac joint. L5 represents the approximate location of the course of the L5 nerve root as it coalesces with the lumbar plexus. *Abbreviations*: GSN, greater sciatic notch; IS, Ischial spine; LSS, lesser sciatic notch; NF, nutrient foramen; OF, obturator foramen.

OSSEOUS ANATOMY

The pelvis is the osseous structure that transfers the weight of the upper axial skeletal structures to the lower extremity via the hip joint. The pelvic ring is comprised of the sacrum and three bones on each side that coalesce during adolescence to form the inominate bone of the adult pelvis. The sacrum connects to the ilium via an irregular joint, the iliosacral joint, which is technically an apophyseal joint. The ilium becomes the pubis anteriorly and the ischium inferiorly. Anteriorly, the two pubic bones connect to one another via the symphysis and thus close the ring.

Acetabulum

The coalescence of the three bones, the ilium, ischium, and pubis, join to each other centrally to form the cotyloid or acetabular cavity. Here, the anlage of the acetabulum develops in utero and as an infant. While not fully developed, alterations or abnormalities can result in conditions of the hip joint such as developmental dysplasia of the hip. The early blood supply to the femoral head traverses through the cotyloid fossa and ligamentum teres. While mostly a vestigial structure in adulthood, this ligament occupies the cotyloid fossa, which is a noncartilagenous, intra-articular portion of the acetabulum. The cartilaginous portion of the acetabulum is a horseshoe-shaped surface that transfers load from the inominate bone to the femur and lower extremity. Its mechanics and vectors of load have been well elucidated and described elsewhere by Olson and Vrahas.

Iliac Wing and Inominate Bone

The external iliac fossa is marked with two semicircular lines dividing it into three zones: posterior (gluteus maximus), middle (gluteus medius), and anterior (gluteus minimus). Within the anterior section, the nutrient artery is found, located near the reflected head of the rectus femoris. The crista glutea is the primary origin of the gluteus maximus and it is located along the border of the posterior superior iliac spine (Fig. 2). The shape of the iliac wing from above is s-shaped as it begins anteriorly with a slight medial oblique orientation. By the time it becomes the posterior iliac spine, it is more sagittally oriented (Fig. 3). The iliac wing is full of hematopoetic and osteogenic marrow elements and is the primary source of autogenous bone graft. Along the crest there is a thickening along which many muscular structures attach. Along the outside are the lower extremity hip motors, while the abdominal (anteriorly) and paraspinal (posteriorly) muscles attach along the top. Along the inner portions the iliacus and obturator internus and pelvic floor musculature attach.

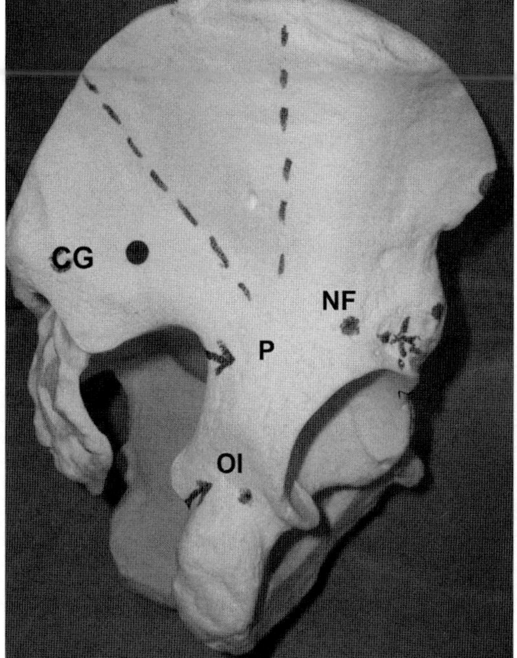

Figure 2 Outer table of the ilium and acetabulum. As noted in text, the ilium can be divided into three anatomic regions. The posterior section, is where the juntional attachments to the sacrum occur. The middle section is a relatively thin area that is mostly for muscle attachment. The anterior segment has the thick anterior pillar of the anterior column. This bone is thick and strong and is primarily where external fixator pins are placed. CG: crista gluteau, origin of gluteus maximus. NF: approximate location of nutrient foramen. Just anterior, in the area of the X is the reflected head attachment of the rectus muscle. OI and arrow: the course and location of the obturator internus tendon within the lesser sciatic notch. P and arrow: the course and location of the piriformis tendon.

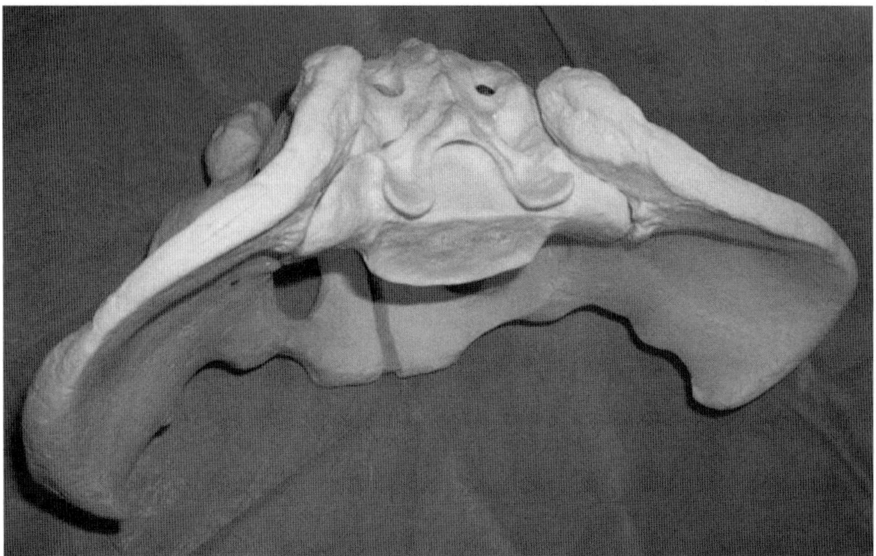

Figure 3 A superior view of the iliac crest. Note the gentle "S" shape which becomes nearly sagittal in its most posterior elements. This is important to know for fixation of screws during anterior and posterior approaches where the "other side" of the bone is not visible.

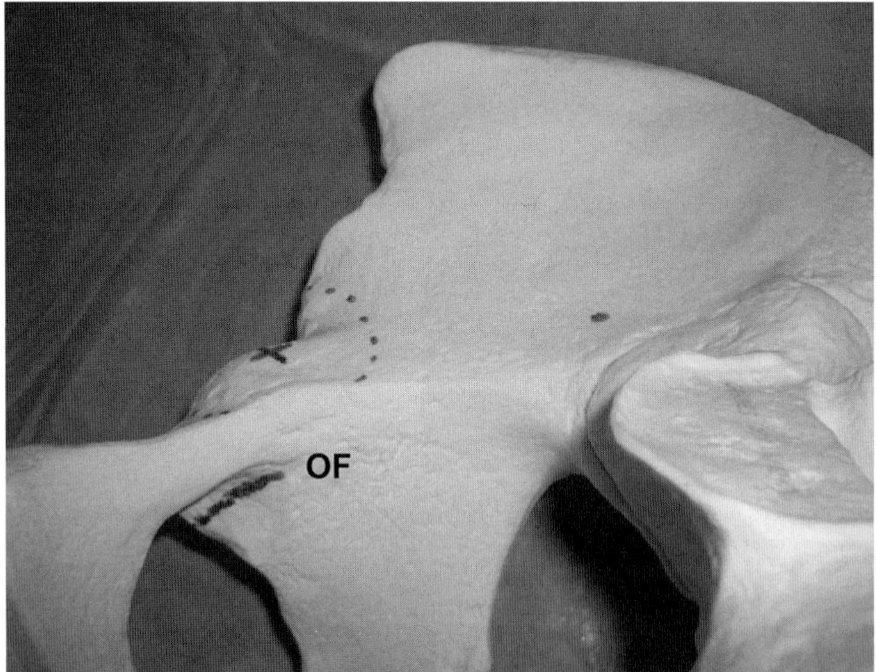

Figure 4 An inside out view of the obturator foramen. This would be similar to the view from the sub-inguinal window of the ilio-inguinal approach.

There are both inner and outer cortices along most of the ilium, except in the most central portion, which thins to a unicortical shell, especially during older age. The posterior inner table, just lateral and anterior to the iliosacral joint contains a major nutrient artery, which is frequently a source of bleeding during surgery in this area. The mechanics of bone and load transfer predicate that there is a strong buttress of bone emanating from the iliosacral joint towards the acetabulum. This structure is termed the sciatic buttress. Nearby structures include the coalescence of the lumbosacral plexus as well as the gluteal vasculature. These vessels are often the source of bleeding during injury and can be reinjured during surgical treatment.

Posteriorly, the posterior superior iliac spine is adjacent to the sacroiliac joint and outer ilium. The sciatic notch is the point at which the neurovascular structures exit the pelvis along with the piriformis muscle. The ischial spine is where the sacrospinous ligament, the gemellus superior, and the levator ani are inserted. On the other side of the ischial spine is the lesser sciatic notch, which contains the obturator internus tendon. The pudendal vessels and nerves pass through this area, first exiting the pelvis and then re-entering it distally.

The anterior-most border of the inominate bone begins with the anterosuperior iliac spine (ASIS), which is the origin of the fascia lata, sartorius, and inguinal ligament. Just below the ASIS is the anteroinferior iliac spine (AIIS) where the direct head of the rectus femoris is inserted. Just medial to the AIIS pass the iliopsoas muscles, under which lies the illiopectineus eminence. Inferior to the AIIS is the indirect head of the rectus femoris and the acetabulum.

The obturator foramen is bordered by the pubis superiorly, the ischium inferiorly, and the anterior horn of the acetabulum posteriorly. Medially, the ischial and pubic rami join to form the symphyseal pubic junction. At its superior–lateral border, the obturator duct is found, which is occupied by obturator vessels and nerve. The foramen is almost circumferentially covered by obturator membrane, which is a thick fascial structure. It is this membrane and the integrity of the inguinal ligament that prevents separation of rami fractures during reduction and fixation of symphyseal plating (Fig. 4).

Sacrum

The sacrum is quadrangular, pyramid-shaped, and forms, together with the last lumbar vertebra, the sacrovertebral angle or promontory. The sacrum is generally wider proximally than distally and has an anterior concavity. The sacrum sits obliquely in the pelvis and is very difficult to interpret radiographically. The sacrum has several major cephalad body segments that can be used for fixation and then tapers in its caudad body segments to become the coccyx. Alongside each vertebral body are the alar roots, which are homogenously connected laterally, contain the sacral foramen, and become the medial aspect of the iliosacral joint. Each foramen is itself obliquely oriented in the sacrum, headed in a posterior–superior–medial direction. The central portion contains the terminal spinal canal and posteriorly is enclosed by confluent laminae that contain posterior foramen. Within this terminal canal are the individual nerve trunks of the filum terminale.

The specific orientation of osseous landmarks of the sacrum and posterior pelvis related to radiographic imaging have only recently been described in detail by Ziran et al. and Ebraheim et al. The S1 ala is where the L5 nerve root lies and this area is of paramount importance when placing iliosacral screws. The superior ala can have various dysmorphisms and be concave or convex. There can also be either a sacralization of the L5 vertebral body, where there is a bony confluence of the alar and vertebral structures, or there can be a lumbarization of the S1 body, wherein there is some separation of the alar and vertebral structures of S1 and S2. In the normal sacrum, the superior ala and iliosacral joint are important to visualize during the placement of percutaneous S1 screws since there can be a risk of injuring the L5 nerve root. The entry point for fixation on the lateral ilium needs to lie inferior and posterior to the superior ala in order to minimize the chance of an in-out-in screw. The opacity seen on fluoroscopy is most likely the confluence of the sacral ala with the iliac cortex, as well as the subchondral bone of the iliosacral joint. It is referred to as the alar slope or iliac cortical density. The orientations of the anterior and superior aspects of the sacrum are important as they are the main landmarks used for directing percutaneous screws into the S1 body.

LIGAMENT ANATOMY—THE JOINTS

The iliosacral joint is covered by fibrocartilage, acts as a dual wedge in axial and anteroposterior directions, and is like a keystone during the transmission of force to the lower limbs. The joint itself has little to no motion due to the strong supporting ligaments anteriorly and posteriorly. The posterior sacro-iliac ligament consists of (*i*) the superficial part going from posterior iliac crest and posterior iliac spines to the posterior tubercles of the sacrum made up of several fascicles, which include Zagals' ligament and Bichat's sacrospinous ligament; and (*ii*) the deep portion or interosseous ligament,

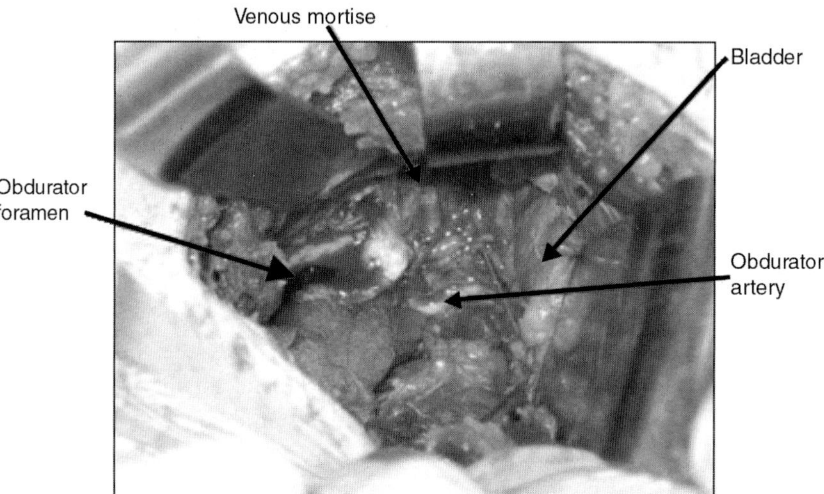

Figure 5 Corona mortise vessels traveling from the iliacs vein and artery toward the obdurator vessels as they exit the obdurator foramen internally.

which is the strongest ligament in human body. The anterior ligaments are mostly capsular and are usually the first to be disrupted with pelvic injury. There are also connections to the lumbar vertebrae via the iliolumbar ligaments going from the L5 transverse process to the iliac crest. These also make up part of the investing fascia covering the lumbar musculature.

The sacrotuberous ligament goes from the posterior iliac spines and sacrum to the ischial tuberosity. The sacrospinous ligament goes from the border of sacrum and coccyx in a plane deep to the sacrotuberous ligament and sciatic spine. This ligament divides the ischial area into two foramen: the greater sciatic foramen and the lesser sciatic foramen. The superior region, or greater sciatic foramen, contains the piriformis muscle, superior glutei nerves, sciatic nerve, ischial vessels, and internal pudendal vessels and nerve. The inferior region, or lesser sciatic foramen, contains the obturator internus muscle and internal pudenda vessels, which have crossed over the sacrospinous ligament (after exiting the pelvis via the greater sciatic foramen) to re-enter the pelvis via the lesser sciatic foramen. Lastly, the lateral sacrolumbar ligaments go from the L5 transverse apophysis down to the sacrum. Put together, these ligaments help withstand rotational and transverse stresses and vertical shearing stresses. In the front, the symphysis pubis is connected via an interosseous ligament.

VASCULAR ANATOMY

In the lower peritoneal region, the aorta bifurcates into the common iliac arteries, with a central ramus that extends in front of the sacrum and becomes the median sacral artery. The common iliac artery is rather short, beginning at around L4 and divides at around the L5–S1 junction into the external and internal arteries. The internal iliac artery or hypogastric artery, branches to form the superior and inferior gluteal vessels, the obturator, the pudendal, and the coccygeal, as well as the sacral and vesicular vessels. The internal pudendal artery goes out from the pelvis underneath the piriformis and re-enters the pelvis through the minor sciatic notch and terminates as the dorsal artery of penis and clitoris and cavernous artery.

The external iliac branches just proximal to the inguinal ligament into the femoral artery. The femoral artery has three rami: urethral inferior, epigastric, and iliac circumflex. The epigastric travels deep and then anastamoses with obturator vessels. When this connection is anomalously large, it is called the corona mortis, or crown of death (Fig. 5).

NEUROLOGIC ANATOMY

There are two important plexus: lumbar and sacrum.

Lumbar plexus consists of the first three lumbar anterior rami and a portion of the anterior ramus of the fourth lumbar nerve. These are commonly contained along the psoas muscle. There are also short collateral rami, which include the hypogastric, ilioinguinal, genitofemoral, and lateral femoral cutaneous nerve. The terminal rami of the lumbar plexus are the femoral and obturator nerve.

The obturator nerve receives contributions from the L2, L3, and L4 trunks, portions from the plexus near the sacro-iliac joint, continues into the pelvis underneath the iliopectineal line, reaches the obturator orifice, and then exits the pelvis together with the obturator vessels. The obturator nerve quickly divides into terminal rami surrounding the brevis muscle, and innervates the adductors and external obturator muscles.

The femoral nerve receives contributions from the L2, L3, and L4 trunks. The main trunk of the femoral nerve continues along the psoas (on its external border) and then passes through the femoral arch. Its terminal branches include the external musculocutaneous, the internal musculocutaneous, the femoral, and the internal saphenous nerves.

The sacral plexus is made by the union of the lumbosacral trunk (L5 anterior ramus with an L4 anasamotic ramus) and the anterior rami of the first four sacral roots. The plexus will ultimately become the major element of the sciatic nerve (posterior tibial and peroneal). There are other viscerally oriented branches that include the hemorrhoidal nerve, anus elevator nerve, and internal pudendal nerves. The posterior branches relevant to orthopedic surgery are the superior gluteal nerve, branches to the external rotators, and inferior gluteal nerve. As the sciatic nerve it exits the greater sciatic notch, courses in front of the piriformis nearly 85% of the time (the other variants include penetration and splitting around the muscle), and then courses behind the obturator internus, under the gluteal sling to enter the thigh. The sciatic nerve is a vital structure that is nearly always noted during posterior approaches to the acetabulum and pelvis. Because of the close proximity of the sciatic nerve and its major branch, the peroneal nerve, to the posterior portion of the acetabulum, fractures and dislocations in this area have a significant incidence of nerve injury.

SUMMARY

The pelvic anatomy is complex and must be understood in three dimensions. The intimacy of vital soft tissue structures such as vessels, nerves, and viscera with the osseous anatomy presents a narrow window of safety for the operating surgeon. Miscalculation of a centimeter during dissection or placement of drills can cause severe hemorrhage or permanent nerve injury. The best strategy for preventing damage during surgery and limiting the damage of the initial injury is having detailed knowledge of every aspect of pelvic anatomy.

BIBLIOGRAPHY

Ebraheim NA, Lin D, Xu R, Stanescu S, Yeasting RA. Computed tomographic evaluation of the internal structure of the lateral sacral mass in the upper sacra. Orthopaedics 1999; 22(12):1137–1140.

Hoppenfeld S, de Boer P. Surgical Exposures in Orthopaedics, 3rd ed. Philadelphia: Lippincott Williams and Wilkins, 2003.

Letournel E, Judet R. Fractures of the Acetabulum, 2nd ed. Berlin, Heidelberg, New York: Springer-Verlag, 1993.

Rohen JW, Yokochi C. Color Atlas of Anatomy, 3rd ed. Igaku-Shoin, Philadelphia: Lippincott Williams & Wilkins, 1993.

Tile M. Fractures of the Pelvis and Acetabulum, 2nd ed. Philadelphia: Lippincott Williams and Wilkins, 1995.

Zinghi GF. Fractures of the Pelvis and Acetabulum. Stuttgart, Germany: Thieme Verlag, 2004.

Ziran BH, Wasan AD, Marks DM, Olson SA, Chapman MW. Fluoroscopic imaging guides of the posterior pelvis pertaining to iliosacral screw placement. J Trauma 2007; 62(2):347–356.

2
Classification of Pelvic Ring Injuries

Johannes K. M. Fakler
Department of Trauma and Reconstructive Surgery, Charité—University Medical School Berlin, Berlin, Germany

Philip F. Stahel
Department of Orthopaedics, Denver Health Medical Center, University of Colorado School of Medicine, Denver, Colorado, U.S.A.

Douglas W. Lundy
Orthopaedic Trauma Surgery, Resurgens Orthopaedics, Atlanta, Georgia, U.S.A.

ANATOMICAL REMARKS

The osseous pelvic ring consists of the bilateral iliac, ischial, and pubic bones, which are posteriorly completed by the sacrum. In combination with the strong ligaments, the pelvis represents the anatomical and functional link between the spine and the lower extremities. During growth, the iliac, ischial, and pubic bones are connected by an inverse y-shaped epiphyseal junction, which is later fused into the osseous hemipelvis by a synostosis in adults. The pelvic ring is closed by the pubic symphysis anteriorly and by the strong sacroiliac ligaments posteriorly. It is divided anatomically by the terminal line into an upper "false pelvis" and a lower "true pelvis," the latter protecting the pelvic organs. The terminal line extends from the promontorium along the arcuatal and ileopectineal lines and ends at the upper pubic crest at the edge of the symphysis. The symphysis consists of an interpubic disk, which is supported ventrocranially by the anterior pubic ligament and dorsocaudally by the arcuate pubic ligaments, thus enabling the pelvis to bear vertical shear forces anteriorly. Posteriorly, the sacroiliacal joints are supported by a strong sacroiliacal ligament complex, consisting of the anterior, interosseous, and posterior sacroiliac ligaments as well as the sacrospinous and sacrotuberous ligaments. The biomechanical stability of the pelvic ring is essentially dependent on the integrity of this ligamentous complex. Aside from neutralizing rotational shear and stress forces on the pelvic ring, the main function of these posterior ligaments consists in bearing the transmission of axial/vertical loading forces from the spine to the lower extremities. Apart from these biomechanical aspects, the pelvic ring functions as a protection for organs of the urogential and gastrointestinal tract as well as vascular and nervous structures. In particular, the posterior presacral and paravesical venous plexus are relevant to surgical considerations, since traumatic injuries may cause severe hemorrhagic shock subsequent to venous mass bleeding. Furthermore, the proximity of the lumbosacral truncus and the sacral and coccygeal nervous plexus to the posterior pelvic ring and sacrum render these important neural structures particularly vulnerable to injuries affecting the posterior pelvic ring. Accordingly, the close topographic relation of urogenital organs to the osseous pelvic ring implicates the high risk of associated vulnerability in case of pelvic ring disruption. Injuries of the vagina, the uterus, or the anorectum by blunt trauma are rare and more frequently associated with open pelvic fractures, for example, due to perineal impalement injuries.

MECHANISMS OF INJURY

The severity of pelvic ring disruption depends on the mechanism of injury: high or low energy impact, direct or indirect forces, blunt or perforating trauma, and the direction or resulting vector of the impacting forces have to be taken into account when estimating the extent of pelvic trauma. The stability of the injured pelvic ring is evaluated based on radiological appearances, physical findings, and the knowledge of the mechanism of injury.

The integrity of the biomechanically pivotal, axial load-transferring posterior pelvic ring complex represents the prime determinant for pelvic ring stability. Thus, fracture patterns considered as fully stable (type A) do not involve posterior pelvic ring

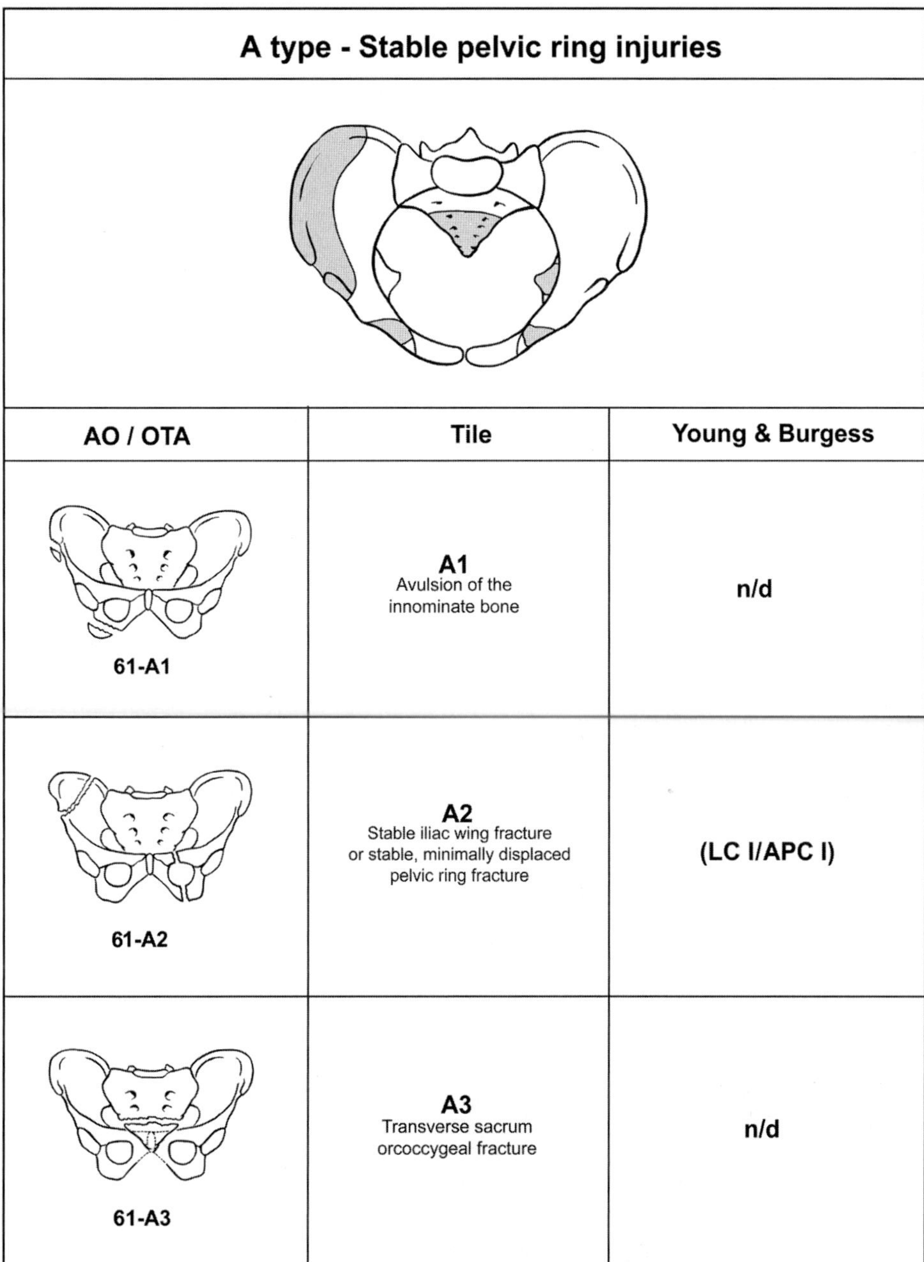

A type - Stable pelvic ring injuries

AO / OTA	Tile	Young & Burgess
61-A1	**A1** Avulsion of the innominate bone	n/d
61-A2	**A2** Stable iliac wing fracture or stable, minimally displaced pelvic ring fracture	(LC I/APC I)
61-A3	**A3** Transverse sacrum orcoccygeal fracture	n/d

Figure 1 Classification of stable pelvic ring injuries (A type). Comparison of injury pattern and mechanism of injury as defined by the three standard classifications. *Abbreviations*: AO, Arbeitsgemeinschaft für Osteosynthesefragen (Association for the Study of Internal Fixation); APC, anterior–posterior compression; LC, lateral compression; OTA, Orthopedic Trauma Association; *Source*: Charts kindly provided by Mrs. M. Peters, University Hospital Benjamin Franklin, Berlin (adapted from Ref. 4).

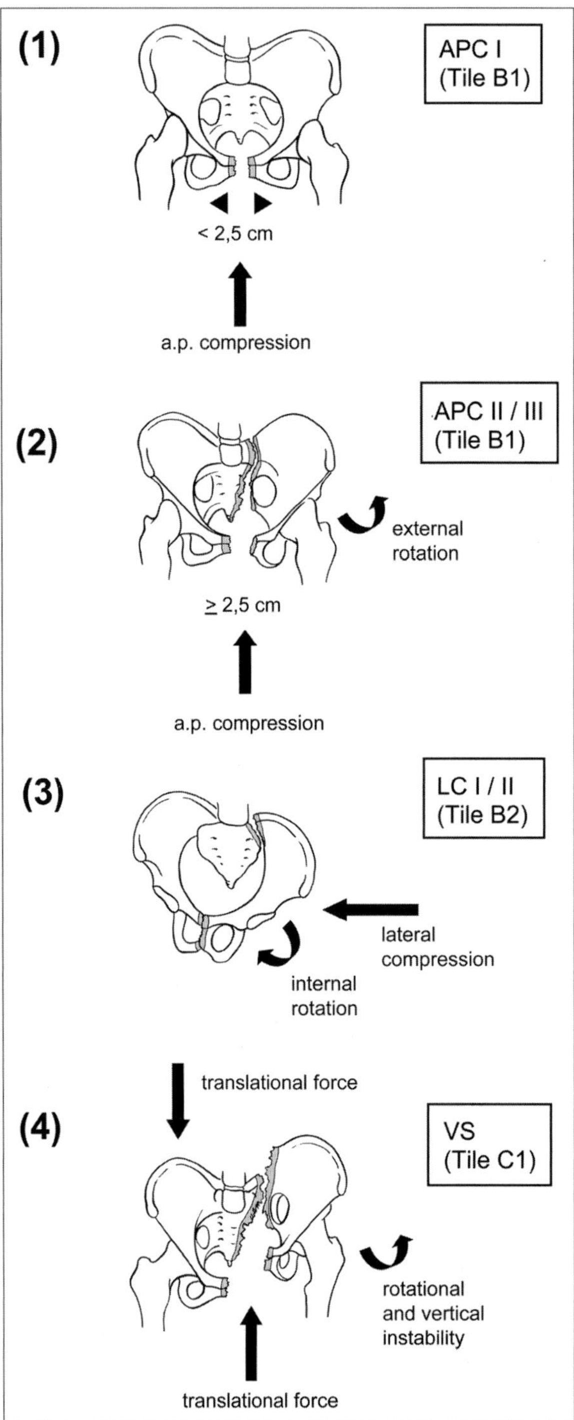

Figure 2 "Classical" mechanisms of injury with resulting fracture patterns. *Abbreviations*: APC, anterior–posterior compression; LC, lateral compression; VS, vertical shear. *Source*: Charts kindly provided by Mrs. M. Peters, University Hospital Benjamin Franklin, Berlin.

elements. Such injuries are usually caused by low-energy trauma in combination with a lateral force vector, typically characterized by pubic rami fractures in elder patients with osteoporosis (e.g., type A2; Fig. 1). In contrast, unstable pelvic ring injuries require a high-energy mechanism of trauma, leading to a partial (type B) or complete (type C) disruption of posterior pelvic ring elements, including sacral fractures and sacroiliac ligament complex injuries. As shown in Figure 2, the mechanism of injury leads to distinct injury patterns with defined archetypes of dislocation of the injured hemipelvis. The knowledge of the exact mechanism of injury and of the resulting force vector represents the basis for pelvic ring fracture classifications. In this regard, four distinct entities of pelvic ring injury patterns have to be differentiated, depending on the resulting force vector on the pelvic ring.

1. Anterior–posterior compression (APC) injuries
2. Lateral compression (LC) injuries
3. Vertical shear (VS) injuries
4. Combined mechanical (CM) injuries

These mechanisms of injury represent the fundamentals for modern classifications of pelvic fractures. Depending on the compressing force, an APC type injury may result in a stable fracture pattern without symphyseal diastasis (<2.5 cm) or in a disruption of the symphysis (≥ 2.5 cm), resulting in an externally rotated hemipelvis (Figs. 2 and 3). In these types of injuries there is no cephalad shift of the injured hemipelvis. The pathology to posterior elements in APC-type injuries depends on the impacting force. Marvin Tile (1) demonstrated that a symphyseal diastasis of ≥ 2.5 cm is usually associated with a disruption of the anterior sacroiliac (SI), sacrospinous, and sacrotuberous ligaments. Complete instability is not achieved until all SI ligaments, that is, anterior and posterior, are affected (APC-III type injury; Fig. 4). In contrast to the externally rotated hemipelvis resulting from APC-type forces, LC force vectors induce an internal rotation of the injured hemipelvis (Figs. 2 and 3) where the anterior SI–ligament complex is affected by crushing rather than by tensile forces. Finally, high-velocity translational forces (Fig. 2) lead to a complete disruption of all posterior pelvic ring elements, thus inducing a combined rotational and vertical instability (type C injuries, Fig. 4).

Lateral and anterior–posterior compression injuries often are associated with traffic accidents (i.e., side or frontal collision of cars or motorcycles), but may also be the consequence of a "roll-over" mechanism or a crush injury. Vertical shear injuries usually result from high-velocity trauma by motorcycle accidents or falls from heights onto the lower limbs where the SI joint and sacrum are subjected to shear stress by massive axial loading. The complete ligamentous and/or osseous disruption of the posterior pelvis leads to cephalad (vertical) displacement of the hemipelvis, accompanied by symphyseal diastasis ≥ 2.5 cm, and/or fractures of the anterior pelvic ring. These shearing injuries are both rotationally and vertically unstable. Finally, since the injuring force vectors cannot always by stratified into one of the above-mentioned mechanistic groups (APC, LC, VS), complex or mixed type injury patterns may occur as a consequence of multiple vectors acting upon the pelvic ring simultaneously (combined mechanical/CM-type injuries, Fig. 4). These mechanisms of injury provide the basis for classification of fractures of the pelvic ring.

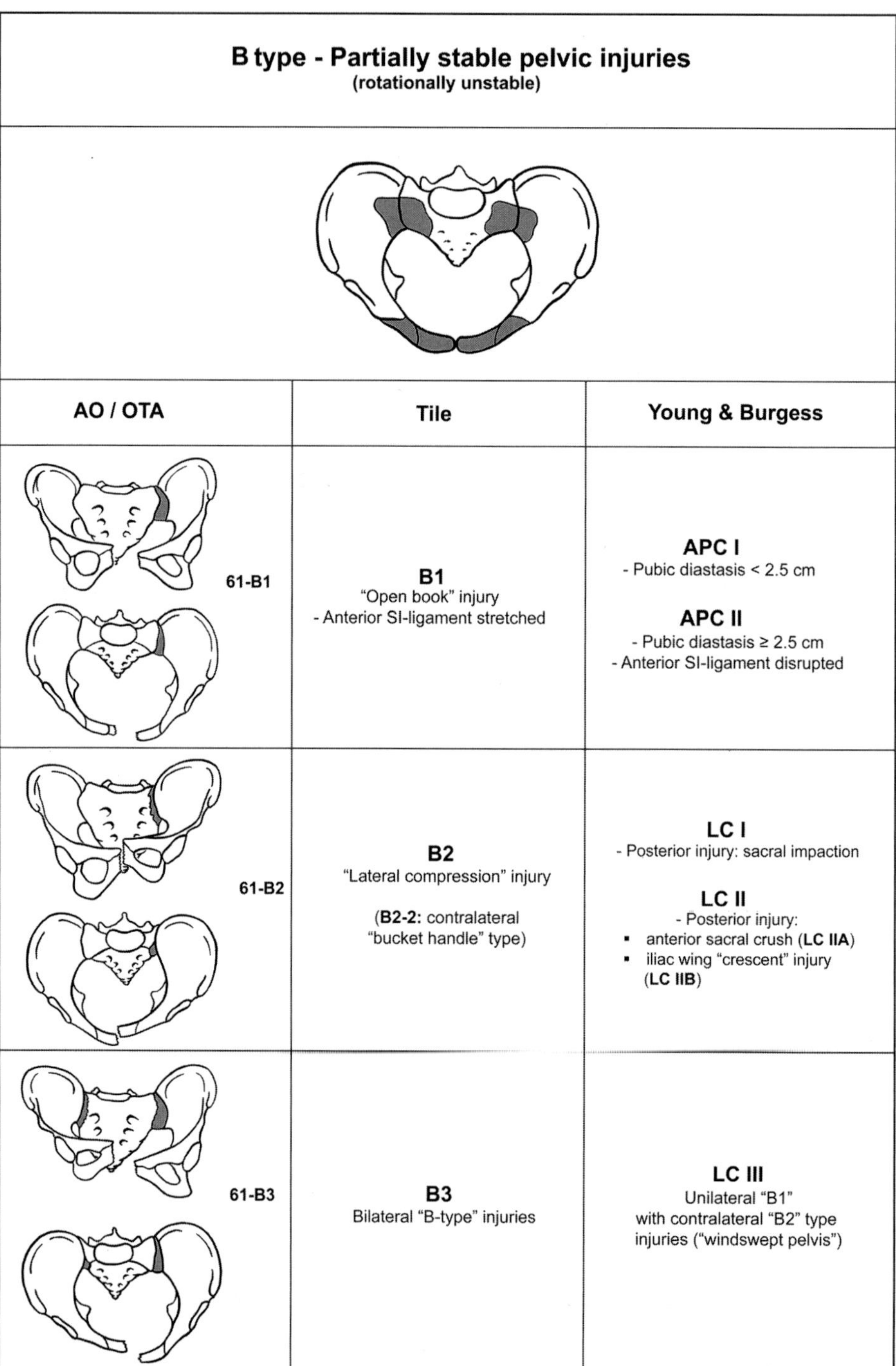

B type - Partially stable pelvic injuries
(rotationally unstable)
AO / OTA
Tile
Young & Burgess
61-B1
B1
"Open book" injury
- Anterior SI-ligament stretched
APC I
- Pubic diastasis < 2.5 cm
APC II
- Pubic diastasis ≥ 2.5 cm
- Anterior SI-ligament disrupted
61-B2
B2
"Lateral compression" injury
(B2-2: contralateral
"bucket handle" type)
LC I
- Posterior injury: sacral impaction
LC II
- Posterior injury:
▪ anterior sacral crush (LC IIA)
▪ iliac wing "crescent" injury (LC IIB)
61-B3
B3
Bilateral "B-type" injuries
LC III
Unilateral "B1"
with contralateral "B2" type
injuries ("windswept pelvis")

Figure 3 Classification of rotationally unstable pelvic ring injuries (B type). Comparison of injury pattern and mechanism of injury as defined by the three standard classifications. *Abbreviations*: AO, Arbeitsgemeinschaft für Osteosynthesefragen (Association for the Study of Internal Fixation); APC, anterior–posterior compression; LC, lateral compression; OTA, Orthopedic Trauma Association. *Source*: Charts kindly provided by Mrs. M. Peters, University Hospital Benjamin Franklin, Berlin (adapted from Ref. 4).

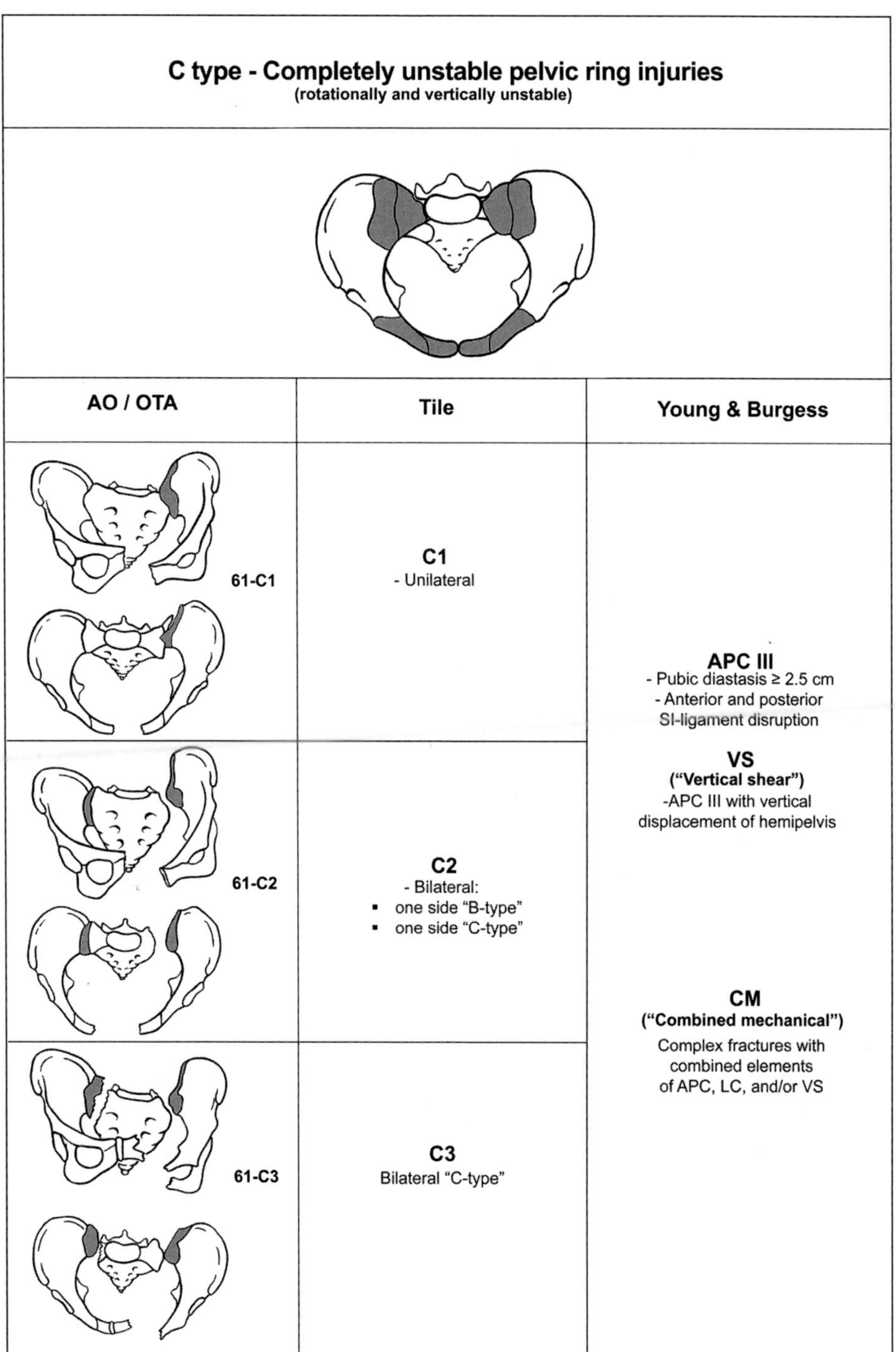

C type - Completely unstable pelvic ring injuries
(rotationally and vertically unstable)
AO / OTA
Tile
Young & Burgess
61-C1
C1
- Unilateral
61-C2
C2
- Bilateral:
one side "B-type"
one side "C-type"
61-C3
C3
Bilateral "C-type"
APC III
- Pubic diastasis ≥ 2.5 cm
- Anterior and posterior
SI-ligament disruption
VS
("Vertical shear")
-APC III with vertical
displacement of hemipelvis
CM
("Combined mechanical")
Complex fractures with
combined elements
of APC, LC, and/or VS

Figure 4 Classification of completely unstable pelvic ring injuries (C type). Comparison of injury pattern and mechanism of injury as defined by the three standard classifications. *Abbreviations*: AO, Arbeitsgemeinschaft für Osteosynthesefragen (Association for the Study of Internal Fixation); APC, anterior–posterior compression; CM, combined mechanical; LC, lateral compression; OTA, Orthopedic Trauma Association; VS, vertical shear. *Source*: Charts kindly provided by Mrs. Peters M, University Hospital Benjamin Franklin, Berlin (adapted from Ref. 4).

CLASSIFICATIONS OF CLOSED PELVIC RING INJURIES

Modern classification systems for pelvic ring injuries represent a key instrument for orthopedic trauma surgeons for evaluating the extent of pelvic trauma and judging the risk for potentially life-threatening injuries. Accurate classification systems should allow an adjusted treatment modality for specific pelvic ring injury patterns and therefore contribute to reduced mortality, particularly due to pelvic hemorrhagic–traumatic shock.

The French surgeon Joseph François Malgaigne (1806–1865) was the first to describe a classification system for pelvic fractures as early as the 19th century. More than 50 different classification systems for pelvic fractures have been proposed and published since then. Most of the early classification systems are based on a purely descriptive nature and are therefore in large part not clinically relevant. The first clinically relevant systematic classification based on the mechanism of injury was introduced by Pennal and Sutherland in 1961 (2). For the first time, classification was based on the force vectors of LC, APC, and VS injury patterns. However, as a drawback, the early Pennal–Sutherland classification did not provide an estimate for the clinically important parameter of pelvic ring stability.

In 1980, Pennal and Tile (3) implemented the aspect of stability into the 1961 classification by incorporating the different conditions of partial and complete instability based on the mechanism of trauma. Since then, the definition of pelvic ring instability has been based on the gradually decreasing osteoligamentous integrity of the posterior pelvic ring (Figs. 2–4). In contrast, a stable pelvic ring has been defined for all cases where the major axial load-transferring structures of the posterior pelvic ring are not affected (Fig. 1). For example, this is the case for low-energy APC or LC trauma leading to fractures of the anterior pelvic ring.

The AO/OTA [Arbeitsgemeinschaft für Osteosynthesefragen (Association for the Study of Internal Fixation)/Orthopedic Trauma Association] (4) classification system for pelvic ring fractures is based on Tile's classification (Figs. 1, 3, and 4). The last substantial revision of the AO/OTA classification was published in 1996 and is based on the main force vector and the determinants of pelvic ring stability.

The classification by Young and Burgess (5) is based on the Pennal and Sutherland (2) classification system from 1961. In this classification, the direction of the force vector (APC and LC) was defined more subtly by quantifying the extent of force applied to the pelvic ring (Figs. 3, 4). In addition to the "classical" force vectors (LC, APC, and VS), a fourth category of complex injuries resulting from diverse force vectors was defined as the "combined mechanical" (CM) injury type (Fig. 4).

Marvin Tile's classification

The Tile classification is alphanumerical and categorized into three main groups according to the extent of pelvic ring instability:

Type A: Stable
Type B: Partial instability (rotationally unstable)
Type C: Complete instability (rotationally and vertically unstable)

Stable injuries of the A type (Fig. 1) imply the osteoligamentous integrity of the posterior pelvic ring. They are most commonly caused by a low-energy trauma. The subgroups are defined as:

Type A1: Rim avulsion fractures of the iliac spine or tuberosity

Type A2: Stable iliac wing fractures or minimally displaced fractures of the pelvic ring

Type A3: Inferior transverse fractures of the sacrum or coccyx

Rotationally unstable injuries of the B type (Fig. 3) are characterized by a complete anterior pelvic ring disruption in conjunction with an incomplete disruption of the posterior elements. This leads to partial instability with respect to rotation, while vertical stability is maintained. The subgroups are defined as:

Type B1: Also referred to as the "open book" injury by Tile. This type of injury is induced by an APC mechanism leading to symphyseal diastasis or obturator ring fractures of the anterior pelvic with partial (anterior) sacroiliac diastasis (*Type B1.1*) or a sacral fracture (*Type B1.2*). This injury pattern is unstable with regard to external rotation, but the posterior sacroiliac ligaments remain partially intact, thus providing vertical stability.

Type B2: The "lateral compression" injury is characterized by Tile as an internal rotation of the hemipelvis with anterior pubic rami fractures and posterior impaction fracture of the sacrum across the sacroiliac joint. The subgroups of B2 type injuries are defined as:

Type B2.1: Ipsilateral injury with two distinct injury patterns: (*i*) dislocation and internal rotation of the pubic rami, potentially causing urogenital lesions, especially in young female patients, are referred to as "tilt fractures;" (*ii*) the "locked symphysis" is characterized by a fixed overlapping dislocation of the symphysis.

Type B2.2: Contralateral injury with fracture of the rami and cranial rotation of the anterior pelvic ring pictorially mimicking a "bucket handle" pattern.

Type B2.3: Incomplete posterior iliac fracture.

Recently, Pol Rommens et al. (6, 7) have suggested that Tile's B1- and B2-type injuries should be classified reciprocally, that is, the "lateral compression" injury as B1 and the "open book" injury as B2. This critique is based on data from a large retrospective study of 100 B-type injuries, where significantly higher complication and mortality rates were found in patients with B1-type injuries as opposed to the B2-type subsets (7). Until present, this re-evaluation of Tile's B-type subsets remains a topic of controversy.

Type B3: Combined bilateral B-type injuries

Type B3.1: Bilateral B1-type injuries

Type B3.2: Bilateral combination of B1- and B2-type injuries

Type B3.3: Bilateral B2-type injuries

The C-type (Fig. 4) injuries are defined as completely unstable pelvic ring disruptions with rotational and vertical instability. Translational high-velocity forces lead to a "vertical shear" mechanism with a complete disruption of the anterior and posterior pelvic rings and a vertical displacement of the hemipelvis.

Type C1: Unilateral injury
Type C2: Unilateral C-type injury, contralateral B-type injury
Type C3: Bilateral C-type injuries

The AO/OTA Classification

The AO/OTA classification system is based on the alphanumerical classification by Tile. In the revised classification, the pelvic ring and acetabulum were defined as bone segments No. 61 and 62, respectively (4). The detailed fracture patterns of stable (A-type), partially unstable (B-type), and completely unstable (C-type) fractures are depicted in Figures 1, 3, and 4.

Young and Burgess Classification

The classification by Young and Burgess (5) is also based on Pennal's 1961 system incorporating the role of the force vector and its direction in pelvic ring injuries. Additionally, LC and APC injuries were split into subgroups depending on the severity of the traumatic impact (Figs. 3 and 4). Similarly to the injury mechanisms defined by Tile, VS injuries represent a different entity in the Young and Burgess classification. In addition to Pennal's system, Young and Burgess classified a fourth group of complex fractures defined as CM injuries (Fig. 4).

- LC injuries occur by direct or indirect lateral impact and lead to internal rotation of the ipsilateral hemipelvis. The anterior pubic rami fractures are typically transverse and the degree of posterior pelvic involvement differentiates the subsets:
  - *LC I*: Anterior transverse fracture patterns of the pubic rami combined with a lateral compression fracture of the ipsilateral sacrum, eventually involving neural foramina. This injury is regarded as stable in most cases.
  - *LC II*: Anterior transverse pelvic fracture patterns with internal rotation of the hemipelvis towards the midline. Posterior injury is typically represented by a crescent iliac wing fracture leaving a small fragment of the posterior ilium firmly attached to the intact posterior sacroiliac ligaments. Stress load on anterior sacroiliac, sacrotuberous, and sacrospinous ligaments is rather relieved than increased. Consequently, this type of injury is vertically, but not rotationally stable.
  - *LC III*: Combination of LC-I or LC-II injuries with contralateral "open-book" (APC) injury. This type of fracture is associated with a high-energy trauma, that is, with high velocity or crush injuries. Combined rotational instability and maintained vertical stability also depicts this injury pattern as a "windswept pelvis."
- APC injuries arise from force impact in the sagittal plane. This type of injury is characterized by a diastasis of the symphysis or a vertical fracture pattern

through one or both sets of pubic rami. Depending on the integrity of the posterior pelvic ligamentous complex, the subgroups are defined as:

- *APC I*: Mild symphyseal diastasis (<2.5 cm) or vertical fracture pattern of the rami and eventually slight widening of the sacroiliac joint. Symphyseal ligaments are disrupted, whereas the anterior sacroiliac, sacrotuberous, and sacrospinous ligaments are stretched, but intact. This type of injury is generally judged as a rotationally and vertically stable fracture.
- *APC II*: Symphyseal diastasis (≥2.5 cm) or anterior vertical fracture pattern and widening of the sacroiliac joint by external rotation of the innominate bone. The anterior sacroiliac, sacrotuberous, and sacrospinous ligaments are disrupted, resulting in rotational instability. On the other hand, the unaffected, strong posterior sacroiliac ligaments provide stability in the vertical plane.
- *APC III*: Symphyseal diastasis or anterior vertical fracture pattern and complete separation of the hemipelvis. Anterior and posterior sacroiliac ligaments are completely disrupted, resulting in rotational and vertical instability. Nevertheless, this type of injury is differentiated from VS injuries by the lack of vertical displacement. Additionally, the direction of the affecting vector (anterior–posterior force) differs from the respective vector in VS-type injuries (translational force; Fig. 2).

- VS type injuries result from massive axial loading. Anteriorly, the VS injury demonstrates a symphyseal diastasis or a vertical fracture pattern of one or both pubic rami. Posterior injury is characterized by a complete disruption of the sacroiliac joint with vertical displacement of the hemiplevis. Occasionally, posterior injury occurs via vertical transsacral or transiliac fractures. As opposed to the Tile classification, unilateral or bilateral VS injuries are not further classified.
- CM injury includes a combination of fracture patterns due to different injuring force vectors. Anterolateral compression with posterior and medial displacement of the hemipelvis represents a possible feature of this particular type of injury.

Denis Classification of Vertical Sacral Fractures

Vertical fractures of the sacrum associated with discontinuity of the pelvic ring are categorized into three groups depending on the location of the vertical fracture line in relation to the neural foramina (Fig. 5).

Type I: The fracture line runs lateral to the neural foramina. Nervous structures are generally are not affected.

Type II: This type incorporates transforaminal fractures of the sacrum, frequently associated with lesions of sacral nerve roots (ca. 25%).

Type III: Central fractures of the sacrum involve the sacral spinal canal and are therefore associated with >50% concomitant neurological injuries.

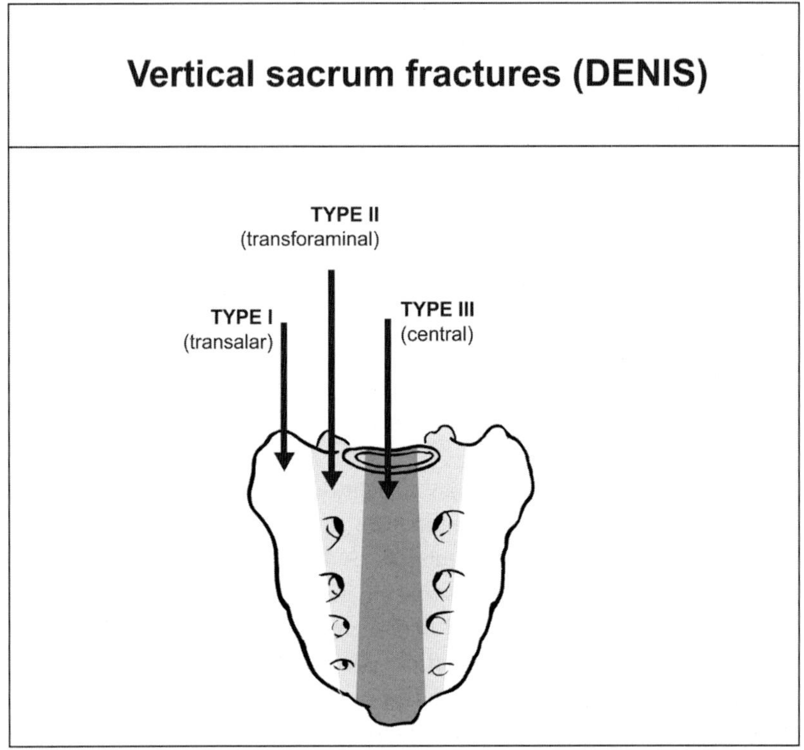

Figure 5 Denis classification of vertical sacrum fractures. *Source*: Chart kindly provided by Mrs. M. Peters, University Hospital Benjamin Franklin, Berlin (adapted from Ref. 17).

CLASSIFICATIONS OF OPEN PELVIC FRACTURES

Open pelvic fractures represent rare injuries accounting for 2% to 4% of all pelvic ring fractures. However, the high rate of mortality (25–50%) and significant morbidity depicts the complexity and severity of these injuries. An open pelvic fracture is defined by a communication to lesions of the integument or the gastrointestinal and urogenital tracts. Classification systems aimed at characterizing open pelvic fractures are associated with prognostic factors, with respect to mortality and morbidity. Furthermore, these classifications should support management decisions and therapeutic modalities for these rare but very severe injuries.

Jones Classification for Open Pelvic Fractures

The Jones classification (8) of open pelvic fractures refers to pelvic ring stability and rectal injury. Based on a retrospective multicenter analysis, three distinct categories were differentiated:

Class 1: Stable open pelvic ring fractures (low mortality)
Class 2: Unstable open pelvic ring fractures without rectal injury (about 33% mortality)

Class 3: Unstable open pelvic ring fractures in combination with rectal injury (up to 50% mortality)

Further stratification of the data revealed a significant correlation between rectal injury and sepsis, implicating the need for an early diverting colostomy.

More recently, the publication by Bircher and Hargrove (9) offered a more subtle and detailed classification of open pelvic fractures.

Bircher and Hargrove Classification of Open Pelvic Fractures

In this new classification, soft tissue injury was divided into three main alphanumerical categories, which were assigned to Tile's classification of pelvic ring fractures. Subsets were defined by the primary skin lesion and associated soft tissue damage.

Type A1: Penetrating trauma, for example, by a bullet. Tile/AO type A fracture.

Type A2: "Outside in" injury of the iliac crest, with minimal soft tissue damage. Tile/AO type A fracture.

Type A3: "Outside in" injury of the iliac crest, with extensive soft tissue damage requiring surgery for soft tissue coverage. Tile/AO type A fracture.

Type B1: "Inside out" injury caused by lateral compression and showing little external damage but possible injury to the genitourinary system (i.e., tilt fracture). Tile/AO type B2 fracture (LC).

Type B2: "Inside out" injury, caused by lateral compression and representing moderate tissue damage. An example would be a rotationally unstable pelvic fracture in combination with extensive degloving (Morel–Lavallé syndrome). Tile/AO type B2 fracture (LC).

Type B3: "Perineal split" following APC injury. Tile/AO type B1 fracture ("open book").

Type C1: "Perineal split" and/or "sacral shear/split" injury with moderate to extensive skin loss, complete genitourinary disruption, and rectal lesions with subsequent fecal contamination. Tile/AO type C fracture.

Type C2: "Hemipelvic destabilization" injury with severe tissue damage, complete urogenital and bowel injury combined with extensive contamination of all tissue layers. Tile/AO type C fracture.

Type C3: "Pelvic crush" with bilateral complex pelvic instability and massive damage to soft tissues and intrapelvic organs. Tile/AO type C fracture.

Since this classification system is new (9), its prognostic value needs to be corroborated in future prospective clinical trials.

REFERENCES

1. Tile M. Acute pelvic fractures: I. Causation and classification. J Am Acad Orthop Surg 1996; 4:143–151.
2. Pennal GF, Sutherland GO. Fractures of the Pelvis. Park Ridge, IL: American Academy of Orthopedic Surgeons, 1961.
3. Pennal GF, Tile M, Waddell J, et al. Pelvic disruption: assessment and classification. Clin Orthop Relat Res 1980; 151:12–21.
4. Orthopedic Trauma Association Committee for Coding and Classification. Fracture and Dislocation Compendium. J Orthop Trauma 1996; 10(suppl 1):1–154.
5. Young JW, Burgess AR, Brumback RJ, et al. Pelvic fractures: value of plain radiography in early assessment and management. Radiology 1986; 160:445–451.
6. Rommens PM, Hessmann MH. Staged reconstruction of pelvic ring disruption: differences in morbidity, mortality, radiologic results, and functional outcomes between B1, B2/B3, and C-type lesions. J Orthop Trauma 2002; 16:92–98.
7. Rommens PM, Gercek E, Hansen M, et al. Mortality, morbidity and functional outcome after open book and lateral compression lesions of the pelvic ring: a retrospective analysis of 100 type B pelvic ring lesions according to Tile's classification [German]. Unfallchirurg 2003; 106:542–549.
8. Jones AL, Powell JN, Kellam JF, et al. Open pelvic fractures: a multicenter retrospective analysis. Orthop Clin North Am 1997; 28:345–350.
9. Bircher M, Hargrove R. Is it possible to classify open fractures of the pelvis? Eur J Trauma 2004; 30:74–79.
10. Burgess AR, Eastridge BJ, Young JW, et al. Pelvic ring disruptions: effective classification system and treatment protocols. J Trauma 1990; 30:848–856.
11. Dalal SA, Burgess AR, Siegel JH, et al. Pelvic fracture in multiple trauma: classification by mechanism is key to pattern of organ injury, resuscitative requirements, and outcome. J Trauma 1989; 29:981–1000.
12. Denis F, Davis S, Comfort T. Sacral fractures—an important problem: retrospective analysis of 236 cases. Clin Orthop Relat Res 1988; 227:67–81.
13. Eastridge BJ, Starr A, Minei JP, et al. The importance of fracture pattern in guiding therapeutic decision-making in patients with hemorrhagic shock and pelvic ring disruptions. J Trauma 2002; 53:446–450.
14. Olson SA, Burgess A. Classification and initial management of patients with unstable pelvic ring injuries. Instr Course Lect 2005; 54:383–393.
15. Resnik CS, Stackhouse DJ, Shanmuganathan K, et al. Diagnosis of pelvic fractures in patients with acute pelvic trauma: efficacy of plain radiographs. Am J Roentgenol 1992; 158:109–112.
16. Sarin EL, Moore JB, Moore EE, et al. Pelvic fracture pattern does not always predict the need for urgent embolization. J Trauma 2005; 58:973–977.
17. Stahel PF, Ertel W. Pelvic ring injuries [German]. In: Rüter A, Trentz O, Wagner M, eds. Unfallchirurgie, 2nd ed. Munich, Germany: Urban & Fischer/Elsevier, 2004:907–934.
18. Stambaugh LE III, Blackmore CC. Pelvic ring disruptions in emergency radiology. Eur J Radiol 2003; 48:71–87.
19. Tscherne H, Pohlemann T, eds. Pelvis and Acetabulum [German]. Berlin, Heidelberg, New York: Springer, 1998.
20. Tscherne H, Pohlemann T, Gänsslen A. Classification, staging, urgency and indications in pelvic injuries [German]. Zentralbl Chir 2000; 125:717–724.
21. Tile M, Helfet DL, Kellam JF, eds. Fractures of the Pelvis and Acetabulum. 3rd ed. Philadelphia, PA: Lippincott Williams & Wilkins, 2003.

22. Young JW, Resnik CS. Fracture of the pelvis: current concepts of classification. Am J Roentgenol 1990; 155:1169–1175.
23. Zwipp H, Dahlen C, Grass R, et al. Injuries of the pelvic girdle—the pathway to exact diagnosis: which imaging methods are indicated [German]? Zentralbl Chir 1986; 160:445–451.

3

Acute Management of Pelvic Fractures: A European Perspective

Axel P. Gänsslen and Christian Krettek
Department of Trauma, Hannover Medical School, Hannover, Germany

Hans-Christoph Pape
Department of Orthopaedic Surgery, University of Pittsburgh Medical School, Pittsburgh, Pennsylvania, U.S.A.

Stefan Machtens
Department of Urology, Hannover Medical School, Hannover, Germany

INTRODUCTION

During resuscitation of polytrauma patients with associated pelvic injuries, a specific subgroup, characterized by unstable pelvic fractures combined with a hemodynamic instability related to the pelvis, requires special attention. In these patients, the cause of death is early exsanguination or the late sequelae of prolonged shock and mass transfusion. For this group we have coined a special term named "complex pelvic trauma," which is defined as pelvic injury combined with a concomitant soft tissue lesion in the pelvic region, which represents injuries to the urogenital system, hollow visceral injuries, neurovascular injuries, and significant damage to the integumentum (1). These injuries represent only about 10% of all pelvic fractures (2). However, this specific group of patients is highlighted by a significant increase in mortality up to 33% when compared to injuries without concomitant soft tissue damage (3).

Acute management primarily focuses on the latter patient group, whereas management in patients without additional peripelvic soft-tissue trauma is addressed to the pelvic bone injury.

PREHOSPITAL EVALUATION AND TREATMENT

During primary resuscitation at the scene of the accident, the severity of a pelvic injury is often underestimated. Open pelvic disruption represents an example. These are, however, rare injuries that lead to spectacular clinical presentations of external massive bleeding and/or severe pelvic deformities. However, the appearance of a highly unstable life-threatening pelvic injury is usually even more inconspicuous when an intact soft tissue envelope is present. Only extended intrapelvic hemorrhage leads to recognizable variations of the external contour. In more than 80% of the mechanically unstable pelvic fractures, the injuries are combined with other severe accompanying injuries. The rate of additional pelvic injuries in polytraumatized patients is around 25% (4). The overall extent of the pelvic trauma is often only realized when a critical blood loss is reached.

Obvious clinical signs for pelvic injuries occur rarely. In polytraumatized patients who sustained high-energy trauma, pelvic injuries always have to be ruled out. Typical accident mechanisms likely to cause a pelvic injury are the following:

- High-speed road traffic accidents
- Side-impact automobile accident with the patient on the side of the impact
- Falls from great heights leading to a combination of side-impact
- Axial forces through the outstretched lower limb
- High-speed trauma in unprotected travellers, such as motorcyclists
- Roll-over-accidents

If the patient is communicable, he has to be asked about pain in the pelvic region. Clinical assessment involves the general inspection of the pelvis for hematomas, open wounds, variations of the external contour, and deformities of the pelvis and/or lower extremities (shortening, external rotation deformities) (Fig. 1), as well as an assessment of the gross neurovascular status as this may often be the last chance before artificial ventilation.

Pelvic stability is investigated by manual compression of the pelvic ring in anterior–posterior and lateral–medial directions. Stability testing should be performed carefully and gently as these measures can result in additional pelvic bleeding. The presence of a pelvic instability is often associated with a high risk of pelvic bleeding.

The treatment at the scene of the injured patient with suspected pelvic injury follows the general Advanced Trauma Life Support (ATLS) guidelines (5). Priority should be given to the treatment of the airway, breathing, and circulatory (ABC) problems. Immediate antishock therapy by intravenous fluid administration is the primary treatment option in all patients with pelvic injuries. The benefit of prehospital intravenous fluids in severe trauma remains unproven. Prehospital intravenous access can be performed without causing a delay in transfer (6,7), but the average volume of fluid preclinically infused is still questionable (8,9). In the recent years, discussion arose if aggressive resuscitation with intravenous fluids may worsen the outcome in patients with hemorrhagic shock. The so-called "hypotensive resuscitation," which is a restoration of the radial pulse indicating a systolic blood pressure of 90 mmHg, was analyzed in penetrating trauma (10) and may probably reduce ongoing hemorrhage due to a decreased pressure gradient across the bleeding site.

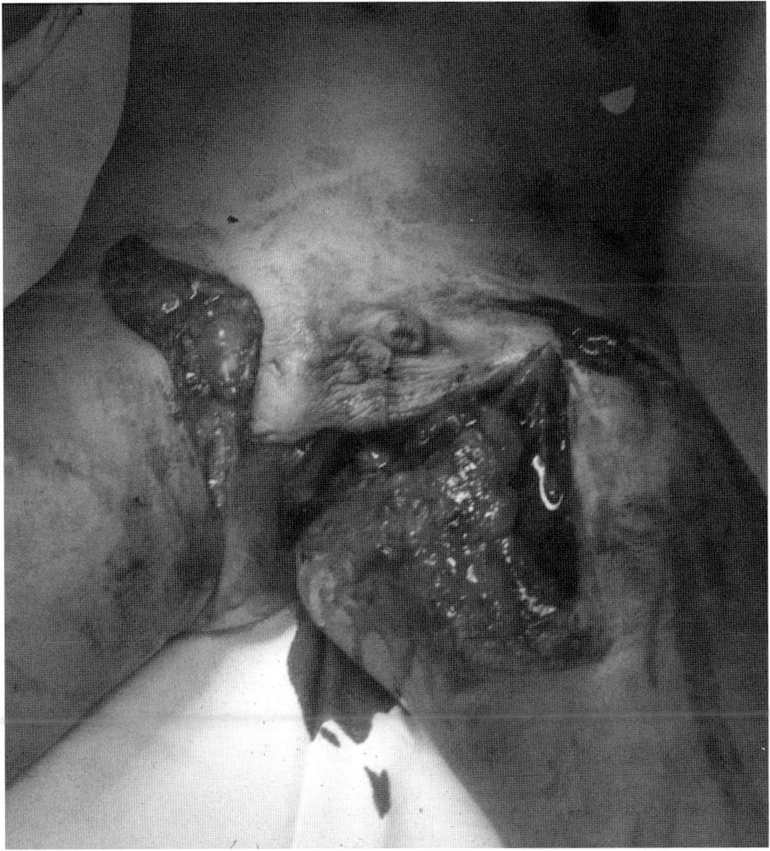

Figure 1 Open pelvic fracture with a large groin wound and injury to the scrotum and penis.

In a recent Cochrane review, there was no evidence from randomized controlled trials to support early or larger volume of intravenous fluid administration in uncontrolled hemorrhage. The best fluid administration strategy in hemodynamic unstable trauma patients is still unknown (11).

Thus, in cases of clinically proven pelvic instability without noticeable gross hemorrhage, intravenous fluid is recommended because even closed unstable pelvic injuries may lead to loss of 2 to 5 L of blood (1,12–15). In the presence of massive external bleeding, direct manual wound compression usually achieves a reduction or cessation of the bleeding (Fig. 2). The latter patients must be treated for shock and transferred immediately to the next trauma center ("load and go").

Reduction is performed in patients with highly unstable open book fractures (external rotation injury) who present with obvious deformities and instability on manual examination by traction, internal rotation, and lateral compression of the pelvis (Fig. 3). Reduction aims at decrease of the pelvic volume and probably assists in hemostasis.

Preclinically, military antishock trousers (MAST) have been used for reduction in pelvic and extremity fractures to increase venous return to the heart. Analysis of two

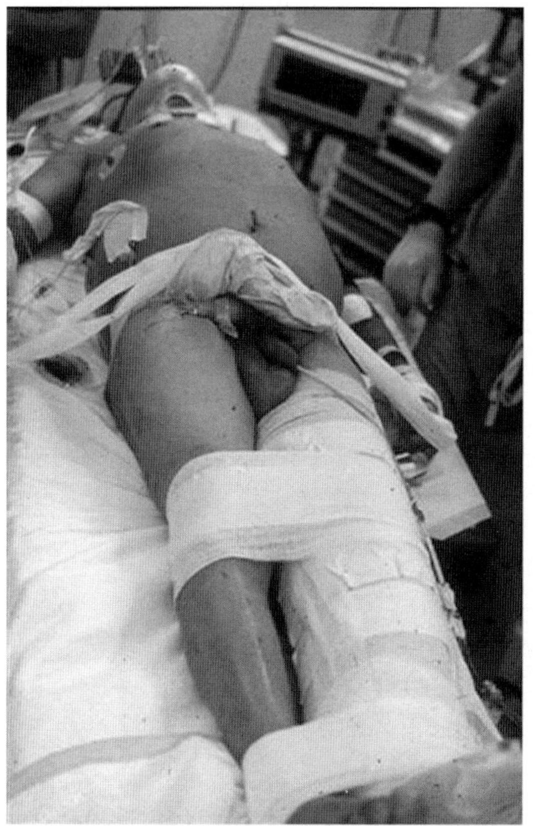

(A)

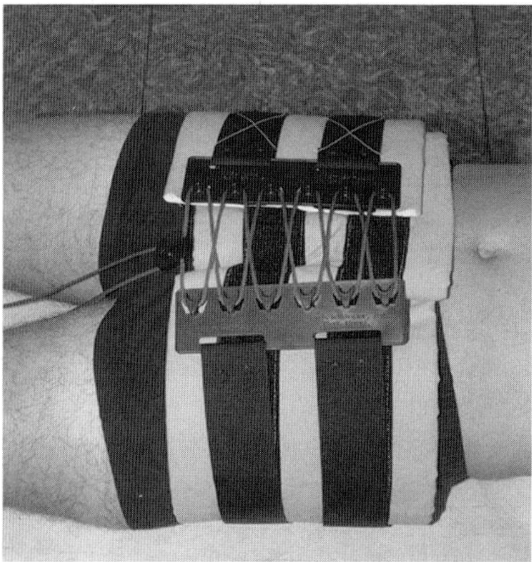

(B)

Figure 2 Prehospital emergency stabilization of the pelvis can be performed by: (**A**) a single bed sling, (**B**) a pelvic sling (*Continued*).

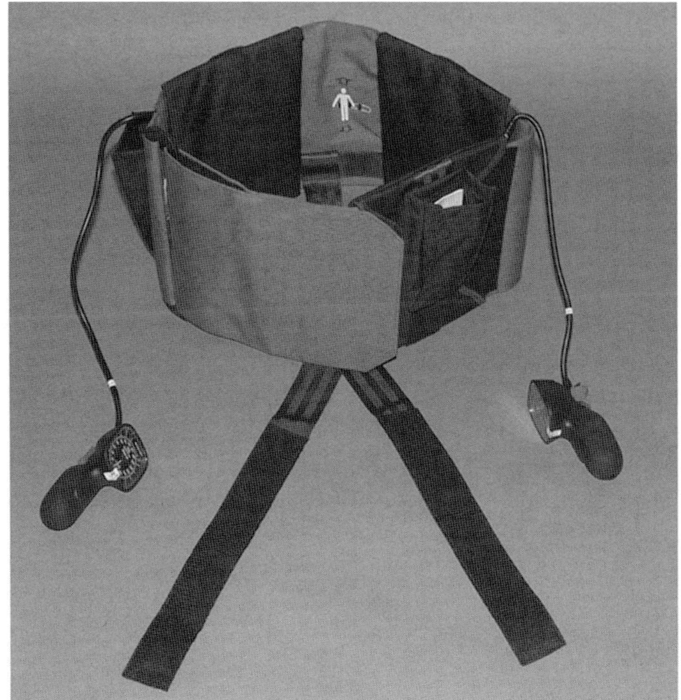

(C)

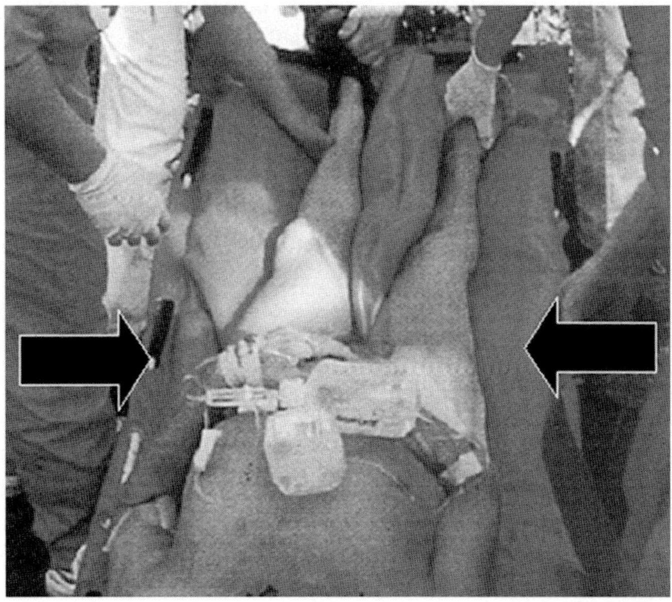

(D)

Figure 2 (*Continued*) (**C**) A pelvic belt that can be tied around the pelvis; (**D**) lateral compression of a bean bag at the pelvis.

randomized trials showed no evidence that MAST application reduces mortality, length of hospitalization, or length of intensive care unit (ICU) stay in trauma patients (16). In Europe, they do not appear to be of help due to extremely short rescue times. Additionally, complications like compartment syndromes, crush syndromes, or electrolyte deficits are not uncommon (17–21).

Alternatively, reduction of unstable pelvic fractures can be held by bean-bags, a bed sheet, or a pelvic sling tied around the pelvis (22–26) (Fig. 2). In contrast to MAST, these new devices reduce the application time, are easier to apply, have a cost advantage (26), and are clinically effective (25). Biomechanical analyses supported their use, as reduction of open-book pelvic fractures was sufficient (22). Even application of a simple bed sheet is reported to be effective (23).

After prehospital stabilization of the patient according to the ATLS guidelines, the transport of the injured patient should be as gentle as possible, preferably by physician-assisted rescue helicopter to a Level I trauma center with facilities for polytrauma treatment. This is particularly true for hemodynamically unstable patients to enable life-saving emergency operations.

INHOSPITAL PRIMARY TREATMENT

Primary inspection of the undressed patient should focus on pelvic asymmetry (Fig. 3), differences in leg length, pelvic soft tissue injury around the complete pelvis, including the perineum, search for urethral or vaginal bleeding (Fig. 4), and search for differences of the color of the feet, probably indicating vascular impairments (Fig. 5).

Besides localization of pain, the clinical examination must investigate the degree of pelvic stability. In lateral compression injuries, the pelvic ring may be quite stable. In open-book injuries, a more severe rotational instability in the horizontal plane may occur with or without additional instability in the craniocaudal direction (Fig. 6). The most severe instability is a combination of a rotational instability in the anterior–posterior and lateral directions and a craniocaudal instability. Repeated maneuvres of stability testing should be avoided as these could increase the danger of bleeding. Stability of the pelvis is graded as clinically stable or unstable.

While the mechanical pelvic instability is thus classified, the severity of additional hemorrhage, the blood loss, and the extent of the soft-tissue injuries remain difficult to assess. Immediate analysis of the primary hemoglobin concentration is performed from capillary, venous, and arterial whole blood by bedside hemoglobinometry (photometry) (27,28). The result is available within 40 seconds. Our observations showed that vital hemorrhage is supposed at a primary hemoglobin concentration of <8 g/dL (15).

The vascular status is analyzed by palpation of the pulses of the lower extremities and inspection of capillary refill. An abnormous capillary refill is defined as more than three seconds. Additionally, in all suspected cases a Doppler examination of the foot pulses is performed.

Neurological screening of the lower extremities is essential and consists of an oriented sensory examination, testing of toe and foot extension, plantar flexion of the

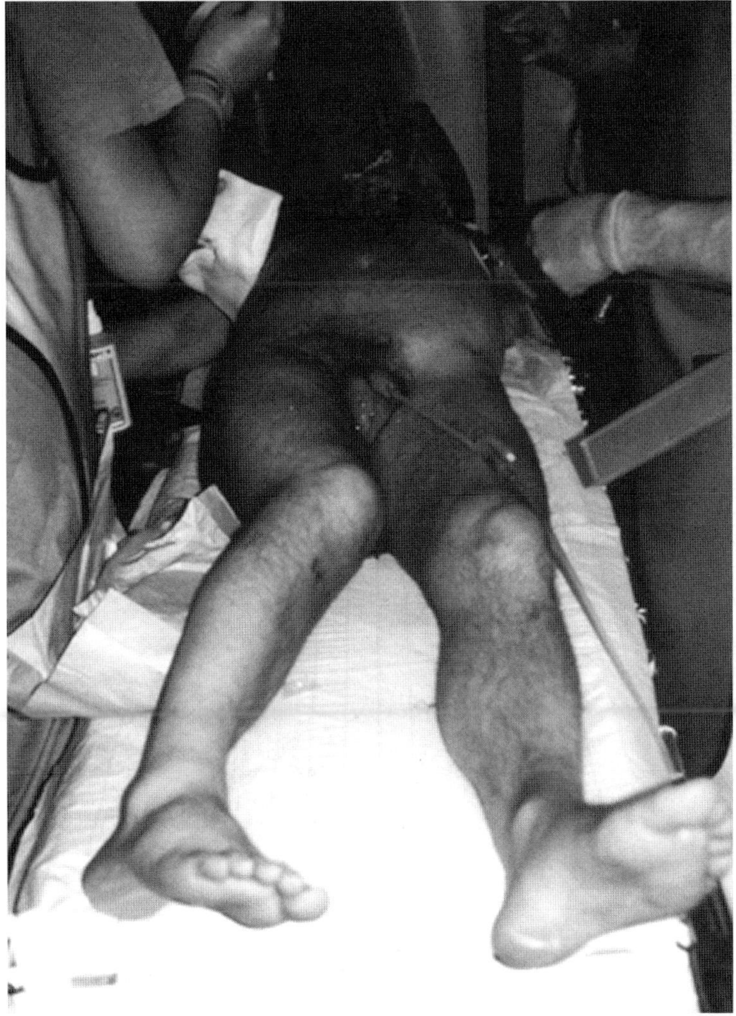

Figure 3 Asymmetry of the right hemipelvis with internal rotation deformity and shortening of the leg indicating an acetabular fracture with hip dislocation or an unstable C-type injury of the right hemipelvis.

foot and knee extension, patellar tendon, and Achilles tendon reflexes in the awake patient. To avoid hypothermia during the diagnostic phase, a connective patient warming system is used (29,30).

Primary radiological evaluation consists of at least an anterior–posterior pelvic X-ray (Fig. 7). As long as the patient is stable, an additional spiral computed tomography (CT) scan consisting of a cranial CT, neck CT, chest, abdominal, and pelvis CT ("trauma scan") with 50 mL iodine contrast medium (Isovist®) given 15 minutes before scanning should be performed as early as possible, depending on the patient's general condition. Inlet and outlet views are no longer taken as these views can be reconstructed from the CT data set (Fig. 8).

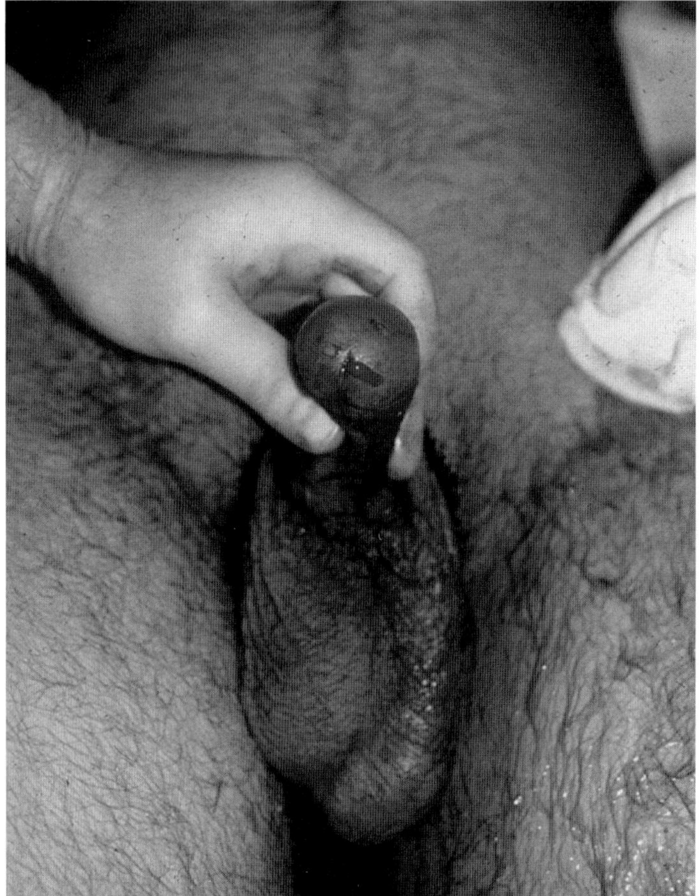

Figure 4 Bleeding at the urethral orificium indicating injury to the urethra or bladder.

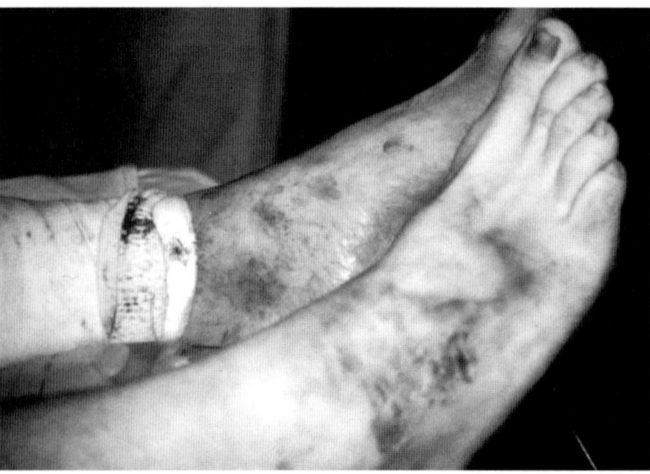

Figure 5 Color difference of the right foot, indicating vascular injury of the right leg or pelvic region.

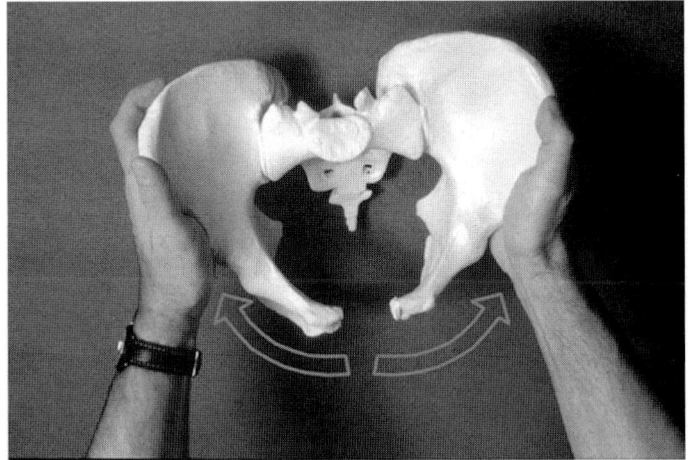

(A)

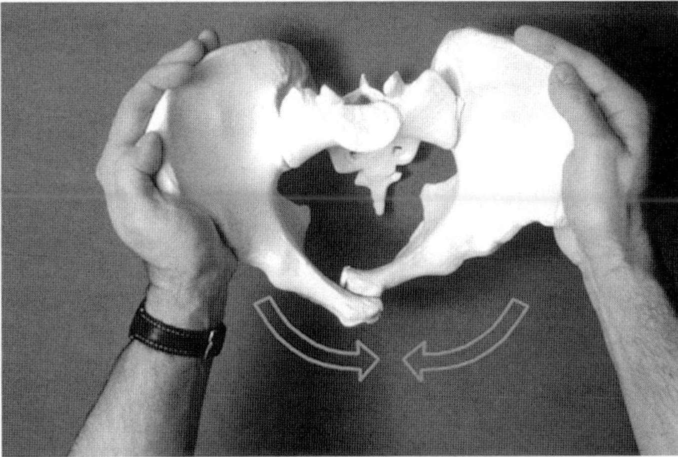

(B)

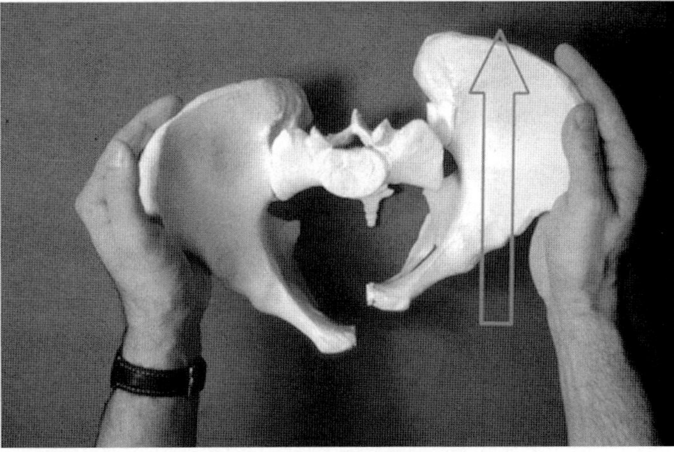

(C)

Figure 6 Stability testing of the pelvis is performed by assessment of rotational instability in the horizontal plane with external rotational stress (**A**) or lateral compression (**B**). Additionally, instability is assessed in the cranio-caudal direction (**C**).

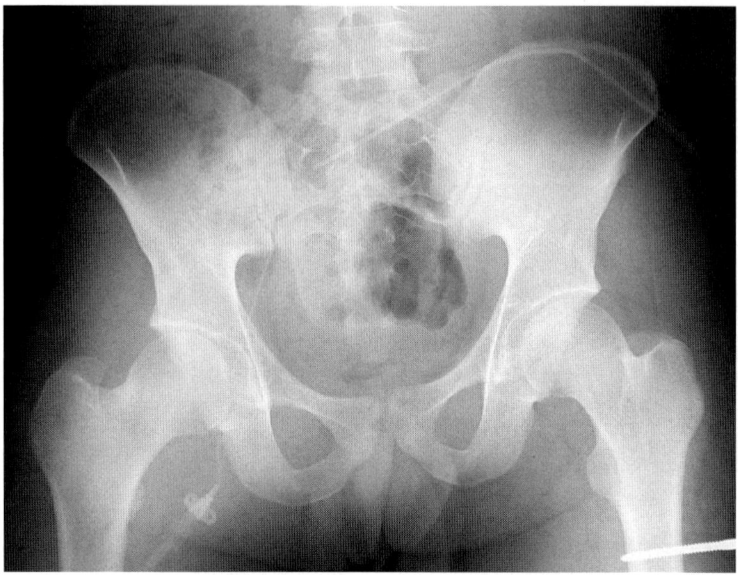

Figure 7 Primary anterior–posterior x-ray of the pelvis, which appears radiographically normal.

Another advantage is that a conventional cystography is not further required for detecting and classification of bladder injuries (31,32). In suspected urethral lesions, a retrograde urethrogram should be performed with 20 mL iodine contrast medium as early as possible for classification of the urological injury (Fig. 9).

Indications for retrograde urethrography are:

- Bleeding from the urethral orifice
- Hematuria
- Anuria
- Perineal hematoma
- Rectal or vaginal bleeding
- Hypermobile prostate during rectal examination
- Extravesical fluid (ultrasonography), and
- Severe displaced fractures of the pubic bones into the small pelvis

The pelvic ring fracture is then classified according to the AO/OTA classification of pelvic injuries and the injury pattern, depending on specific fracture locations, to evaluate the exact indication for operation (33,34).

Within the AO/OTA classification three different grades of stability/instability are differentiated (Fig. 10):

- Type A: Stable fractures, with the mechanical ring structure of the pelvic ring remaining intact (incidence 50–70% of the patients).
- Type B: Partially unstable injuries with partial posterior, rotational instability after anteroposterior or lateral compression (incidence 20–30% of the patients).
- Type C: Unstable injuries with combined anterior and posterior vertical instability (incidence 10–20% of the patients).

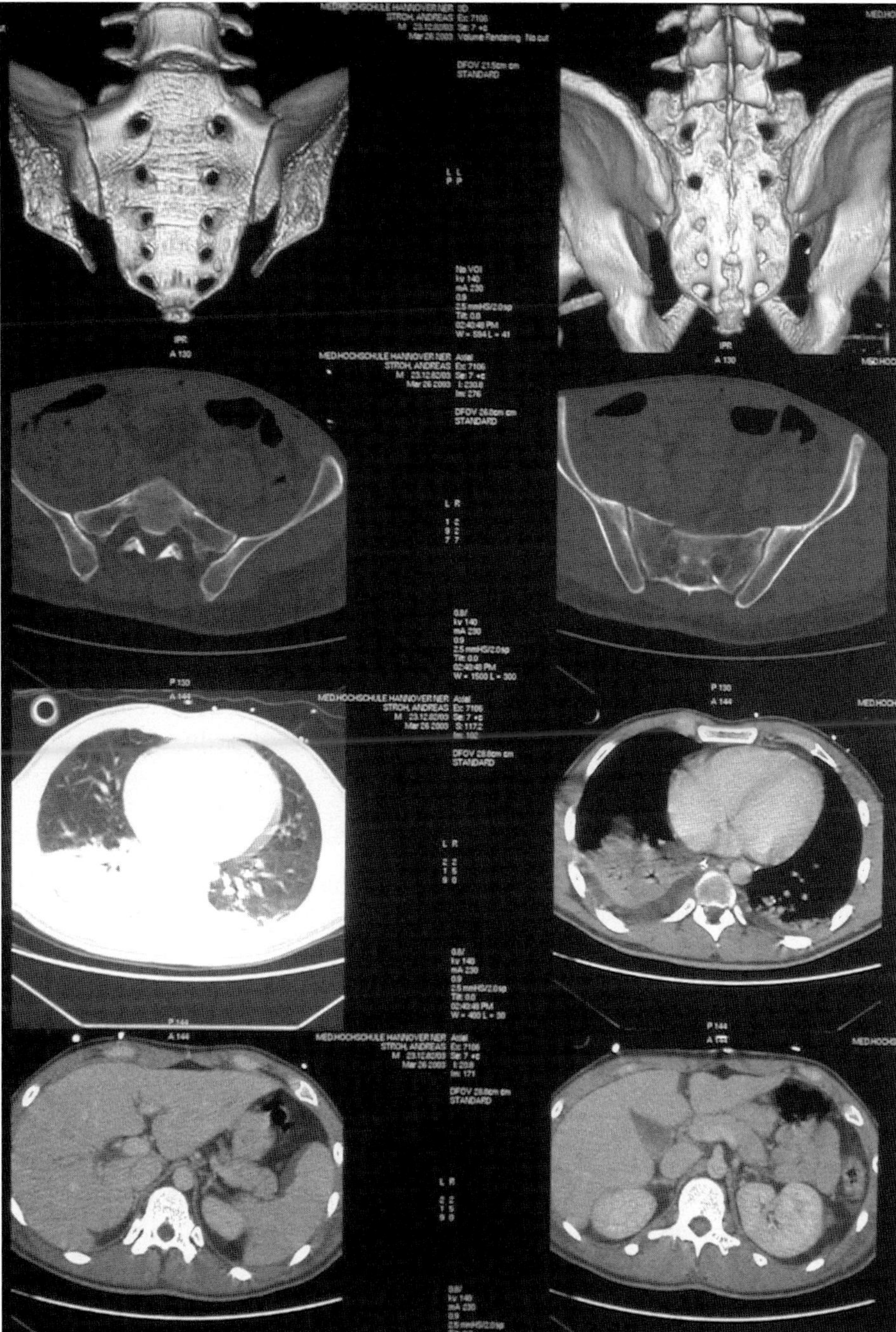

Figure 8 Summary of the "Trauma-Scan" (cranial, neck, chest, abdominal, and pelvic CT-scan) of the patient from Fig. 9 showing a right sacral fracture, right lung contusion with hematothorax and free fluid at the spleen.

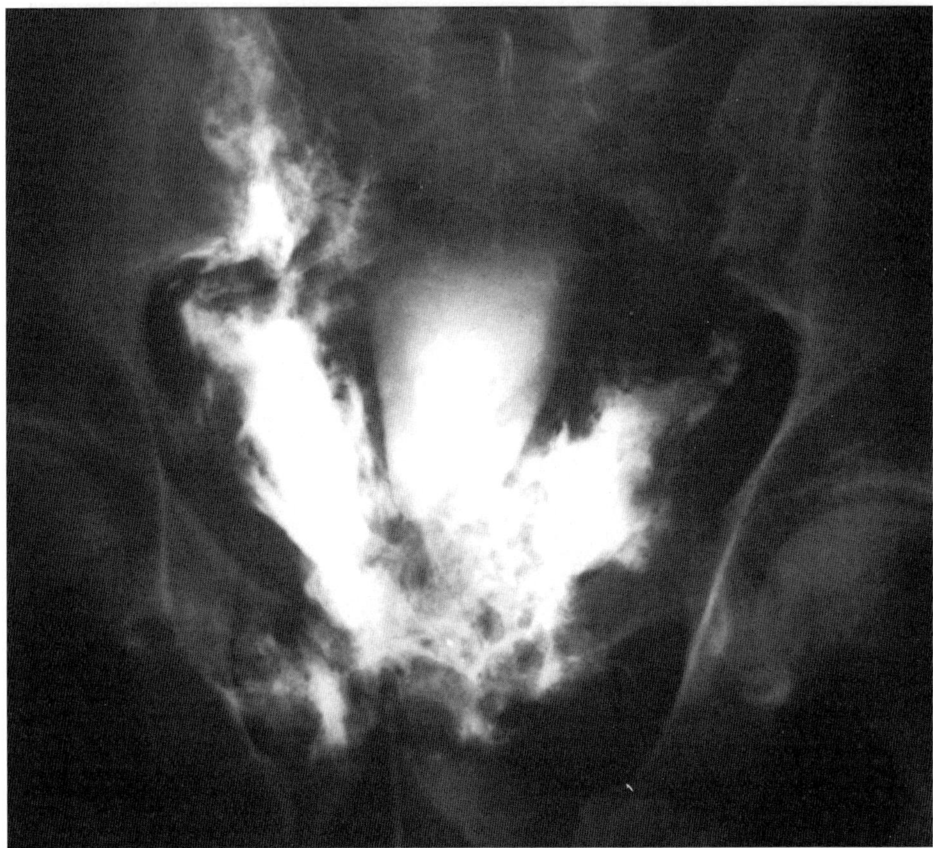

Figure 9 In suspected urological lesions, a retrograde urethrogram is performed, in this case showing an extraperitoneal bladder laceration.

For emergency classification of these injuries and to facilitate the identification of life-threatening pelvic injuries, the following definitions have been shown to be useful, practicable, and of relevance as far as a prediction of mortality is concerned (34) (Table 1):

- *Simple* pelvic fractures with little soft tissue injury and pure osteoligamentous instability. This group covers about 90% of pelvic fractures (2,35).
- *Complex pelvic trauma*: Pelvic fracture combined with a serious soft tissue lesion in the pelvic region (1).
- *Fractures with pelvic and hemodynamic instability*: Mechanically unstable pelvic fractures (type B or C) combined with hemodynamic instability related to the pelvic injury with a systolic blood pressure of <70 mmHg and/or a hemoglobin concentration of <8 g/dL on admission (15,36).
- *Traumatic hemipelvectomy*: A total or subtotal dislocation of one or both hemipelvises with complete disruption of the vascular and neural structures of the pelvis (37,38).

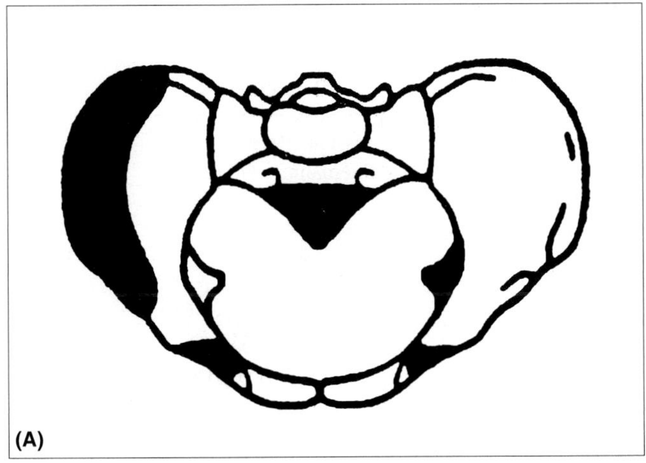

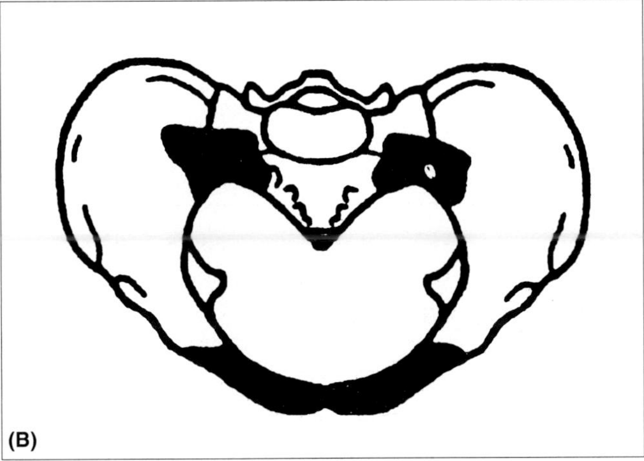

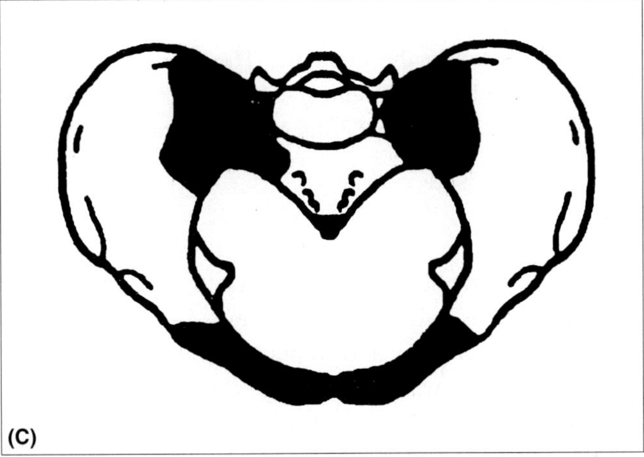

Figure 10 Classification of pelvic ring injuries according to the OTA-classification. (**A**) Stable A-type injuries not involving the pelvic ring, (**B**) rotational unstable B-type injury with partial disruption of the posterior pelvis, and (**C**) completely unstable C-type injuries with complete disruption of the posterior elements. *Source*: Reprinted from Ref. 148.

Table 1 Mortality Depending on the Type of Pelvic Injury

Pelvic injury	Definition	References	Mortality (%)
Simple pelvic fracture	Pelvic fracture with minor soft tissue injury and pure osteoligamentous instability	Gänsslen, 1996 (35) Pohlemann, 1998 (2)	7.9–10.8
Complex pelvic trauma	Pelvic fracture combined with a serious soft tissue lesion in the pelvic region (1)	Bosch, 1992 (1) Pohlemann, 1994 (4) Gänsslen, 1996 (35) Pohlemann, 1998 (2)	21.3–34.8
Pelvic and hemodynamic instability	Mechanically unstable pelvic fractures (type B or C) combined with haemodynamic instability	Pohlemann, 1996 (15)	58
Traumatic hemipelvectomy	Total or subtotal dislocation of one or both hemipelvises with complete disruption of the vascular and neural structures of the pelvis	Pohlemann, 1996 (37)	63.6

Source: From Refs. 1, 2, 4, 15, 35, 37.

TREATMENT OPTIONS IN PATIENTS WITH PELVIC AND HEMODYNAMIC INSTABILITY

Injuries with mechanical and hemodynamic instability are rare with a reported incidence even in trauma centers of 1% to 2% of all pelvic injuries (34). The treatment is highly case-dependent and a delay in diagnosis and adequate treatment dramatically reduces the patient's chance of survival.

Several treatment options are reported in the literature. The available treatment protocols for emergency hemostasis range between waiting for *self-tamponade*, MAST, spica casts, angiography, embolization, and emergency internal stabilization (Table 2) (1,4,18,19,21–26,39–59).

Self-Tamponade

In the majority of patients with pelvic fractures without circulatory instability, the concept of retroperitoneal self-tamponade is valid (13). In contrast, in unstable pelvic fractures, especially C-type fractures, frequently a disruption of all retroperitoneal muscle compartments (60) (e.g., gluteus medius–minimus compartment, gluteus maximus compartment, and iliopsoas compartment) may lead to a phenomenon named *chimney effect* (61), where the pelvic hemorrhage creeps cranially above the psoas muscle or along the gluteal muscles with the risk of pelvic and abdominal compartment syndromes (Fig. 11). Clinically, these cases often present as abdominal injuries. As the retroperitoneum is not a closed space, pressure induced tamponade is not of clinical importance (60).

Table 2 Treatment Options in Patients with Pelvic and Hemodynamic Instability

Type of treatment	Advantage	Disadvantage	Effectivity
Self tamponade	None	Only in hemodynamic stable patients valid Disruption of all compartimental borders	None
MAST	Direct compression of the pelvic ring and the lower extremities	Access to the traumatised region is limited Possible hazardous complications	None
Ligation hypogastric artery	None	Collateral supply	None
Pelvic sling/belt	Direct pelvic compression without access limitations Biomechanical effective	Unknown	Possible
Angiography/embolization	Open access to retroperitoneal space unnecessary Isolated arterial bleedings may be controlled without surgical intervention	Arterial bleeding source in only 10% to 20% Time consuming	Possible
Temporary aortic occlusion	Acute effectivity	Only temporary measure	Yes
External fixation	Easy and fast handling Control of blood loss by direct pressure on bleeding vessels or prevention of repeated insults to already clotted vessels	Patient access impaired Critical in C-type injuries	Yes
Direct bleeding control	Control of major vascular injuries	Time consuming	Yes
C-clamp	Posterior pelvic stabilization Basis for tamponade	Special indications Knowledge of anatomy Possible complications	Yes
Internal fixation	Biomechanical most effective	Time consuming Special indications	Yes

Abbreviation: MAST, military antishock trousers.

Military Antishock Trousers

MAST achieves direct compression of the pelvic ring and the lower extremities (20). Thus, the pelvis is immobilized, and systemic circulation is supported (19). In contrast, access to the traumatized region is limited, and assessment and treatment of concomitant injuries will be impaired (Fig. 12). Major complications such as compartment syndromes and impaired perfusion leading to amputations are reported particularly after long-term application (18,19,21,62).

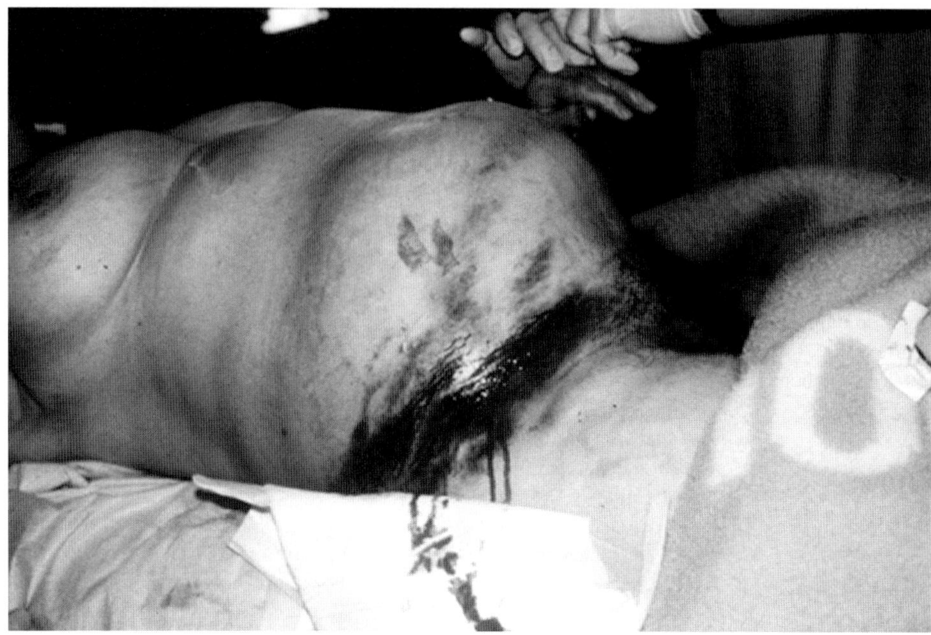

Figure 11 Pelvic injury with complete disruption of all retroperitoneal muscle compartments, clinically presenting as an abdominal compartment syndrome.

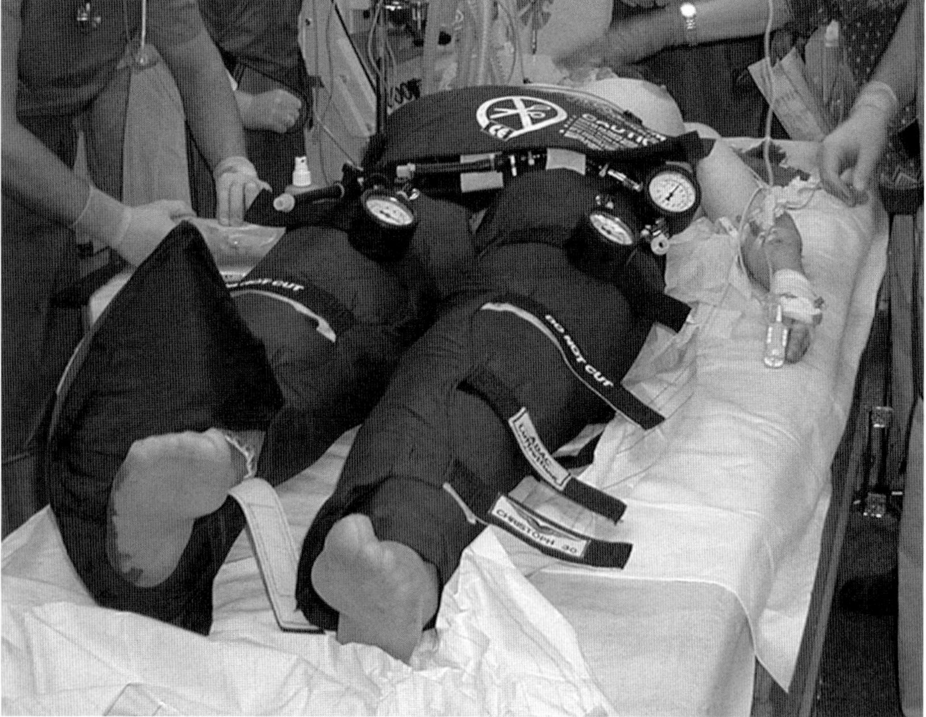

Figure 12 Patient after application of the MAST with disadvantage of impaired access to the pelvis and lower extremities.

Pelvic Sling

A simple alternative to the MAST is the pelvic bed sheet, pelvic sling, or pelvic belt tied around the pelvis (Figs. 2 and 13), which allows direct satisfactory pelvic compression without major limitations of patient accessibility (22–26,42). Prophylactic application of this device at the scene of the injury or in the emergency department has to be considered as biomechanical analyses showed positive effects on the stabilization of external rotation injuries of the pelvis (22,42).

Embolization

Arterial bleeding is associated with hemodynamically unstable pelvic fractures in only 10% to 20% of the patients (15,63,64). Therefore, the efficacy of angiographic embolization of pelvic vessels remains controversial. Also, angiographic embolization has been reported to have severe complications. Some authors even reported a mortality of 50% despite effective bleeding control in the majority of the cases (65,66). Simultaneous treatment of the patient's further injuries is limited during this time, even though better time-saving technology has improved the role of angiography as a therapeutic tool (15,40,48,67).

Several authors have reported on their experience with angiographic embolization of pelvic hemorrhage. Some of them are given below.

Chaufour et al. (68) embolized nine patients after 8 to 24 hours postinjury (average 17.8 hours). All embolizations were effective and no complications were observed. The average amount of packed red blood cells (PRBC) prior to the procedure was 13,9 PRBC, indicating a rate of 0.78 PRBC/hr. One patient died due to respiratory failure and myocardial dysfunction two hours after embolization.

Hölting et al. (69) analyzed 20 patients with pelvic hemorrhage. The time from injury to embolization decreased from 17 to 13.5 hours (1–38 hours). The average amount of PRBC before embolization was 28 PRBC (2.1 PRBC/hr). Despite immediate stabilization of circulation after embolization, mortality rate was 55% due to septic–toxic multiple organ failure and multifactorial causes.

Piotin et al. (49) analyzed six patients with pelvic fractures, embolized one to six days postinjury (average 44 hours). Prior to embolization the average PRBC was 11.3 PRBC, indicating a rate of 0.25 PRBC/hr.

Agolini et al. (39) retrospectively investigated 15 patients with pelvic angiography and embolization. All embolizations were successful, No deaths resulted from ongoing hemorrhage. Embolization was performed between 50 minutes and 19 hours after arrival of the patient. The average time to perform angiography was 90 (50–140 minutes). Patients who were embolized within three hours of arrival had a significantly greater survival rate. No data was given for pelvic ring instability and hemodynamic instability. The authors concluded that embolization is effective, but only a small percentage of patients with pelvic fractures require embolization.

Perez et al. (48) reviewed all patients with angiographic embolization of pelvic bleeding over a 10-year period. In eight patients the time until embolization was 5.7 hours and the average amount of preangiographic PRBC was 10.6 PRBC, indicating a rate of 1.8 PRBC/hr. Mortality rate was 25%. During the clinical course, sepsis was common. The authors concluded that standardized parameters of a successful intervention are yet to be defined.

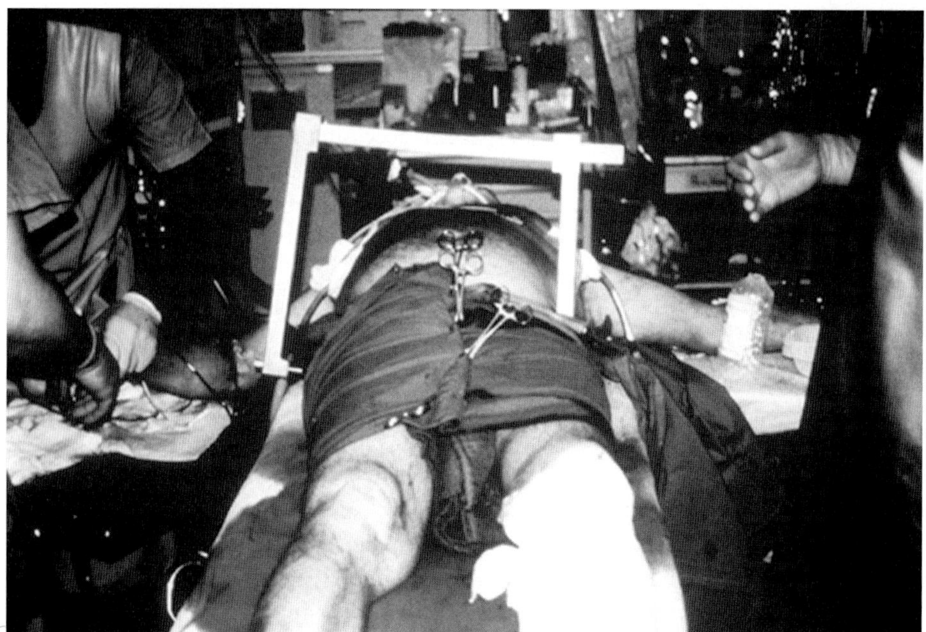

Figure 13 Simple pelvic bed sheet tied around the pelvis prior to application of the emergency C-clamp for immediate stabilization of the pelvis.

Hamill et al. (66) retrospectively analyzed 76 patients with more than six units of blood transfusion within the first 24 hours after admission. Twenty of them underwent pelvic embolization with a primary success rate of 90%. The average time from injury to angiography was five hours (2.3–23 hours). The average amount of PRBC given before embolization was 14 (2.8 PRBC/hr). In eight patients (40%), a second angiography due to ongoing hemorrhage was required, and four of these patients died.

The embolized patients were of older age and had a higher pelvic AIS. ISS was comparable in both groups. Fracture patterns indicative of an increased pelvic volume [anterior–posterior compression type II + III, lateral compression type III, vertical shear, and combined mechanism according to Burgess (70)] showed significant higher rate of embolization compared to other injury mechanisms. The overall mortality rate was 45%.

Velmahos et al. (71) analyzed 30 patients with angiographic embolization of bilateral internal iliac arteries. Thirteen patients first had laparotomies with unsuccessful control of the bleeding. In the remaining 17 patients, embolization was performed as the primary treatment for hemorrhage control. The overall success rate was 97% for patients with blunt pelvic trauma. The authors concluded that this concept seems to be useful in selected patients.

Cook et al. (65) analyzed 150 patients with unstable B- and C-type injuries. In 23 of these, angiographic embolization was performed because of persistent hemodynamic instability (systolic blood pressure <90 mmHg). Vertical shear injuries were associated

Table 3 Analysis of Different Embolization Studies

Author	Number of patients	Time to embolization (hr)	PRBC pre-embolization	PRBC/hr	Mortality rate (%)
Chaufour 1986 (68)	9	17.8	13.9	0.78	11.1
Grabenwöger 1989 (72)	6	—	24	—	50
Hölting 1992 (69)	20	13.5	28	2.1	55
Piotin 1995 (49)	6	44	11.3	0.25	0
Perez 1998 (48)	8	5.7	10.6	1.8	25
Hamill 2000 (66)	20	5	14	2.8	45
Cook 2002 (65)	23	3.7	—	—	43
Average	92	10.6	18.3	1.65	39.1

Abbreviation: PRBC, packed red blood cells.
Source: From Refs. 48, 49, 65, 66, 68, 69, 72.

with the highest rate of angiographic intervention. No correlation was found between fracture morphology and arterial injury. The average time to embolization was 3.7 hours and the average time for angiography was 102 minutes. The average amount of PRBC during the first 24 hours was 25 PRBC. Two complications were described: one gluteal infarction and one false aneurysm of the external iliac artery. Overall, 10 patients died (43%); six of these had their angiography as the first therapeutic intervention. Five of these had a fracture which could have been stabilized by an external fixator. The authors recommended external pelvic fixation prior to fore pelvic angiography.

Whereas the availability of interventional angiography is normally present in Level I trauma centers, the average time to intervention is reported as up to 17 hours (48,49,68,69,72), but with a decrease to five hours during the last few years (48).

In summary (Table 3), the average time between admission and performed angiographic embolization was 10.7 hours. During this time, 17.7 PRBC was administered on average, indicating a rate of 1.65 PRBC/hr.

Ligation of Hypogastric Artery

Due to the remarkable collateral supply within in the small pelvis, ligation of the hypogastric artery does not lead to satisfactory reduction in arterial bleeding (73–77).

Temporary Aortic Occlusion

Occlusion of the aorta is a temporary measure to control disastrous massive hemorrhage, either as a direct cross clamping, or via percutaneous or open by inserted balloon catheter, which helps in regaining intraoperative access to the bleeding site (78).

External Fixation

Pelvic emergent stabilization with an external fixator is the most widely accepted measure (45,47,50,51,55,57,59,79,80) due to relatively easy handling and the ready availability in trauma departments. From a mechanical point of view, the stability of simple constructions for type C injuries is critical, but external fixation does not help to control pelvic bleeding by generating pelvic tamponade (60). Application of an external fixator can only control blood loss by inducing hemorrhage control from the fracture site by direct pressure on bleeding vessels or by prevention of repeated insults to already clotted vessels. Additionally, the access to the patient, particularly for laparotomies, is reduced with almost every construction.

In a recent analysis, external fixation was shown to be helpful in the acute phase of resuscitation, whereas single treatment of unstable type-C injuries and type-B open-book injuries with symphyseal disruption showed a high rate of secondary displacement (81).

Pelvic C-Clamp

Application of the pelvic C-clamp has the biomechanical advantage of direct and improved stabilization of the posterior pelvic ring compared to the external fixator, giving the basis for effective pelvic tamponade (15,82,83). Clinical series support these results (15,44,46,52,58). Disadvantages are their special indications (not applicable in fractures of the ilium and transiliac fracture dislocations), potential injury to adjacent organs and the gluteal neurovascular structures, and overcompression with the risk of secondary nerve compression in sacral fractures, as well as pin tract infections in cases of prolonged application, and perforation into the small pelvis with the risk of additional organ damage.

Internal Fixation

Definitive reduction and internal fixation is the procedure of choice for pelvic ring fixation as various biomechanical studies revealed a higher stability compared to external fixation (84–86). The quality of the reduction is usually superior and normally there is no requirement for further acute measures. In the acute management, symphyseal plating, anterior plating of the SI joint, and application of transiliosacral screws are feasible only when the patient is in a stable condition (4,87–89).

Direct Bleeding Control

Direct surgical hemostasis is possible by vascular ligation, vascular clips (clamps), and, rarely, by a vascular reconstruction of major vessels, and is the principal aim of every hemostasis in the pelvic region (46,54,74,83,90–92). The more common venous bleedings from large ruptured venous plexus have the disadvantage of a time-consuming bleeding control with sometimes additional blood loss. Uncontrolled circumferential stitching and/or clip application due to insufficient visualization, especially in the area of the plexus, may lead to iatrogenic nerve injuries. Therefore, in exsanguinating diffuse pelvic bleeding, especially major venous bleeding, pelvic tamponade is proposed under a condition of emergent posterior pelvic ring stabilization (46,54,74,83,91,92).

Immediate posterior pelvic ring stabilization with the pelvic C-clamp or an external fixator provides the required mechanical stability to perform for pelvic tamponade, as fracture reduction leads to reduction of fracture hemmorrhage (60,90). The presacral and paravesical regions are packed from posterior to anterior using standard surgical tamponades. Thus, pelvic hemorrhage can be controlled effectively during the primary resuscitation period (46,54).

We have previously analyzed 15 patients "in extremis" with pelvic instability (C-type pelvic ring injuries) and hemodynamic instability with a primary hemoglobin concentration of less than 8 g/dL (54). The average ISS was 37.4 points (range: 20–66). Parameters indicating severe hemorrhagic shock were a mean systolic blood pressure of 63 mmHg (range: 10–100) and a mean primary hemoglobin level of 5.6 g/dL. Traumatic shock was additionally indicated by a mean base deficit of −10.1 mmol/L. During the first hour after admission, the mean amount of given units of blood was 7.9 (range: 2–12), equivalent to 1970 mL of blood.

In six patients, pelvic C-clamp stabilization was performed in the emergency department within 30 minutes after admission. Primary operative treatment was indicated in 13 patients, all including pelvic tamponade. The remaining two patients were directly transferred to the ICU. Twelve of the 13 patients needed additional laparotomy due to concomitant intra-abdominal injury in 11 cases and severe retroperitoneal bleeding in four cases. At the end of lapartotomy, external fixation of the anterior pelvic ring was performed in two patients. One patient without intra-abdominal injury had initial anterior SI-plating via anterolateral approach. For the 12 patients surviving the first six hours after admission, the mean amount of blood replacement with PRBC was 37.4 units (range: 11–89), equivalent to 9340 mL of blood, indicating a rate of 3.1 PRBC/hr. No angiographic embolization was performed.

Overall mortality rate was 66.6%. According to the TRISS method (93,94), a mean survival rate of 17.5% was expected. The observed survival rate of these patients was doubled at 33.3%.

Ertel et al. (46) prospectively analyzed 20 consecutive patients with pelvic ring disruption and hemorrhagic shock. All patients were treated with immediate pelvic C-clamp followed by laparotomy and pelvic packing in persistent or massive hemorrhage. The overall mortality rate was 25%. Hemorrhagic shock was indicated when blood lactate levels at admission were of 5.1 mmol/L; 33.2 units of blood transfusions were required on average within the first 12 hours, indicating a rate of 2.8 PRBC/hr.

In a further analysis, Ertel et al. (95) analyzed 41 patients "in extremis," defined as patients with either absent vital signs or with severe shock due to torrential hemorrhage which needed mechanical resuscitation or repeatedly catecholamines despite complete blood volume replacement within 120 min (more than 12 blood transfusions in two hours) (96). The average ISS was 40 points, the average amount of transfused blood units was 33.9. Ten patients had stable A-type pelvic fractures, 12 rotational unstable B-type injuries, and 19 C-type injuries. Concomitant injuries were common with additional 66% head injuries, 73.2% chest injuries, 61% additional abdominal injuries, and 88% musculoskeletal injuries. Emergency treatment consisted of nine crash thoracotomies, 23 crash laparotomies, nine aortic clampings to control hemorrhage (hemorrhage control in one patient), and two pelvic C-clamp applications. Effective angiographic embolization was performed in one patient. Overall, mortality rate of these patients "in extremis" was 90.2%. The majority of patients (56%) died within 24 hours due to persistent hemorrhagic shock.

EMERGENCY TREATMENT ALGORITHMS

There are various algorithms to simplify the decision making of treatment modalities in cases of pelvic fractures with hemodynamic instability (40,54,70,96,97–104). Due to the variability of the injury itself and the number of possible treatment options, emergency algorithms are often complex and therefore often not applicable in the common emergency situation.

Therefore, an algorithm for pelvic injuries must fulfill the following criteria:

- *Precision* (inclusion criteria)
- *Simplicity* (few decisions criteria)
- *Flexibility* (consideration of other injuries by integration into the general polytrauma algorithm)

Based on these criteria, the decisionmaking for mechanically unstable pelvic injuries with hemodynamic instability was reduced to three decisions within the initial 30 minutes following admission (34,54). The most important aims are:

- Localization of the source of hemorrhage
- Identification of mechanical pelvic ring instability

Proposed Emergency Treatment Protocol

A standardized protocol for prehospital and primary clinical treatment is used for all polytrauma patients (105–108). For patients with suspected severe pelvic injuries, the general polytrauma protocol is expanded by a *complex pelvic fracture module* based on three decisions all to be made within 30 minutes after admission (34,54) (Fig. 14).

First Look

During the "first look" of the trauma algorithm, the vital functions of the patient are judged (first five minutes after admission), analyzing for impairments of ventilation (dyspnea and cyanosis), the central nervous system (unconsciousness), and circulatory (bleeding) parameters. The first look results are used for intubation decisions as well as decisions on stopping pelvic or other external bleeding by manual compression, and/or immediate aggressive blood-fluid substitution. In cases of massive pelvic hemorrhage or a pelvic rollover/crush injury, immediate transport to the operation room is performed for hemorrhage control. If the patient is not in extremis (<3 PRBC/1 hr), resuscitation is performed according to the general polytrauma algorithm.

Shock Treatment

In the second period (about 5–15 minutes after admission), shock treatment is performed with a minimum of two large-bore venous lines. In the case of massive bleeding, universal donor blood (group O, rhesus negative) is administered immediately. Blood samples are taken from the femoral artery and analyzed for a blood-gas check and basic laboratory screening. A urinary catheter, a central venous catheter, an artery line, and monitoring equipment are inserted.

If the patient's general condition is stable, further treatment is oriented according to the general polytrauma algorithm. Simultaneously, basic diagnostic measures including clinical assessment, radiographs of the chest and pelvis, and an additional abdominal ultrasound are performed to focus on massive hemorrhage.

With remaining hemodynamic instability, massive blood replacement (PRBC) with noncross-matched blood is continued. The pelvic ring is latest reduced by traction

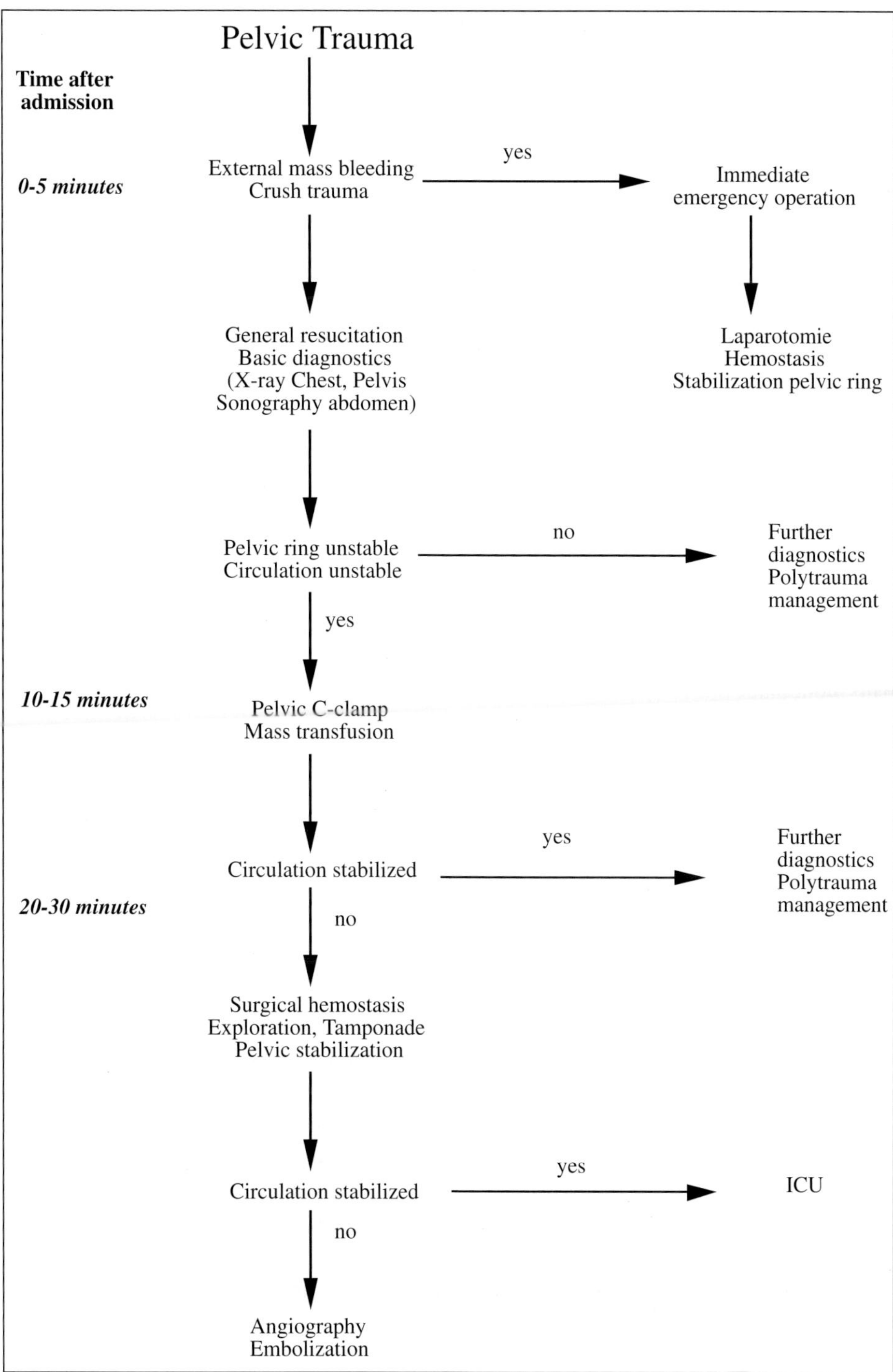

Figure 14 Emergency algorithm for pelvic trauma with three decisions within the first 30 minutes after admission.

and manual compression, and an emergency stabilization of the pelvic ring is considered depending on the fracture type. In type C injuries, a pelvic C-clamp (82) has proved to be useful (54). In rare occasions, a pelvic sling is tied around the pelvis.

With persistent hemodynamic instability lasting more than 15 minutes after application of the clamp, surgical revision of the pelvic retroperitoneum is required.

Technique of Pelvic C-Clamp Application (82)

Indication

The use of the emergency pelvic C-clamp is indicated in patients with unstable pelvic ring fractures classified as type B or C injuries (AO/OTA classification) (33) in combination with persistent unstable hemodynamics despite blood substitution estimated by a hemoglobin concentration of <8 g/dL who are too critical for a primary open reduction internal fixation (ORIF) (15,54).

Application

The pelvic C-clamp consists of two sidearms that move along a crossrail. The free end of each sidearm has an opening that accepts a threaded tube with an inner bore that allows a Steinmann pin with a minimum length of 250 mm to pass through it (Fig. 15). The Steinmann pin allows the device to be anchored to the obliquely oriented surface of the posterior ilium.

In the supine position the pelvic region is iodized. According to the radiograph, the displaced site is reduced by applying manual traction and internal rotation to the lower leg. A stab incision of about 1.5 to 2 cm length is performed on both sides at the recommended entry point (crossing of two lines, one parallel to the longitudinal axis of the femur, and a vertical line from the anterior iliac spine posteriorly) (Fig. 16). The outer ilium is prepared and sometimes palpation with a Steinmann pin or the scissors is helpful for orientation. The change of the orientation of the bony surface analyzed, allowing the identification of a *groove* directly opposite to the first sacral body (Fig. 17).

The sidearms of the pelvic clamp are then inserted with fixation into the ilium by hammering under fluoroscopic C-arm control, followed by connection of these with the crossbar (Fig. 18). Manual compression of the bars and tightening of the threads leads to correct application, which is checked by an anteroposterior (AP) pelvic radiograph.

Possible errors are perforation of the iliac bone and possible organ damage by too anterior application of the sidearms, the risk of posterior malplacement into the greater sciatic notch by too posterior placement of the sidearms with resulting damage to the gluteal neurovascular structures, and the risk of overcompression of the posterior pelvic ring, especially in sacral fractures, possibly resulting in iatrogenic nerve injury.

Technique of Pelvic Packing

The patient is positioned supine on a standard operating table. A heated blanket should be applied. The extremities and, if possible, the thorax as well are covered by blankets or a blowing forced-air patient warming system to avoid hypothermia. Temperature control is essential as hypothermia is associated with impairments of hemostasis.

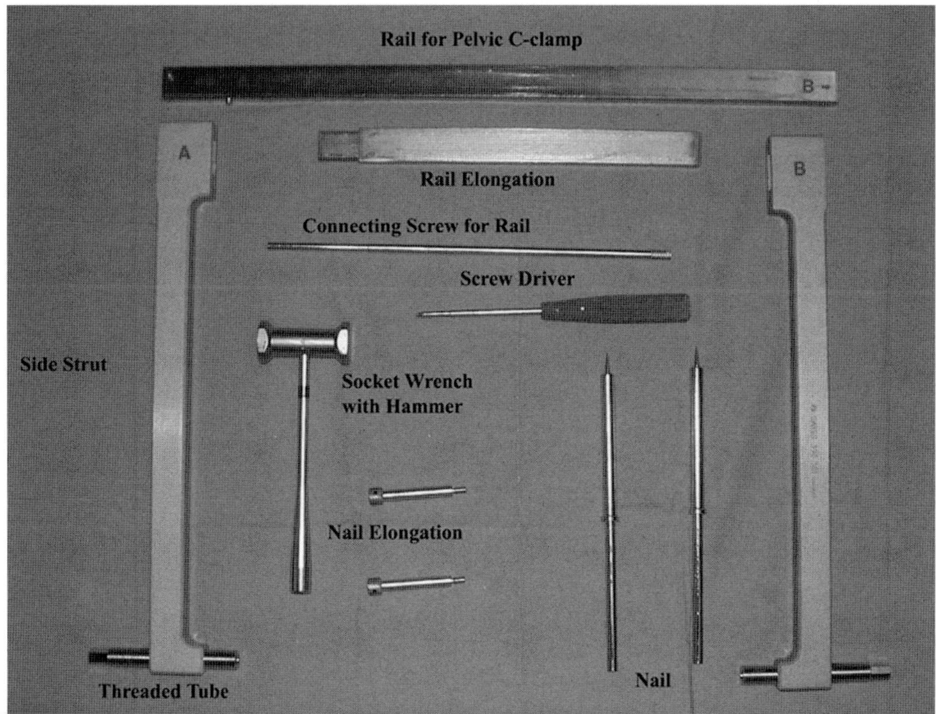

Figure 15 Pelvic C-clamp set.

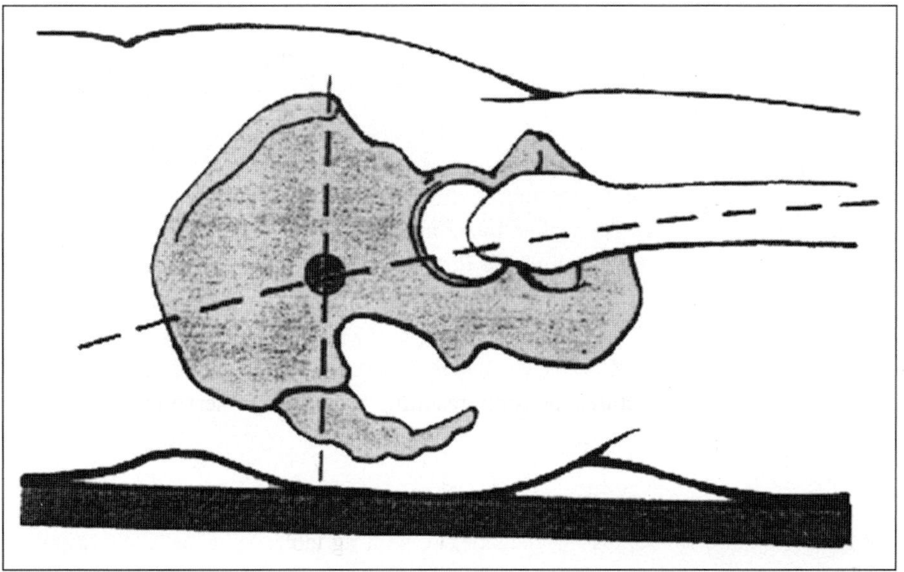

Figure 16 The entry point for the C-clamp nails is at the crossing of a line along the longitudinal femoral axis and a vertical line from the anterior superior iliac spine.

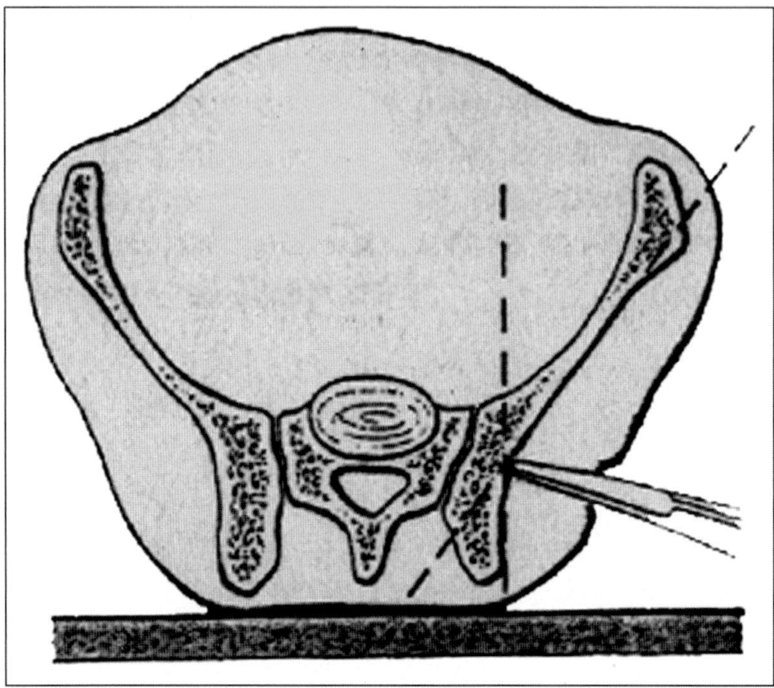

Figure 17 By preparing the outer ilium, a change of the orientation of the bony surface is found, identifying a *groove* directly opposite to the first sacral body.

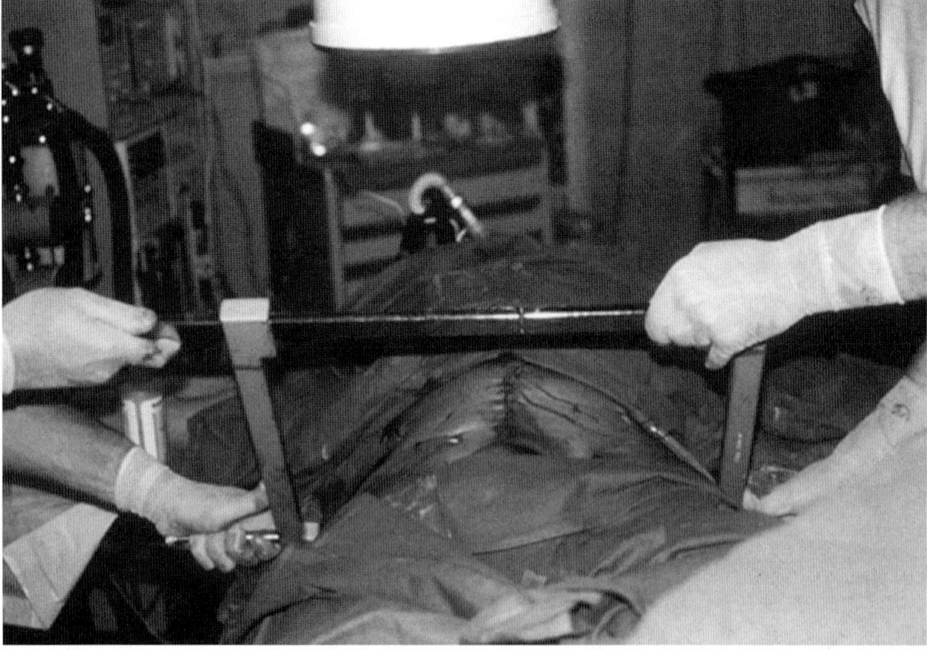

Figure 18 Connection of the side struts with the crossrail and manual compression of the side struts for optimal stability of the C-clamp.

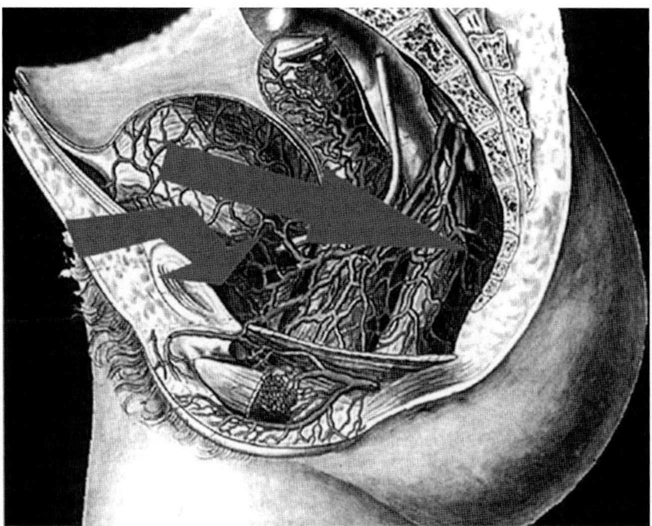

Figure 19 Localization of the pelvic tamponade. The packing is performed at the presacral region following anterior packing perivesical.

Preoperative retrograde fill-up of the bladder minimizes the risk of injury to urological structures during preparation. Additionally, a C-arm should be in place for possible support during pelvic fixation.

Incision

The abdomen is draped from the pubic symphysis up to the xyphoid process. In cases with suspected chest hemorrhage, the draping is extended to the chest to allow anterior or lateral thoracotomy. The choice of the incision depends on the ultrasound findings. In the presence of a large volume or a rapidly increasing volume of intraperitoneal fluid a median laparotomy is performed. General surgical rules are applied to treat intraperitoneal organ injuries. In the presence of multiple massive hemorrhages, tamponade of the areas or even aortic compression is performed. Temporary aortic clamping can be considered. Initial general assessment is gained by step-by-step attention to the various potential organ injuries present. Complex reconstructive procedures in the abdomen are avoided in the presence of additional pelvic hemorrhage. In the presence of major splenic ruptures, splenectomy is usually required. In the presence of hepatic injuries, attention is paid only to major vessels and a hepatic tamponade is applied. Bowel injuries are clamped and covered, and treatment is performed after the hemodynamic situation is stabilized (damage control surgery) (109–116).

When the origin of bleeding is clearly localized in the pelvic region, a midline incision is made in the lower abdomen, leaving the peritoneum intact. In most cases, the parapelvic fasciae are already disrupted. Direct manual access through the right or left paravesical space down to the presacral region can be achieved without further soft tissue dissection. The primary goal is to rule out or treat arterial bleeding by clamping, ligation, or by vascular repair. In massive bleeding, transient clamping of the infrarenal part of the aorta can be helpful. In most cases a specific source of bleeding cannot be identified. The origin of hemorrhage is mostly diffuse either from the venous plexus or

(A)

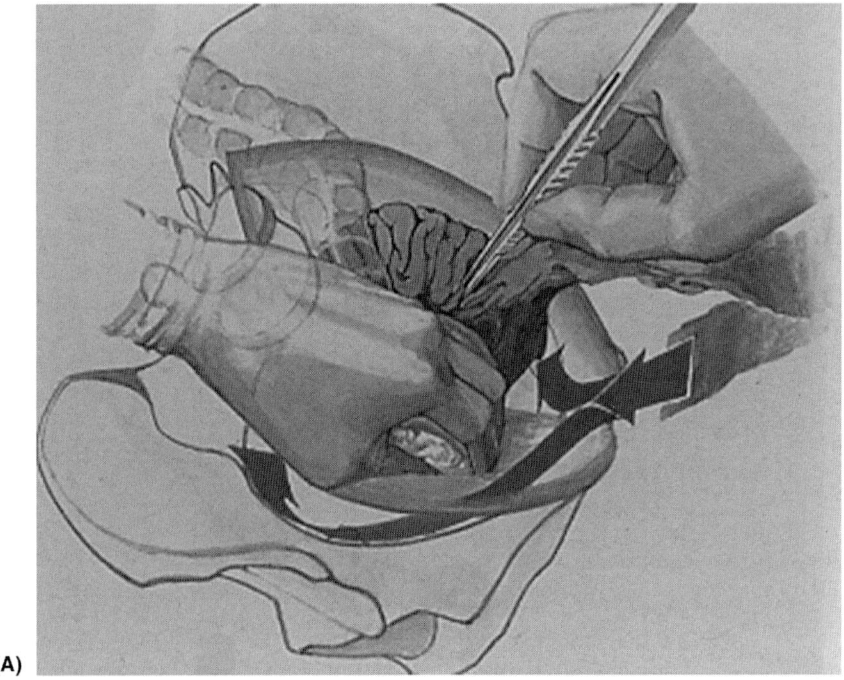

(B)

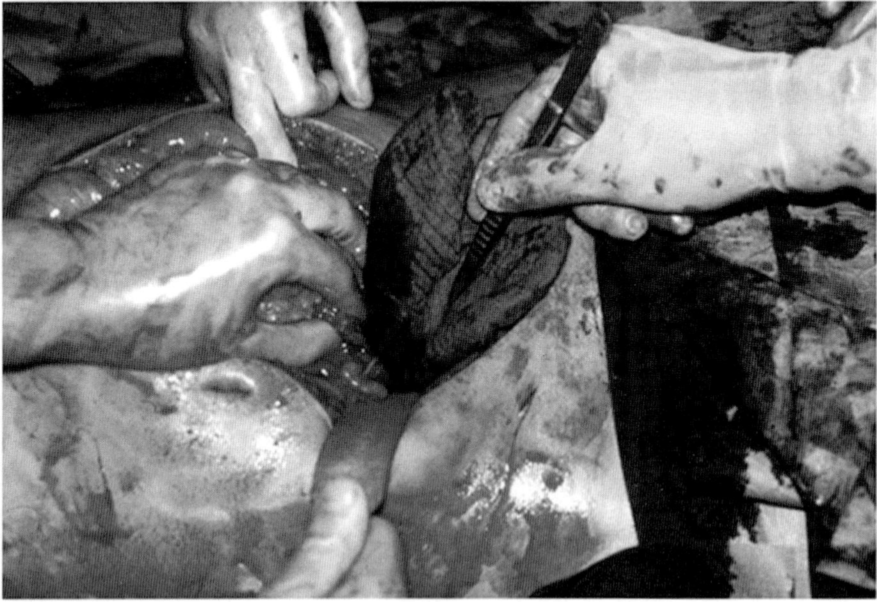

Figure 20 Schematic (**A**) and intraoperative (**B**) view of pelvic packing. Normally, four to eight surgical tamponades are necessary for sufficient compression inside the small pelvis.

the fracture site. In external-rotation-type injuries, the source of bleeding is generally located close to the anterior pelvic ring. In this region, control of bleeding by surgical hemostasis, closure of the pelvic ring, and paravesical packing is relatively easy. With a greater degree of pelvic instability, especially in C-type injuries, bleeding is usually located in the presacral region. With all compartmental borders disrupted, this space can generally be entered easily. The presacral and paravesical regions are packed from posterior to anterior using standard surgical tamponades (Fig. 19). About four to eight surgical tamponades will be necessary for sufficient compression inside the small pelvis (Fig. 20). When the acute bleeding is under control, the integrity of the bladder and urethra is inspected. Urological repair should be adequate to the patients general condition and is generally restricted to suprapubic drainage of urine, insertion of a transurethral catheter, and suture of the bladder.

The effectiveness of the tamponade is then re-evaluated, and all now identifiable bleedings are controlled by direct surgical means. If the quality of reduction of the posterior ring is unsatisfactory, it should now be improved to minimize bleeding from the fracture site. This is done by a short period of loosening of the clamp, manual traction, and internal rotation of the leg. Radiographic analysis by fluoroscopy should reveal proper reduction of the posterior pelvic ring. Therefore, specific landmarks have to be analyzed (Fig. 21). After re-tightening of the pelvic C-clamp the definitive packing is applied. Because of soft tissue swelling and the need for revision, the abdomen has frequently to be left open. The extraperitoneal fascia can be partially closed to improve the tamponade effect. The patient is then transferred to the ICU for further stabilization.

With still active bleeding and need for blood substitution, first the body temperature has to be normalized as soon as possible for stabilization of the intrinsic hemostatic system. When the body temperature is normal, a second attempt for hemorrhage control by changing the packing is performed.

When the hemodynamic situation is stabilized, packing is left in place for 24 to 48 hours. During a planned "second look" operation, there is usually a better view and the bleeding has completely stopped, or can be controlled by local surgical hemostasis. With a persistent bleeding, new tamponades are inserted and a "third look" is planned 24 to 48 hours later.

Depending on the patient's general condition, the anterior pelvic ring injury is stabilized. In symphyseal disruptions, an open reduction and internal fixation with a plate is performed, isolated transpubic instabilities are stabilized with a simple anterior supra-acetabular external fixator.

Treatment of Additional Pelvic Injuries

Bladder Injuries

There is as yet no consensus on whether extraperitoneal bladder ruptures should be treated surgically. Of all extraperitoneal bladder ruptures, 90% to 100% are associated with pelvic fractures (Fig. 9), whereas only 5% to 10% of all pelvic fractures are combined with bladder ruptures (117–119). Whereas some authors support the conservative therapy of single, small lesions by catheterization for at least 10 days, others promote a mandatory surgical repair (117,120). We use surgery, with a formal repair

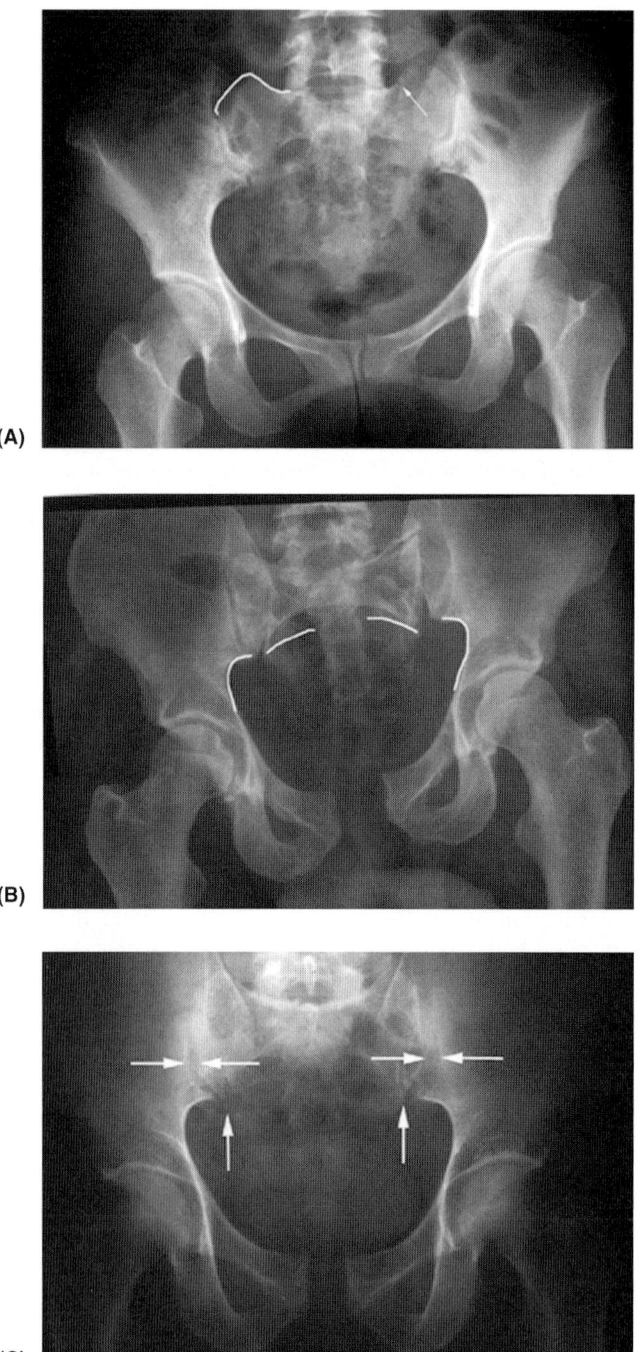

Figure 21 Reduction is radiographically controlled by analyzing specific landmarks: (**A**) sacral alar, (**B**) iliopectineal line to the second sacral arcuate line, (**C**) parallelism and width of the sacroilac-joint lines.

in all patients except those in a critical general condition that prohibits a surgical procedure. This practical approach is supported by the observation that the degree of extravasation in preoperative cystograms does not correlate with the size of rupture, so that a diagnostic stratification into larger and smaller bladder injuries is unreliable (117,119).

From a lower abdominal midline incision, the dome of the bladder is opened and the lesion repaired intravesically with 3/0 absorbable sutures. To avoid secondary complications such as urinary incontinence or erectile dysfunction (ED), injuries of the bladder neck, the proximal urethra, the prostate, or the vagina must be excluded. These injuries should be carefully reconstructed intravesically via the bladder dome incision. If the vagina is affected, a formal repair from a transvaginal approach is necessary.

An intraperitoneal rupture, which accounts for 35% to 40% of all bladder injuries, requires formal repair. After a midline incision, a complete inspection of the entire intraperitoneal abdomen is mandatory to exclude intraperitoneal injuries. Any injury at the bladder dome should be used to inspect the entire bladder lumen, and thus repair possible further ruptures intravesically. Later, this usually large tear is repaired with a double-layer suture. In cases of extensive ruptures of the bladder wall with subsequent risk of urine extravasation, additionally, 6-10Ch splints are introduced in a retrograde fashion from the bladder into the ureters, fixed at the region of the orifices and tunneled through the abdominal wall to a urostomy. Just before the removal of the ureteric stents at 10 to 12 days, a cystography should rule out leakage of contrast fluid.

Combined extra- and intraperitoneal bladder ruptures are present in 5% to 10%; penetrating injuries should be explored surgically. All such patients should undergo a formal repair with a combination of the appropriate procedures as detailed above.

Injuries to the Urethra

The incidence of urethral lacerations in complex pelvic injuries appears to be very similar to bladder ruptures. In suspected urethral injuries (particularly bleeding from the urethral meatus), a retrograde urethrogram should be obtained. In most cases, there is a shearing injury through the membranous urethra. Pelvic fractures are present in >90% of patients with urethral ruptures, and most are associated with posterior bony or ligamentous injuries around the sacroiliac joint, in addition to anterior bony disruption, causing instability.

Experience either in the acute treatment of patients with complex pelvic fractures and complete urethral ruptures, or the handling of late complications, have shown that an interdisciplinary therapeutic approach is necessary. This concept considers the vital functions of the patient, accompanying further bony and soft-tissue injuries, the extent of the retropubic and perivesical hematoma, and the need for operative exploration for other indications close to the urethral lesion.

If there is a complete urethral rupture in an unstable patient, with an extensive retropubic or perivesical hematoma, a suprapubic catheter is inserted and the urethra reanastomosed after at least three months of complete urinary drainage, or when the osseous lesions and possible infections have healed. This concept of delayed urethral bulboprostatic end-to-end anastomosis via a perineal approach represents the current "gold standard" of treatment (121,122). The incidence of urethral strictures and ED for this kind of therapeutic approach is reportedly lower than for any other treatment (123–125). Primary repair is still recommended if there is bladder neck laceration, severe prostatomembranous dislocation, and concomitant vascular or rectal injury (118,126,127).

If surgical exploration close to the urethral injury is necessary because of other surgical or traumatic indications, we try to achieve an antegrade or retrograde realignment with an indwelling catheter. We avoid prolonged manipulations so that the incidence of bleeding, infection, ED, and incontinence is minimized.

Additional Gynecological Injuries

Gynecological injuries are predominantly caused by direct injury forces to the perineal region with direct injury to the labias or vagina. Injury to the nonpregnant uterus is extremely rare. Additionally, pelvic injuries during pregnancy are rare with a high risk of maternal and especially fetal death due to the general injury severity (128,129).

A detailed primary evaluation of the female patient is mandatory to avoid ignoring occult gynecological injuries. Therefore, vaginal palpation is recommended in every female patient with suspected pelvic injury.

The amount of vaginal or vulval reconstruction depends on the general patient status. In combination with a gynecologist, the therapeutic regimen is focused on the control of bleeding and local debridement. In massive injuries to the perineal region, a colostoma is applied, and an antegrade washout is performed. Secondary soft-tissue reconstruction is then performed dependent on the general status of the patient.

In pregnant women, the interdisciplinary approach (gynecologist, perinatologist) is of fundamental importance for the probable indication of an emergency section for optimization of the treatment of the newborn.

Abdominal Aortic Rupture

In cases with complete disruption of the abdominal aorta, emergency laparotomy to obtain bleeding control is of primary priority (130–132). In incomplete ruptures, first pelvic stabilization (C-clamp) and pelvic packing are performed. Systolic blood pressure should be less than 120 mmHg. In the latter cases, reconstruction of the aorta is performed after stabilization of the patient.

Severe Liver Rupture

In cases of severe liver rupture, this injury is treated with first priority. The pelvic C-clamp should be applied in the emergency department during extended shock therapy. Prior to definitive treatment of the liver injury, a pelvic packing should be performed. Temporary aortic compression, perihepatic packing, or a Pringle maneuver helps to gain better overview of the hepatic bleeding localization (111,133).

Massive Trauma to the Lower Extremities

Patients with additional massive lower extremity injuries, often after roll-over or crush injuries, have severe soft-tissue lesions with release of several mediators, indicating a high risk of development of multiple organ failure (105).

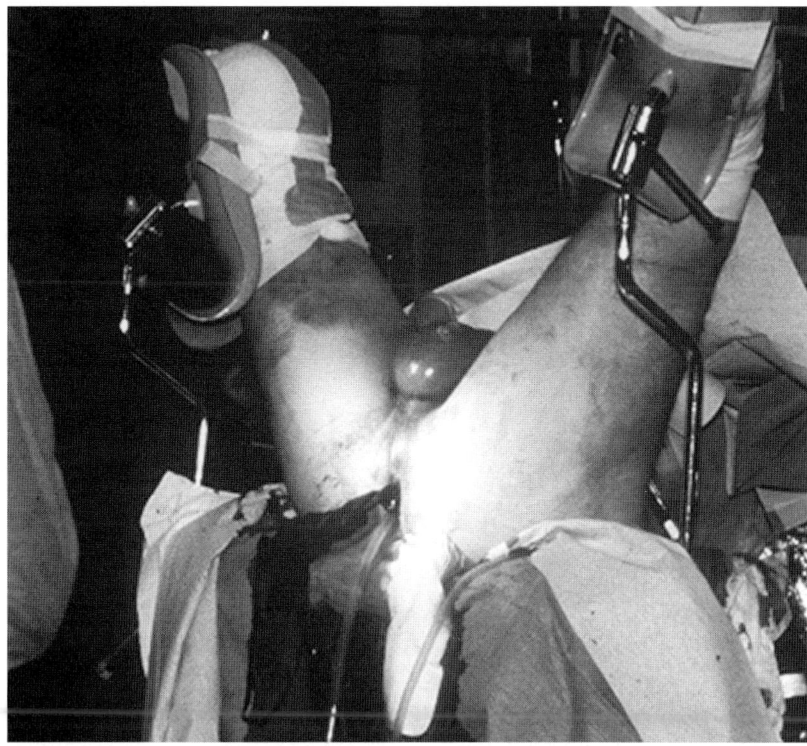

Figure 22 In open pelvic fractures, especially combined with rectal lesions, a thorough washout is performed.

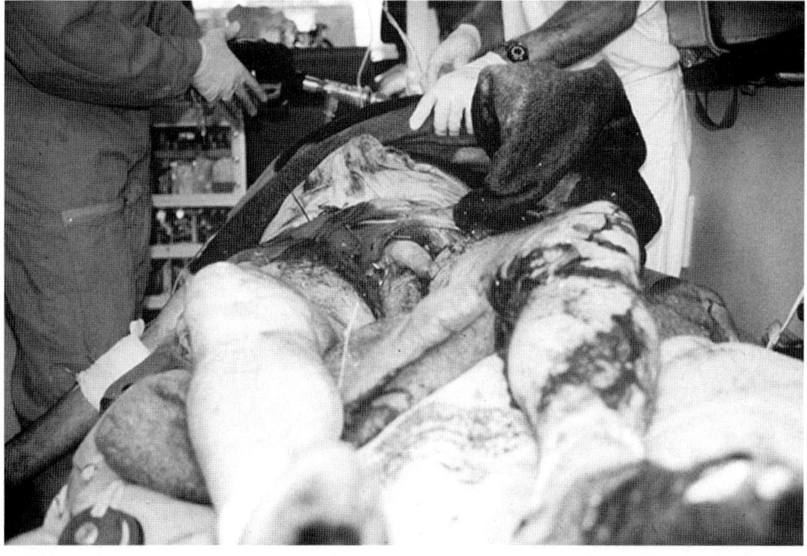

Figure 23 Clinical view of a patient with right-sided traumatic hepipelvectomy with a large open inguinal wound.

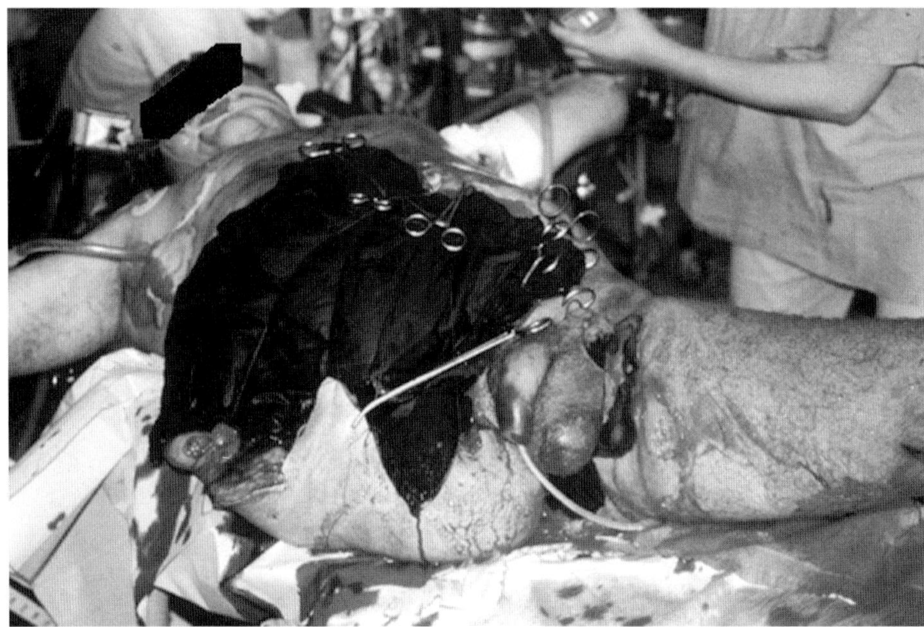

Figure 24 Hemipelvectomy is completed immediately, as attempts at pelvic reconstruction showed an increase of mortality.

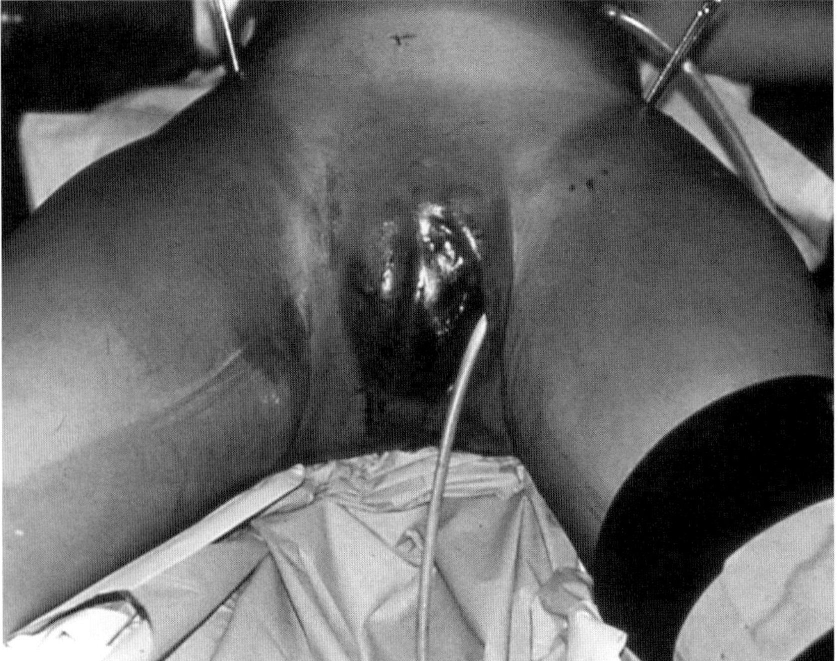

Figure 25 An expanding hematoma within the small pelvis leads to severe swelling in the perianal region with the risk of skin perforation.

If the bleeding is uncontrollable, the pelvis is temporarily stabilized with the pelvic C-clamp and a pelvic packing is performed. The extremity hemorrhage is then controlled by tourniquet. Often, an amputation is necessary in these extreme cases.

Open Pelvic Fractures

Open pelvic fractures (Fig. 1) are characterized by a high mortality (134–142). Mortality is predominantly related to massive bleeding and septic complications (143). The main treatment concept is comparable to closed complex pelvic injuries. After initial control of blood loss, the search and optimal treatment of additional rectal, vaginal, or urogenital injuries is essential for avoiding septic complications. The indication for a colostoma and thorough washout in case of severe rectal lacerations or extended perineal injuries should be addressed generously (Fig. 22). Basic treatment principle is the extended debridement of severely injured soft-tissues, open wound management, and adequate second-look operations to avoid development of muscle necrosis, especially of the gluteal and psoas muscles. Early detection and treatment of a pelvic compartment syndrome (gluteal/psoas compartment) is mandatory.

Traumatic Hemipelvectomy

Traumatic hemipelvectomy is defined as total dislocation of the hemipelvis with complete disruption of the vascular and neural structures of the pelvis (e.g., the hypogastric vessels and lumbosacral plexus) (37).

The severity of the soft tissue involvement varies from complete (with no attachment or near complete detachment of the soft tissue connection) to incomplete (Fig. 23). There are frequently associated internal organ injuries (colon, rectum, or genitourinary system). These injuries are rare with an incidence reported between 0.19% and 0.6% (37,38).

An immediate completion of the hemipelvectomy is necessary (Fig. 24). Attempts at pelvic reconstruction showed an increase of mortality.

The question of wound closure is certainly controversial. Some authors close the wound primarily for better future prosthetic fitting, others find it difficult to determine the zone of injury primarily or prefer frequent and generous débridements followed by flap coverage. In all cases, consideration should be given to the retrieval and preservation of skin from the amputated extremity for future wound coverage.

Pelvic Compartment Syndrome

Pelvic compartment syndrome is a rare complication after severe pelvic injury (144–146). The pelvic injury itself is a rare reason for development of a compartment syndrome as in unstable pelvic fractures the retroperitoneal and gluteal fascias are often disrupted. However, with extended soft-tissue lacerations, expanding hematomas can lead to severe swelling of the complete pelvic region (Fig. 25). Muscular compartments around the pelvis are the iliopsoas compartment, the glutaeus medius and minimus compartment, and the glutaeus maximus compartment.

The significance of pelvic compartment syndromes is due to compression induced ischemic damage to nerves (sciatic, femoral, obturator nerve) and secondary organ failure due to crush syndrome of the large muscle mass and the skin. Treatment consists of early fasciotomy with removal of the hematoma, identification and control of the

(A)

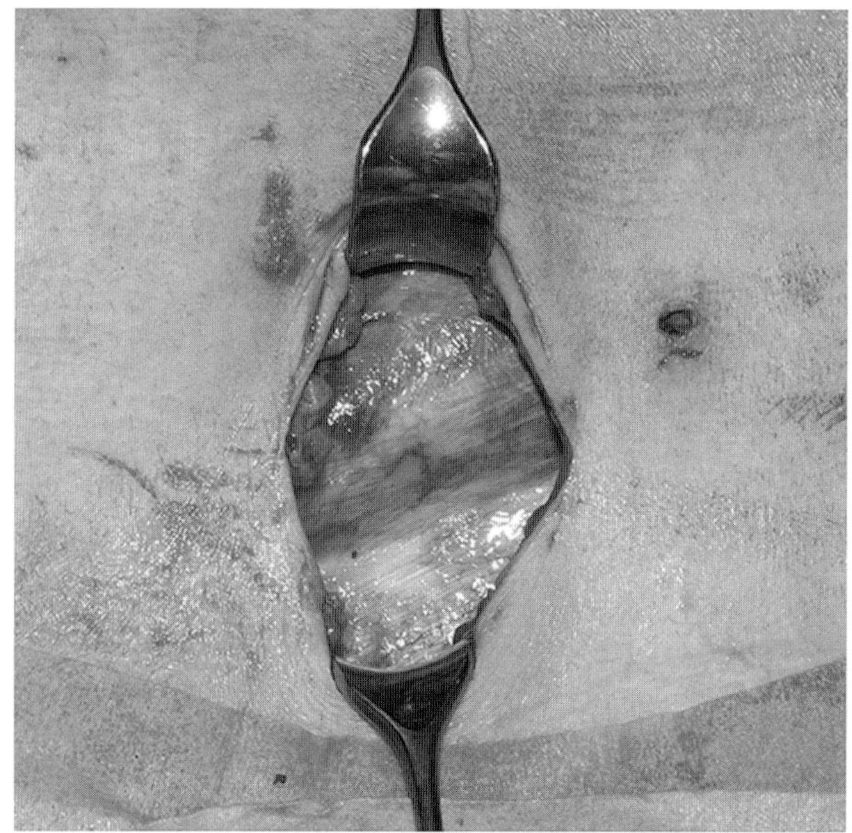

(B)

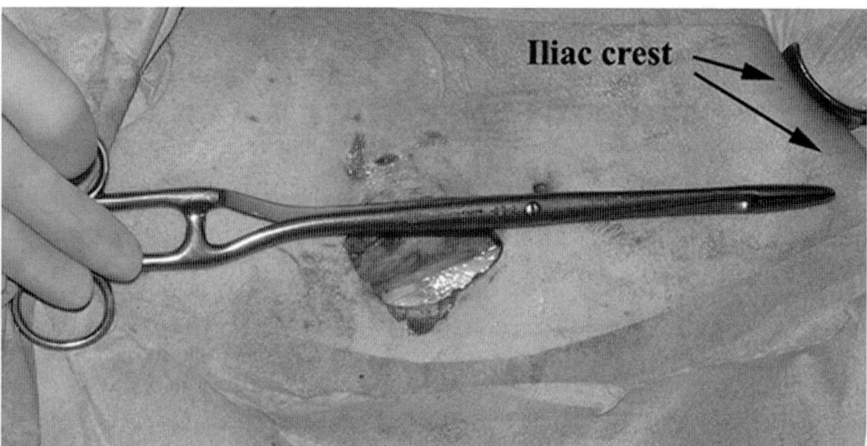

Figure 26 Morel-Levallé lesion of the anterolateral fascia of the thigh (**A**) extending to the pelvic region (**B**).

bleeding source, and extensive debridement of necrotic muscles. Gluteal compartments are approached via a Kocher–Langenbeck incision and iliopsoas compartments via an anterolateral approach to the pelvis. Depending on skin retraction, temporary wound closure is often required with vacuum-assisted wound closures.

Morel Lavallé Lesions

An extended decollement of the anterolateral fascia of the thigh and pelvis is rarely combined with pelvic injuries (Fig. 26). Due to lymphatic fluid intake, extended seromas are possible. Secondary infections are reported despite closed soft-tissues (147). Spontaneous healing of these lesions is rarely seen, whereas extended skin necroses with secondary soft-tissue infections are frequent. An open wound management after an extended debridement in these lesions is recommended. Pelvic stabilization should be performed as soon as possible due to potential infection. Drainage should be performed with vacuum-assisted techniques.

CONCLUSION

Damage control orthopedics currently appears to be the treatment of choice for polytraumatized patients with unstable pelvic fractures and additional hemodynamic instability who are at high risk to develop systemic complications, such as multiple organ failure. The authors feel that the following principles are relevant: the procedure can be conceived as part of the resuscitation effort by maintaining blood volume and tissue oxygenation, thus minimizing the damage induced by the procedure while utilizing the surgical treatment options to maintain the benefits of pelvic fracture stabilization.

Immediate external fixation of the unstable pelvis with pelvic packing to control pelvic hemorrhage seems to be a useful approach in patients in extremis and borderline patients. Angiographic embolization is only recommended in the more stable patient.

REFERENCES

1. Bosch U, Pohlemann T, Haas N, Tscherne H. Klassifikation und management des komplexen beckentraumas. Unfallchirurg 1992; 95:189–196.
2. Pohlemann T, Gänsslen A, Hartung S. Für die arbeitsgruppe becken: beckenverletzungen/pelvic injuries. Hefte zu "Der Unfallchirurg" 1998; Heft 266.
3. Pohlemann T, Tscherne H, Baumgärtel F, et al. Beckenverletzungen: epidemiologie, therapie und langzeitverlauf. Übersicht über die multizentrische studie der arbeitsgruppe becken. Unfallchirurg 1996; 99:160–167.
4. Pohlemann T, Bosch U, Gänsslen A, et al. The Hannover experience in management of pelvic fractures. Clin Orthop 1994; 305:69–80.
5. Advanced Trauma Life Support for Doctors, ATLS, Instructor Course Manual. Chicago: American College of Surgeons, 1997.
6. O'Gorman M, Trabulsy P, Pilcher D. Zero time prehospital IV. J Trauma 1989; 29:84–86.
7. Pons P, Moore E, Cusick J. Prehospital venous access in an urban paramedic system: a prospective on-scene analysis. J Trauma 1988; 28:1460–1463.
8. Dalton A. Prehospital intravenous fluid replacement in trauma: an outmoded concept. J R Soc Med 1995; 88:213–216.
9. Kaweski S, Size M, Virgilio R. The effect of prehospital fluids on survival in trauma patients. J Trauma 1990; 30:1215–1219.
10. Bickell W, Wall M, Pepe P. Immediate versus delayed fluid resuscitation for hypotensive patients with penetrating torso injuries. N Engl Med J 1994; 331: 105–1109.
11. Kwan I, Bunn F, Roberts I. Committee obot WP-HTCS: Timing and volume of fluid administration for patients with bleeding following trauma (Cochrane Review). In: The Cochrane Library, Issue 2. Oxford: Update Software, 2003.
12. Brotman S, Soderstrom C, Oster-Granite M, et al. Management of severe bleeding in fractures of the pelvis. Surg Gynec Obstet 1981; 153:823–826.
13. Downs AR, Dhalla S. Hemorrhage and pelvic fractures. Can J Surg 1988; 31:89–90.
14. Moreno C, Moore EE, Rosenberger A, et al. Hemorrhage associated with major pelvic fracture: a multispecialty challenge. J Trauma 1986; 26:987–994.
15. Pohlemann T, Culemann U, Gänsslen A, et al. Die schwere Beckenverletzung mit pelviner massenblutung: ermittlung der blutungsschwere und klinische erfahrung mit der notfallstabilisierung. Unfallchirurg 1996; 99:734–743.
16. Dickinson K, Roberts I. Medical anti-shock trousers (pneumatic anti-shock garments) for circulatory support in patients with trauma (Cochrane Review). In: The Cochrane Library, Issue 2. Oxford: Update Software, 2003.
17. Ali J, Qi W. Fluid and electrolyte deficit with prolonged pneumatic antishock garment application. J Trauma 1995; 38:612–615.
18. Christensen KS. Pneumatic antishock garments (PASG): Do they precipitate lower-extremity compartment syndromes? J Trauma 1986; 26:1102–1105.
19. Clarke G, Mardel S. Use of MAST to control massive bleeding from pelvic injuries. Injury 1993; 24:628–629.
20. Frank LR. Is MAST in the past? The pros and cons of MAST usage in the field. J Emerg Med Serv JEMS 2000; 25:38–41,44–45.
21. Vahedi M, Ayuyao A, Parsa M, Freeman H. Pneumatic antishock garment-associated compartment syndrome in injured lower extremities. J Trauma 1995; 38:616–618.
22. Bottlang M, Simpson T, Sigg J, et al. Noninvasive reduction of open-book pelvic fractures by circumferential compression. J Orthop Trauma 2002; 16:367–373.
23. Duxbury M, Rossiter N, Lambert A. Cable ties for pelvic stabilisation. Ann R Coll Surg Engl 2003; 85:130.

24. Routt M, Falicov A, Woodhouse E, Schildhauer T. Circumferential pelvic antishock sheeting: a temporary resuscitation aid. J Orthop Trauma 2002; 16:45–48.
25. Simpson T, Krieg JC, Heuer F, Bottlang M. Stabilization of pelvic ring disruptions with a circumferential sheet. J Trauma 2002; 52:158–161.
26. Vermeulen B, Peter R, Hoffmeyer P, Unger PF. Prehospital stabilization of pelvic dislocations: a new strap belt to provide temporary hemodynamic stabilization. Swiss Surg 1999; 5:43–46.
27. Morris LD, Pont A, Lewis SM. Use of a new HemoCue system for measuring haemoglobin at low concentrations. Clin Lab Haematol 2001; 23:91–96.
28. Rippmann CE, Nett PC, Popovic D, et al. Hemocue, an accurate bedside method of hemoglobin measurement? J Clin Monit 1997; 13:373–377.
29. Schroeder F, Horn EP, Redmann G, Standl T. Intraoperative normothermia with partial warming of patients undergoing orthopedic procedures. Anasthesiol Intensivmed Notfallmed Schmerzther 1999; 34:475–479.
30. Smith CE, Desai R, Glorioso V, et al. Preventing hypothermia: convective and intravenous fluid warming versus convective warming alone. J Clin Anesth 1998; 10: 380–385.
31. Lis L, Cohen A. CT cystography in the evaluation of bladder trauma. J Comput Assist Tomogr 1990; 14:386–389.
32. Sandler C, Hall J, Rodriguez M, Corriere J. Bladder injury in blunt pelvic trauma. Radiology 1986; 158:633–638.
33. OTA. Fracture and dislocation compendium. J Orthop Trauma 1996; 10:71–75.
34. Tscherne H, Pohlemann T. Tscherne Unfallchirurgie: Becken und Acetabulum. Berlin, Heidelberg, New York: Springer-Verlag, 1998.
35. Gänsslen A, Pohlemann T, Paul C, et al. Epidemiology of pelvic ring injuries. Injury 1996; (suppl 1):13–20.
36. Bone L. Emergency treatment of the injured patient. In: Browner B, Jupiter J, Levine A, Trafton P, eds. Skeletal Trauma. Vol. I. Philadelphia, London, Toronto, Montreal, Sydney, Tokyo: Saunders, 1992.
37. Pohlemann T, Paul C, Gänsslen A, et al. Die traumatische hemipelvektomie. erfahrungen aus 11 fällen. Unfallchirurg 1996; 99:304–312.
38. Rieger H, Dietl KH. Traumatic hemipelvectomy: an update. J Trauma 1998; 45:422–426.
39. Agolini S, Shah K, Jaffe J, et al. Arterial embolization is a rapid and effective technique for controlling pelvic fracture hemorrhage. J Trauma 1997; 43:395–399.
40. Bassam D, Cephas GA, Ferguson KA, et al. A protocol for the initial management of unstable pelvic fractures. Am Surg 1998; 64:862–867.
41. Batalden D, Wickstorm P, Ruiz E, Gustilo R. Value of the G suit in patients with severe pelvic fracture. Arch Surg 1974; 109:326–328.
42. Baumgaertel F, Wilke M, Gotzen L. Experimentelle Erprobung eines pneumatischen Gürtels zur äußeren Beckenkompression. Swiss Surgery 1996; (suppl 2): 42.
43. Ben-Menachem Y. Exploratory angiography and transcatheter embolization for control of arterial hemorrhage in patients with pelvic ring disruptions. Tech Orthop 1995; 9:271–274.
44. Buckle R, Browner B, Morandi M. Emergency reduction for pelvic ring disruptions and controll of associated hemorrhage using the pelvic stabilizer. Techniques in Orthopaedics 1995; 9:258–266.
45. Bühren V, Marzi I, Trentz O. Indikation und technik des fixateur externe in der akutversorgung von polytraumen. Zentbl Cir 1990; 115:581–591.
46. Ertel W, Keel M, Eid K, et al. Control of severe hemorrhage using C-clamp and pelvic packing in multiply injured patients with pelvic ring disruption. J Orthop Trauma 2001; 15:468–474.

47. Kellam J. The role of external fixation in pelvic disruptions. Clin Orthop 1989; 241:66–82.
48. Perez JV, Hughes TM, Bowers K. Angiographic embolisation in pelvic fracture. Injury 1998; 29:187–191.
49. Piotin M, Herbreteau D, Guichard J, et al. Percutaneous transcatheter embolization in multiply injured patients with pelvic ring disruption associated with severe haemorrhage and coagulopathy. Injury 1995; 26:677–680.
50. Poka A, Libby E. Indications and techniques for external fixation of the pelvis. Clin Orthop 1996; 329:54–59.
51. Riska E, von Bonsdorf H, Hakkinen S, et al. External fixation of unstable pelvic fractures. Intern Orthop 1997; 3:183–188.
52. Schütz M, Stöckle U, Hoffmann R, Südkamp N, Haas N. Clinical experience with two types of pelvic C-clamps for unstable pelvic ring injuries. Injury 1996, (suppl 1):46–50.
53. Stock J, Harris W, Athanasoulis A. The role of diagnostic and therapeutic angiography in trauma to the pelvis. Clin Orthop 1980; 151:31–40.
54. Tscherne H, Pohlemann T, Gansslen A, et al. Crush injuries of the pelvis. Eur J Surg 2000; 166:276–282.
55. Tucker MC, Nork SE, Simonian PT, Routt ML Jr. Simple anterior pelvic external fixation. J Trauma 2000; 49:989–994.
56. Velmahos GC, Toutouzas KG, Vassiliu P, et al. A prospective study on the safety and efficacy of angiographic embolization for pelvic and visceral injuries. J Trauma 2002; 53: 303–308; discussion 308.
57. Vrahas MS, Wilson SC, Cummings PD, Paul EM. Comparison of fixation methods for preventing pelvic ring expansion. Orthopedics 1998; 21:285–289.
58. Witschger P, Heini P, Ganz R. Beckenzwinge zur Schockbekämpfung bei hinteren Beckenringverletzungen. Orthopäde 1992; 21:393–399.
59. Yang A, Iannacone W. External fixation for pelvic ring disruptions. Orthop Clin North Am 1997; 28:331–344.
60. Grimm M, Vrahas M, Thomas K. Pressure–volume characteristics of the intact and disrupted pelvic retroperitoneum. J Trauma 1998; 44:454–459.
61. Trentz O, Bühren V, Friedl H. Beckenverletzungen. Chirurg 1989; 60:639–648.
62. Williams T, Knopp R, Ellyson J. Compartment syndrome after anti-shock trouser use without lower-extremity trauma. J Trauma 1982; 22:595–597.
63. Huittinen V, Slätis P. Postmortem angiography and dissection of the hypogastric artery in pelvic fractures. Surgery 1973; 73:454–462.
64. Kadish L, Stein J, Kotler S. Angiographic diagnosis and treatment of bleeding due to pelvic trauma. J Trauma 1973; 13:1083.
65. Cook RE, Keating JF, Gillespie I. The role of angiography in the management of haemorrhage from major fractures of the pelvis. J Bone Joint Surg Br 2002; 84:178–182.
66. Hamill J, Holden A, Paice R, Civil I. Pelvic fracture pattern predicts pelvic arterial haemorrhage. Aust N Z J Surg 2000; 70:338–343.
67. Stephen DJ, Kreder HJ, Day AC, et al. Early detection of arterial bleeding in acute pelvic trauma. J Trauma 1999; 47:638–642.
68. Chaufour J, Melki JP, Riche MC, et al. Complications vasculaires hémorragiques des fractures du bassin. Presse Med 1986; 15:2097–2100.
69. Hölting T, Buhr H, Richter G, et al. Diagnosis and treatment of retroperitoneal hematoma in multiple trauma patients. Arch Orthop Trauma Surg 1992; 111:323–326.
70. Burgess A, Eastridge B, Young J, et al. Pelvic ring disruption: effective classification systems and treatment protocols. J Trauma 1990; 30:848–856.

71. Velmahos GC, Chahwan S, Hanks SE, et al. Angiographic embolization of bilateral internal iliac arteries to control life-threatening hemorrhage after blunt trauma to the pelvis. Am Surg 2000; 66:858–862.
72. Grabenwöger F, Dock W, Ittner G. Perkutane embolisation von retroperitonealen blutungen bei beckenfrakturen. RÖFO 1989; 150:335–338.
73. Hauser C, Perry J. Control of massive hemorrhage from pelvic fractures by hypogastric artery ligation. Surg Gynec Obstet 1964; 121:313.
74. Platz A, Friedl H, Kohler A, et al. Chirurgisches management bei schweren beckenquetschverletzungen. Helv Chir Acta 1992; 58:925–929.
75. Ravdin I, Ellison E. Hypogastric artery ligation in acute pelvic trauma. Surgery 1964; 56:601–602.
76. Saueracker AJ, McCroskey BL, Moore EE, Moore FA. Intraoperative hypogastric artery embolization for life-threatening pelvic hemorrhage: a preliminary report. J Trauma 1987; 27:1127–1129.
77. Seavers F, Robinson R. Hypogastric artery ligation for uncontrollable hemorrhage in acute pelvic trauma. Surgery 1964; 55:516.
78. Bühren V, Trentz O. Intraluminäre ballonblockade der aorta bei traumatischer massivblutung. Unfallchirurg 1989; 92:309–313.
79. Bellabarba C, Ricci WM, Bolhofner BR. Distraction external fixation in lateral compression pelvic fractures. J Orthop Trauma 2000; 14:475–482.
80. Bircher M. Indications and techniques of external fixation of the injured pelvis. Injury 1996; 27:3–19.
81. Lindahl J, Hirvensalo E, Bostman O, et al. Failure of reduction with an external fixator in the management of injuries of the pelvic ring. Long-term evaluation of 110 patients. J Bone Joint Surg Br 1999; 81:955–962.
82. Ganz R, Krushell R, Jakob R, et al. The antishock pelvic clamp. Clin Orthop 1991; 267:71–78.
83. Pohlemann T, Gänsslen A, Bosch U, et al. The technique of packing for control of hemorrhage in complex pelvic fractures. Techniques in Orthopaedics 1995; 9:267–270.
84. Pohlemann T, Angst M, Schneider E, et al. Fixation of transforaminal sacrum fractures: a biomechanical study. J Orthop Trauma 1993; 7:107 –117.
85. Stocks G, Gablel D, Noble P, et al. Anterior and posterior internal fixation of vertical shear fractures of the pelvis. J Orthop Research 1991; 9:237–245.
86. Tile M, Helfet D, Kellam J. Fractures of the Pelvis and Acetabulum, 3rd ed. Philadelphia: Lippincott, Williams and Wilkins, 2003.
87. Barei DP, Bellabarba C, Mills WJ, Routt ML Jr. Percutaneous management of unstable pelvic ring disruptions. Injury 2001; 32:SA33–SA44.
88. Kregor PJ, Routt ML Jr. Unstable pelvic ring disruptions in unstable patients. Injury 1999; 30:B19–B28.
89. Routt ML Jr, Nork SE, Mills WJ. High-energy pelvic ring disruptions. Orthop Clin North Am 2002; 33:59–72, viii.
90. Beard J, Davidson C. Pelvic injuries associated with traumatic abduction of the leg. Injury 1988; 19:353–356.
91. Finan MA, Fiorica JV, Hoffman MS, et al. Massive pelvic hemorrhage during gynecologic cancer surgery: "pack and go back." Gynecol Oncol 1996; 62:390-395.
92. Flory P, Trentz O, Bühren V, et al. Management der komplexen beckenverletzung. Akt Traumatol 1985; 15:139–144.
93. Boyd CR, Tolson MA, Copes WS. Evaluating trauma care: the TRISS method. Trauma Score and the Injury Severity Score. J Trauma 1987; 27:370–378.

94. Osterwalder JJ, Riederer M. Quality assessment of multiple trauma management bu ISS, TRISS or ASCOT? Schweiz Med Wochenschr 2000; 130:499–504.
95. Ertel W, Eid K, Keel M, et al. Therapeutical strategies and outcome of polytraumatized patients with pelvic injuries—a six-year experience. Eur J Trauma 2000; 26(6):278–286.
96. McMurtry R, Walton D, Dickinson D, et al. Pelvic disruption in the polytraumatized patient: a management protocol. Clin Orthop 1980; 151:22–30.
97. Agnew S. Hemodynamically unstable pelvic fractures. Orthop Clin North Am 1994; 25:715–721.
98. Allen CF, Goslar PW, Barry M, Christiansen T. Management guidelines for hypotensive pelvic fracture patients. Am Surg 2000; 66:735–738.
99. Coppola PT, Coppola M. Emergency department evaluation and treatment of pelvic fractures. Emerg Med Clin North Am 2000; 18:1–27, v.
100. Evers BM, Cryer HM, Miller FB. Pelvic fracture hemorrhage: priorities in management. Arch Surg 1989; 124:422–424.
101. Failinger M, McGanity P. Unstable fractures of the pelvic ring. J Bone Joint Surg 1992; 74-A:781–791.
102. Gruen G, Leit M, Gruen R, et al. The acute management of hemodynamically unstable multiple trauma patients with pelvic ring fractures. J Trauma 1994; 36:706–711.
103. Malangoni MA, Miller FB, Cryer HM, et al. The management of penetrating pelvic trauma. Am Surg 1990; 56:61–65.
104. Nerlich M, Maghsudi M. Algorithms for early management of pelvic fractures. Injury 1996; (suppl 1):29–37.
105. Krettek C, Simon R, Tscherne H. Management priorities in patients with polytrauma. Langenbecks Arch Surg 1998; 383(3–4):220–227.
106. Pape HC, Giannoudis P, Krettek C. The timing of fracture treatment in polytrauma patients: relevance of damage control orthopedic surgery. Am J Surg 2002; 183:622–629.
107. Pape HC, Krettek C. Management of fractures in the severely injured—influence of the principle of "damage control orthopaedic surgery." Unfallchirurg 2003; 106:87–96.
108. Tscherne H, Regel G. Tscherne Unfallchirurgie: Trauma-Management. Springer-Verlag, 1997:257–297.
109. Bowley DM, Barker P, Boffard KD. Damage control surgery—concepts and practice. J R Army Med Corps 2000; 146:176–182.
110. Kouraklis G, Spirakos S, Glinavou A. Damage control surgery: an alternative approach for the management of critically injured patients. Surg Today 2002; 32:195–202.
111. Krige JE, Bornman PC, Terblanche J. Therapeutic perihepatic packing in complex liver trauma. Br J Surg 1992; 79:43–46.
112. Little JM, Fernandes A, Tait N. Liver trauma. Aust N Z J Surg 1986; 56:613–619.
113. Parreira JG, Solda S, Rasslan S. Damage control: a tactical alternative for the management of exanguinating trauma patients. Arq Gastroenterol 2002; 39:188–197.
114. Shapiro MB, Jenkins DH, Schwab CW, Rotondo MF. Damage control: collective review. J Trauma 2000; 49:969–978.
115. Stagnitti F, Mongardini M, Schillaci F, et al. Damage control surgery: the technique. G Chir 2002; 23:18–21.
116. Zacharias SR, Offner P, Moore EE, Burch J. Damage control surgery. AACN Clin Issues 1999; 10:95–103; quiz 141–142.
117. Carroll P, McAninch J. Major bladder trauma: mechanisms of injury and a unified method of diagnosis and repair. J Urol 1984; 132:254–257.
118. Corriere J. Trauma to the lower urinary tract. In: Gillenwater J, Grayhack J, Howards S, et al., eds. Adult and Pediatric Urology. St. Louis, Baltimore, Boston: Mosby, 1991:499–521.

119. Corriere JJ, Sandler CM. Mechanisms of injury, patterns of extravasation and management of extraperitoneal bladder rupture due to blunt trauma. J Urol 1988; 139:43–44.
120. Kotkin L, Koch M. Morbidity associated with nonoperative management of extraperitoneal bladder ruptures. J Trauma 1995; 38:895–898.
121. Morey A, MacAninch J. Reconstruction of posterior urethral disruption injuries: outcome analysis in 82 patients. J Urol 1997; 157:506–510.
122. Webster G, Ramon J. Repair of pelvic fracture posterior urethral defects using an elaborated perineal approach: experience with 74 cases. J Urol 1991; 145:744–748.
123. Carr L, Webster G. Genitourinary trauma. Current Opinion in Urology 1996; 6:140–143.
124. Mundy A. The role of delayed primary repair in the management of pelvic fracture injuries of the urethra. Br J Urol 1991; 68:273–276.
125. Mundy A. Pelvic fracture injuries of the posterior urethra. World J Urol 1999; 17:90–95.
126. Devine C, Jordan G, Schlossberg S. Surgery of the penis and urethra. In: Walsh P, Retik AB, Stamey TA, et al., eds. Campbell's Urology. 6th ed. Philadelphia: WB Saunders, 1992:2957–3032.
127. Herschorn S, Thijssen A, Radomski S. The value immediate or early catheterisation of the posterior urethra. J Urol 1992; 148:1428–1431.
128. Drost T, Rosemurgy A, Sherman H, et al. Major trauma in pregant women: maternal/fetal outcome. J Trauma 1990; 30:574–578.
129. Pape HC, Pohlemann T, Gansslen A, et al. Pelvic fractures in pregnant multiple trauma patients. J Orthop Trauma 2000; 14:238–244.
130. Brathwaite CE, Rodriguez A. Injuries of the abdominal aorta from blunt trauma. Am Surg 1992; 58:350–352.
131. Reisman JD, Morgan AS. Analysis of 46 intra-abdominal aortic injuries from blunt trauma: case reports and literature review. J Trauma 1990; 30:1294–1297.
132. Roth SM, Wheeler JR, Gregory RT, et al. Blunt injury of the abdominal aorta: a review. J Trauma 1997; 42:748–755.
133. Pachter H, Feliciano D. Complex hepatic injuries. Surg Clin North Am 1996; 76: 763–782.
134. Faringer P, Mullins R, Feliciano P, et al. Selective fecal diversion in complex open pelvic fractures from blunt trauma. Arch Surg 1994; 129:958–964.
135. Govender S, Sham A, Singh B. Open pelvic fractures. Injury 1990; 21:373–376.
136. Jones A, Powell J, Kellam J, et al. Open pelvic fractures. A multicenter retrospective analysis. Orthop Clin North Am 1997; 28:345–350.
137. Perry J. Pelvic open fractures. Clin Orthop 1980; 151:41–45.
138. Richardson JD, Harty J, Amin M, et al. Open pelvic fractures. J Trauma 1982; 22: 533–538.
139. Rieger H, Winde G, Brug E, et al. Open pelvic fracture—an indication for laparotomy? Chirurg 1998; 69:278–283.
140. Rothenberger D, Velasco R, Strate R, et al. Open pelvic fractures: a lethal injury. J Trauma 1978; 18:184–187.
141. Sinnott R, Rhodes M, Brader A. Open pelvic fractures: an injury for trauma centers. Am J Surg 1992; 163:283–287.
142. Woods RK, O'Keefe G, Rhee P, et al. Open pelvic fracture and fecal diversion. Arch Surg 1998; 133:281–286.
143. Michel JM, Peter RE, Roche B, et al. Primary surgical care of pelvic fractures associated with perineal laceration. Swiss Surg 1999; 5:33–37.
144. Bosch U, Tscherne H. The pelvic compartment syndrome. Arch Orthop Trauma Surg 1992; 111:314–317.

145. Hessmann M, Rommens P. Bilateral ureteral obstruction and renal failure caused by massive retroperitoneal hematoma: is there a pelvic compartment syndrome analogous to abdominal compartment syndrome? J Orthop Trauma 1998; 12:553–557.
146. Hessmann M, Rommens P. Does the intrapelvic compartment syndrome exist? Acta Chir Belg 1998; 98:18–22.
147. Kottmeier S, Wilson S, Born C, et al. Surgical management of soft tissue lesions associated with pelvic ring injury. Clin Orthop 1996; 329:46–53.
148. Orthopaedic Trauma Association/committee for Coding and Classification. Fracture and dislocation compendium. J Orthop Trauma 1996; 10(1):66.

4

Indications for Surgery in Pelvic Fractures and Dislocations

Ian Pallister
Department of Trauma and Orthopaedics, Morriston Hospital, University of Wales Swansea, Morriston, Swansea, U.K.

INTRODUCTION

Discussion of indications for surgery in pelvic injuries is often dominated by the biomechanical considerations of the pattern of pelvic injury. A clear understanding of the pattern of injury is key to planning and executing surgical reconstruction of pelvic injuries (1). However, the surgeon caring for the patient in an acute service must, first and foremost, clearly understand the indications for emergency surgical intervention. At this early stage, clarity of thought and good communication are essential, as planning subsequent "semielective" reconstruction can begin from the moment the patient is first encountered in the emergency room. Furthermore, life-threatening complications of severe local or multiple injuries may mean that ideal surgical reconstruction cannot be executed in the acute phase. Similar problems may also be encountered in casualties sustaining injuries in war zones or developing countries without access to advanced medical care.

Thus, indications for surgery in pelvic injuries may be considered in three broad groups. First, emergency, or damage-control surgery, is the surgical intervention required in order to keep the patient alive (2). The second group is surgery to reconstruct fresh pelvic injuries (1,3,4). This planned reconstruction forms the bulk of the workload for those specialized in this field of orthopedic trauma. Finally, the third group is encountered when, due to local or systemic problems, initial planned reconstruction surgery may not be feasible. To some extent this group merges with malunions and nonunions (5–8). Salvage surgery for such problems is a major challenge.

EMERGENCY SURGERY

The emergency surgical management of patients with mechanically unstable pelvic injuries and hypovolemic shock begins in the emergency room. Advanced trauma life-support teaching is now widely applied (9). Shock recognition is followed by search for the source of hemorrhage while volume resuscitation is initiated. Clues to the nature of pelvic injuries are obtained from the history of injury (e.g., a fall from a height or a motorcyclist sustaining a straddle injury) and physical examination.

Conscious patients with intact sensation will have no doubt that they have an unstable pelvic injury. Stressing the pelvis is inhumane as well as unnecessary. A plain AP radiograph of the pelvis is a rapid and reliable means of diagnosing most unstable pelvic injuries. Injuries resulting in an increase in intrapelvic volume can result in massive hemorrhage. Reducing the intrapelvic volume is analogous to pressing upon an open external wound. This must be done immediately. Hence, application of external fixators in the emergency room has several obvious potential pitfalls. First, they cannot be applied to conscious patients. Second, the equipment must be complete and readily at hand. Finally, the surgeon skilled in its application must also be right there, exactly when needed. If any of these requirements are not met, disastrous delays can result.

Experience now indicates that application of a pelvic binder (whether improvised or a commercially available orthosis) is easy and effective (10–12). It can be applied to a conscious patient in the following manner (Fig. 1). Having identified the need for a binder, a pillow should be folded in two to make a bolster and secured with sticky tape. A cotton sheet is then slid under the patient's buttocks to the level of the greater trochanters and tied with a single throw of a wreath knot at the front. Three cable ties should then be passed under this single throw. The bolster is placed behind the patient's knees, and two assistants then lean towards each other, pressing firmly on opposite trochanters. The single throw can then be pulled tight and secured with cable ties, and six-inch crepe bandages applied around the lower thighs (not the knees) and ankles, suitably padded (13). A radiograph must then be taken to confirm reduction, and when desired, inlet and outlet views also. Properly applied as described, laparotomy, anterior external fixation, or even posterior sacroiliac screw fixation can be carried out without difficulty. The binder should be replaced with external or internal fixation soon to relieve pressure on the soft tissues.

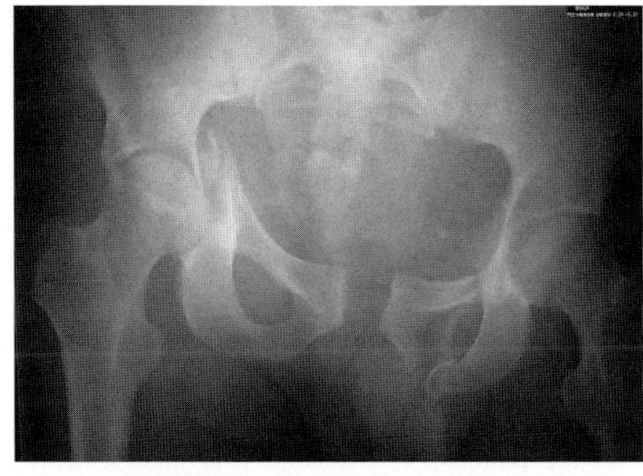

(A)

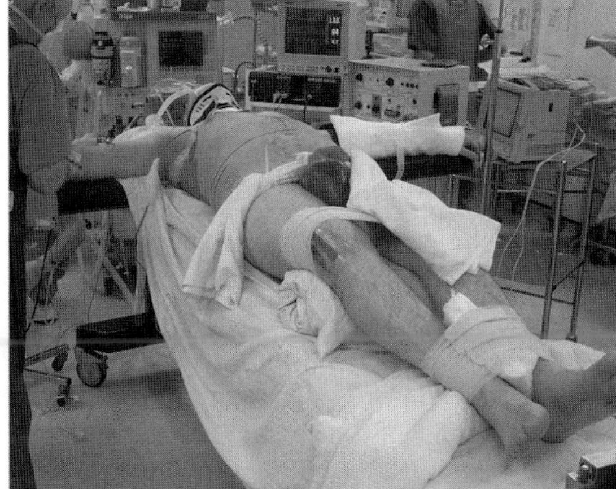

(B)

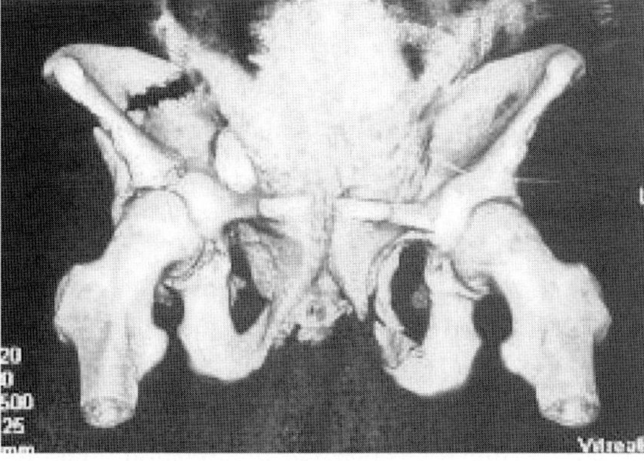

(C)

Figure 1 Application of an improvised pelvic binder. Admission plain radiograph (**A**) illustrating combined pelvic ring and acetabular fracture sustained in head on motor vehicle accident. The patient was hypotensive at presentation. A binder was applied immediately with good effect, (**B**) and postbinder-application contrast CT shows excellent reduction with an associated complete bladder rupture (**C**). Posterior sacroiliac screw fixation was performed with the binder in place, followed by anterior plating and bladder repair. Because of raised intracranial pressure from a cerebral contusion, the acetabular fracture was operatively stabilized via a posterior approach several days later.

To summarize, the presence of hypovolemic shock in a patient with a pelvic injury resulting in an increase in intrapelvic volume is an indication for immediate reduction of the pelvis using a pelvic binder. This is a means to buy time and should be replaced with an external fixator or C-clamp at the earliest opportunity.

Further management of continued hemodynamic instability can appear controversial. Additional thoracoabdominal sources of hemorrhage should already have been identified and will therefore require surgical control in their own right. Intra-abdominal injuries cannot be managed nonoperatively in the presence of hypovolemic instability. Continued hemorrhage associated with the pelvic injury itself can be managed either with packing or angiography. Which of these is preferable is best determined upon the basis of the patients response, requirements for further surgical intervention, and the familiarity of the radiologists available with therapeutic trauma angiography (10,14).

PLANNED RECONSTRUCTION

The definitive surgical reconstruction of pelvic ring injuries hinges upon clear understanding of the injury pattern itself. Clothed as the pelvis is in thick, highly vascular muscle, provided the patient survives, fractures of the pelvis are likely to heal in whatever position they come to rest in. On the other hand, ligamentous injuries, particularly involving the posterior pelvis, do not heal well, and anatomical reduction with surgery directed towards achieving fusion is the goal (15–17). As with fractures in general, operative management is indicated for those injuries that require reduction in order to afford the best chance of optimal functional outcome.

Sufficient published data exist to provide rational indications for operative reduction and stabilization of certain patterns of pelvic injuries. Open fractures, plus those associated with vascular and visceral injuries, clearly require aggressive management (18,19). Definitive reduction and stabilization of the skeletal component of such injuries is the only rational course of action to be taken, both to protect the soft-tissue repairs and afford the greatest chance of uncomplicated recovery.

The pelvic injury pattern, degree of displacement, and associated injuries are factors that determine the need for and method of reduction and stabilization. Rotational displacement can often be reduced with closed indirect methods, however, maintenance of such a reduction with external fixation can be problematic particularly in the obese or noncompliant patient. Conversely open reduction and stabilization are likely to be problematic in those with extensive, closed, degloving injuries (19). In such circumstances indirect reduction and minimally invasive stabilization may provide attractive options.

The association between residual displacement and outcome as far as pelvic fractures is concerned is difficult to quantify in absolute terms. More severe injury patterns (typified by type C injuries) do carry a worse prognosis; however, it needs to be noted that these are also associated with greater chance of neurological injury, bladder and erectile dysfunction, and dyspareunia (17,20,21). Thus, despite achieving a good reduction, the patient's quality-of-life may be deeply affected by associated injuries.

Useful information can be gleaned from studies of the late surgical reconstruction of pelvic deformity. Long-term problems occur due to residual translational and rotational displacement of the injured hemipelvis (4,6–8,16). Both posterior translation (in type C injuries) and internal rotation (type B injuries) lead to prominence of the posterior ilium. Impingement of the hip with loss of external rotation can also occur with type B rotational displacement. Vertical translation results in limb-length inequality and also problems with sitting balance. Anterior displacement at the symphysis may be associated with local problems such as visceral entrapment or herniation and pain. The extent of anterior diastasis reflects the severity of major ligamentous damage and residual posterior instability.

Residual pelvic instability is associated with significant pain whether deformity is present or not (5–8). Much of the pain experienced originates from the posterior pelvic ring, and can be relieved by stabilization and bony union. Pure sacroiliac joint dislocations carry a poor prognosis if not anatomically reduced and stabilized. Similarly, displaced sacral fractures are associated with poor prognosis but these injuries in particular can be associated with a high incidence of neurological injury, which is also associated with poor outcome.

Stable pelvic injuries (type A) do not usually warrant operative management. Partially stable pelvic ring injuries (type B) may require operative management in terms of reduction and stabilization depending on the extent of displacement (1,3,4). Type B1 open book injuries can, provided symphyseal diastasis is 2.5 cm or less, be managed nonoperatively. A good outcome cannot always be assured. Anatomical studies have indicated that the symphysis can separate by up to 2.5 cm with disruption at the symphyseal ligaments alone, with the anterior sacroiliac, sacrospinous, and sacrotuberous ligaments remaining intact. Provided this is the case, the prognosis will be good. However, instances can occur where operative stabilization is required at a later date due to SI and anterior pain (Fig. 2). Anterior plating in acute injuries will close the diastasis and prevent visceral herniation. Perhaps more important still is the effect of closing the posterior pelvic ring in a tension band manner. In most cases this is sufficient to restore SI joint congruency and stability. However, posterior pain can still occur, which, if localized to the SI joints, may require fusion at a later date.

Type B2 lateral compression injuries may result in ipsilateral disruption to the anterior and posterior pelvic ring (Type B2-1) or contra-laterally (B2-2). In either instance, the pelvic floor remains intact unless penetrated by one of the fragments of the pubic rami. Careful evaluation of the posterior ring is required as it is possible for complete disruption of the SI joint to have occurred. Type C injuries can masquerade as type B injuries and obviously carry a poor prognosis if not addressed. It is possible for the pubic bones to override each other anteriorly and lock (Fig. 3). These may be associated with significant lower urinary tract injuries but in either instance the dislocated anterior joint is likely to remain symptomatic and should be reduced and stabilized. Internal rotational deformity can result in loss of external rotation at the hip due to acetabular impingement. Bilateral injuries, the B3 group, should be approached in much the same way as the B1 injuries, but with particular care taken to ensure that there is not in fact complete SI dislocation on one or both sides.

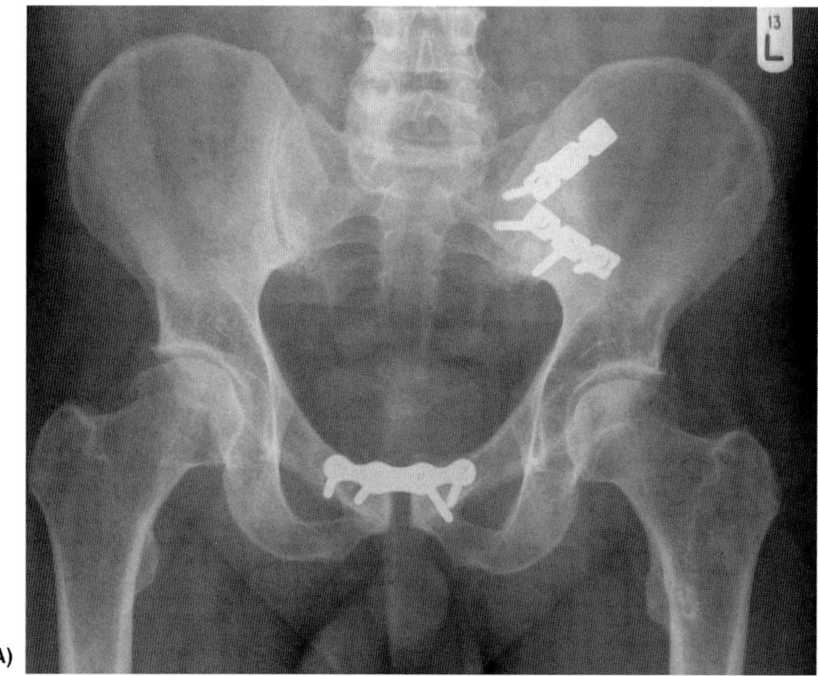

(A)

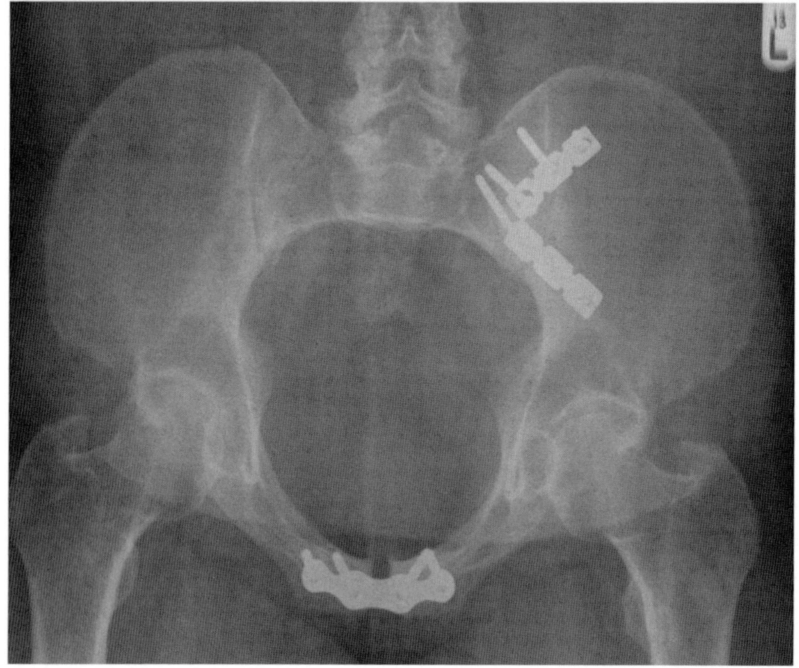

(B)

Figure 2 Late problems in "stable" rotational type B1 injuries. Anteroposterior plain radiograph (**A**) and inlet view (**B**) of the pelvis of a male patient who sustained this apparently stable AP compression (type B1) injury in a fall from a height. Once the pain from associated rib fractures settled, he mobilized well on crutches and was discharged. Over the following months, he experienced worsening anterior and posterior pelvic pain. Open reduction of the diastasis with sacroiliac joint bone grafting and plating achieved sound fusion and relieved his pain.

Completely unstable pelvic injuries, the type C group, carry the worst prognosis and the highest risk of association with massive bleeding, neurological, and visceral injuries. Even in the presence of anatomical reduction and stable fixation, persisting pain and associated disability can be a major problem.

Prominence of the posterior ilium can lead to discomfort sitting and sleeping. Pelvic obliquity from vertical displacement not only alters limb length when walking, but can also make sitting balance difficult (8). Compensatory lumbar scoliosis is a further source of associated long-term pain. Retrospective series have indicated the greater chance of problems returning to work and leisure activities for posterior displacements of greater than 1.4 cm (22).

Particular, rare variants include bilateral C3 injuries with an intact anterior arch (Fig. 4). These injuries are largely ligamentous and require accurate reduction and surgical stabilization with a view to achieving fusion of the SI joints. Pelvic ring disruptions associated with acetabular fractures present a further group for which very careful strategic planning is required. Depending on the patient's overall condition, a staged procedure may be required, first to restore the integrity of the pelvic ring, and then restore the acetabulum in continuity with this.

As far as neurological injuries are concerned, there is a trend toward improved outcome for neurological injuries provided anatomic reduction and stabilization can

(*Text continues on page 84.*)

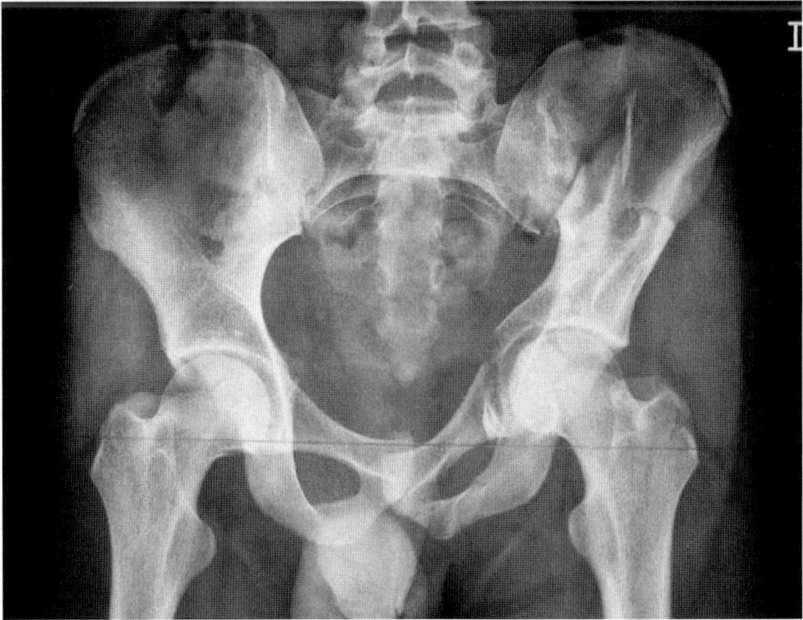

Figure 3 Rotational type B2 injuries. Admission plain radiograph illustrating a lateral compression (type B2) pelvic ring fracture sustained in a motor cyclist struck by an automobile from the left side. Despite the locked symphysis anteriorly, there was no lower urinary tract injury in this case. The extent of the internal rotation of the left hemipelvis can be appreciated by comparing the line of the posterior wall of the acetabulum in the injured and intact sides. The line of the posterior wall bisects the head of the femur in the right hip, but lies at a subcapital level on the left side. The pelvic ring injury and the associated juxtatectal acetabular fracture were reduced and stabilized via an ilio-inguinal approach.

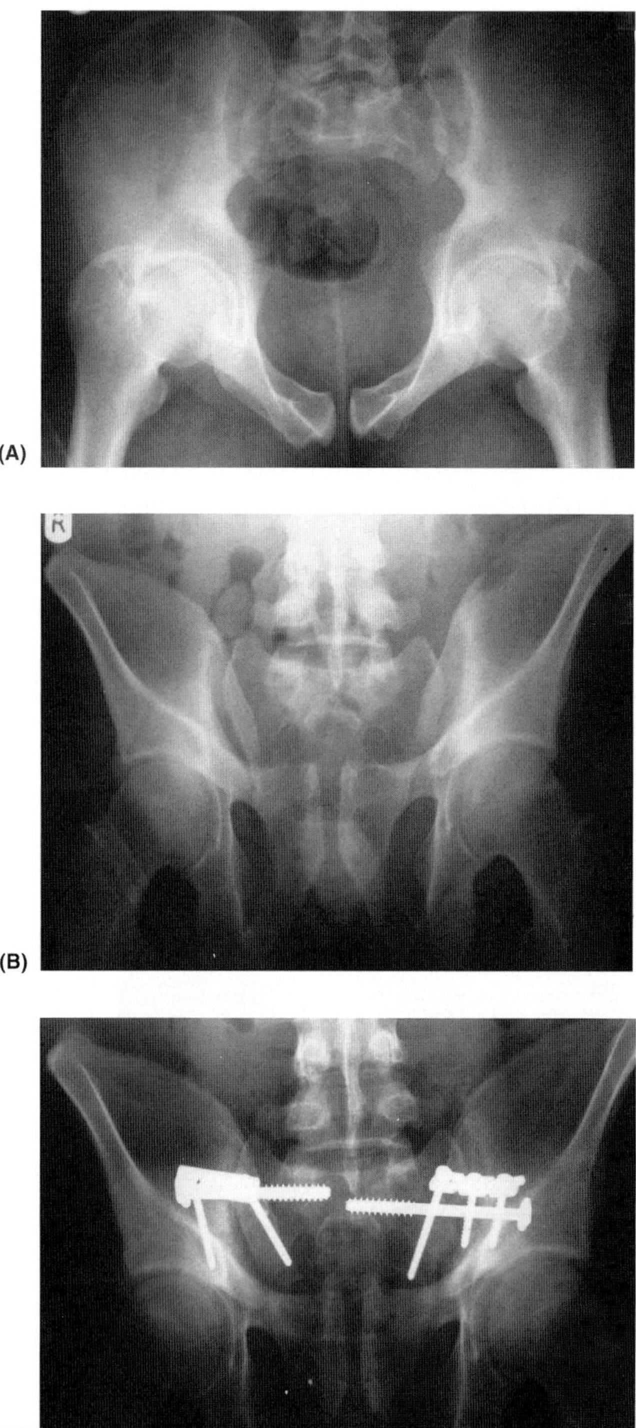

Figure 4 Bilateral C3 injuries with an intact anterior arch. Admission inlet (**A**) and outlet (**B**) radiographs illustrating bilateral sacroiliac joint dislocations sustained by a driver involved in a head-on motor vehicle accident. The SI joints were reduced via bilateral lateral windows and stabilized with plating and SI screws after open bone grafting (**C**). Sound union and good function was achieved.

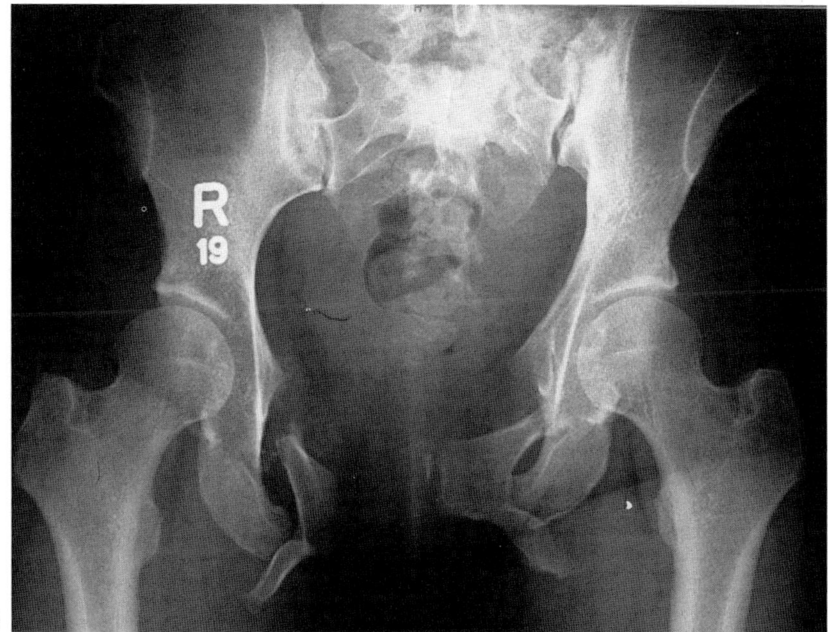

(A)

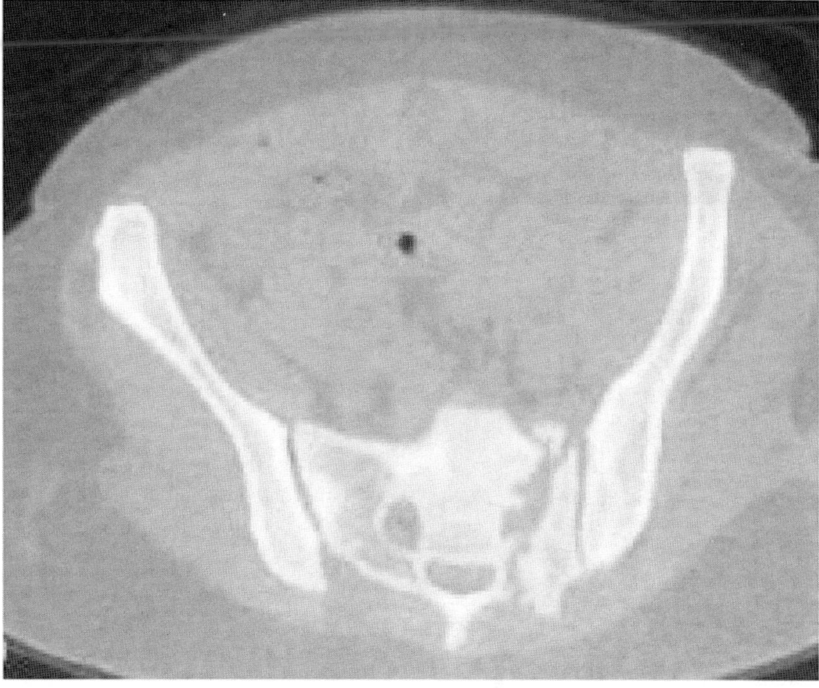

(B)

Figure 5 Untreated type C injury. Anteroposterior plain radiograph (**A**) of the pelvis plus CT scan of the posterior elements (**B**) of a female patient injured three months earlier in a bus crash in a developing country. There were 20 fatalities, and this patient survived without any specific intervention. Despite a 2 cm leg-length inequality, a wide diastasis, sciatic nerve parasthesia on the left side, and sacral and pubic ramus nonunions, she had resumed physically demanding work by applying a firm corset. Her sciatic nerve symptoms improved, and she declined surgery.

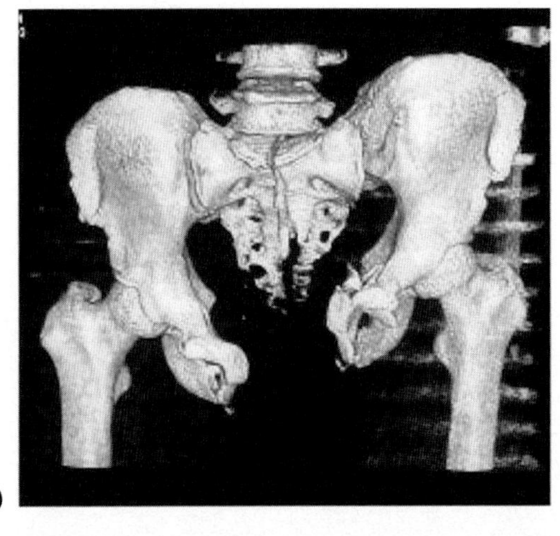

(a)

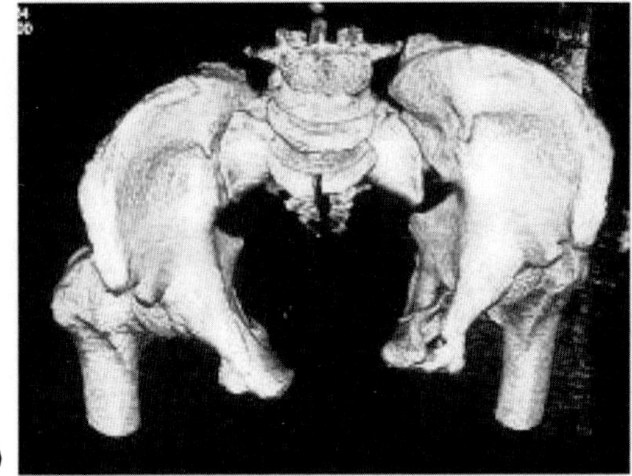

(b)

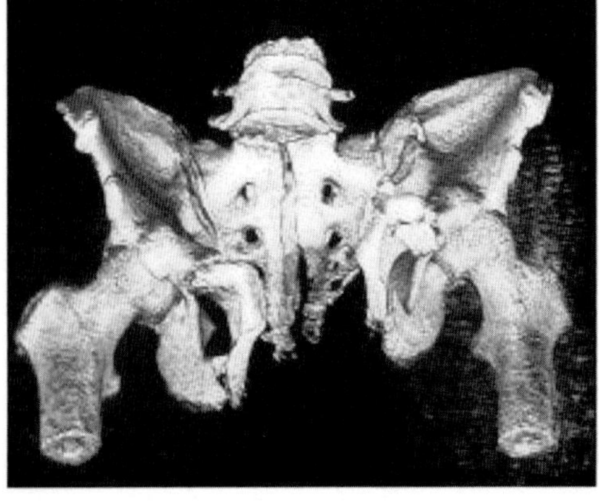

(A) (c)

Figure 6 (**A**) Staged-surgical reconstruction in severe infection. Admission AP (a), inlet (b) and outlet (c) 3D CT reconstructions of an obese male motorcyclist admitted in severe hypovolemic shock exsanguinating through a perineal wound. A binder was applied and exchanged for an iliac-crest external fixator, with packing of the perineal wound and ileostomy for fecal diversion. Plain radiographs confirmed severe persisting displacement anteriorly and posteriorly. (*Continued*)

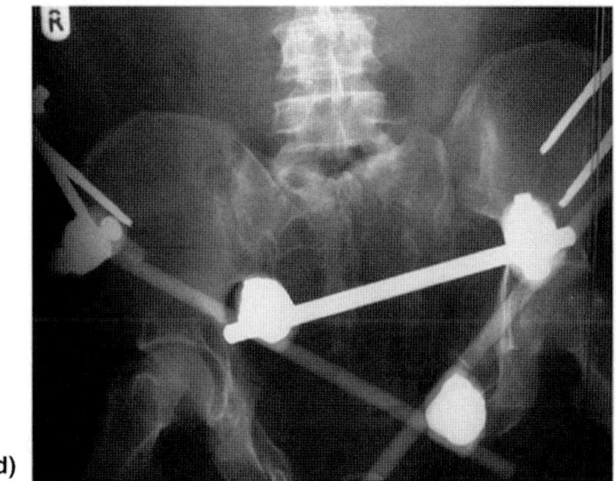

(d)

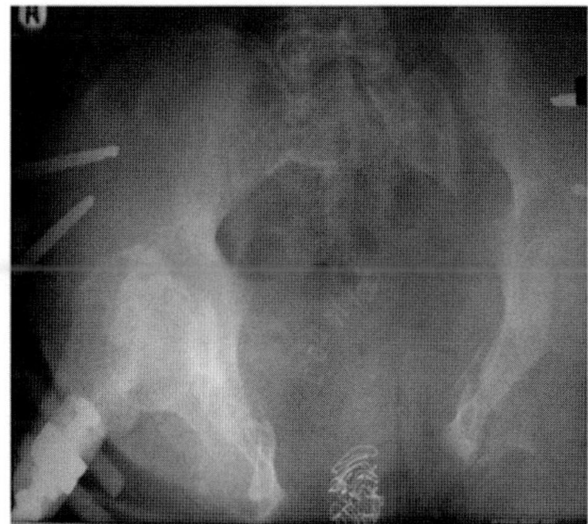

(e)

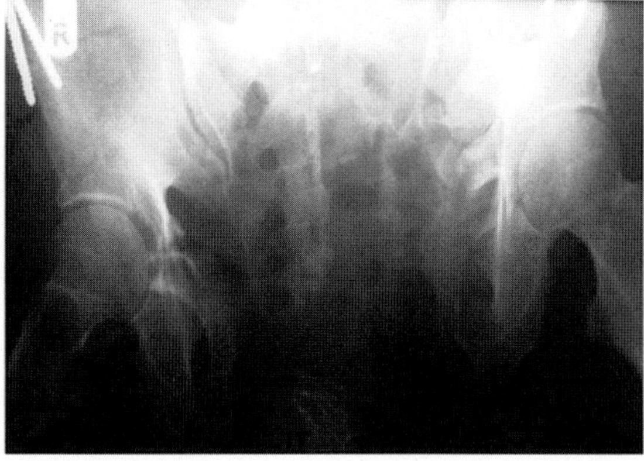

(A) (f)

Figure 6 *(Continued)*

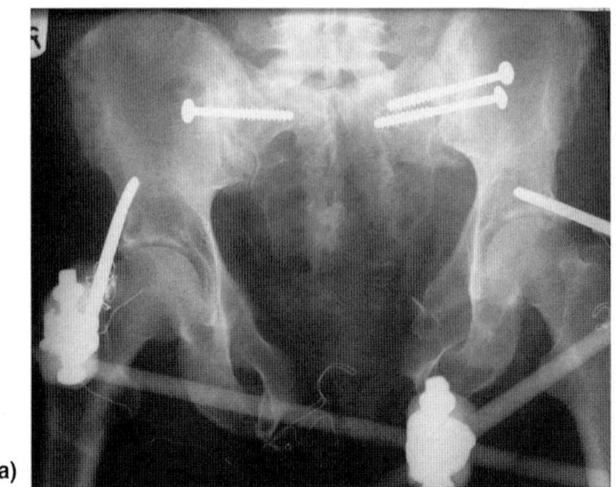

(a)

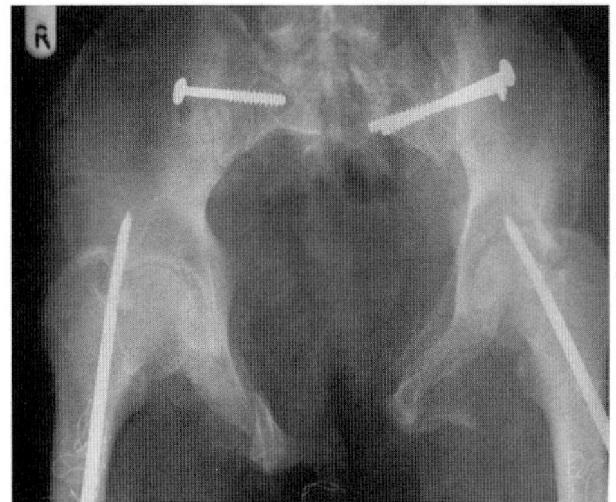

(b)

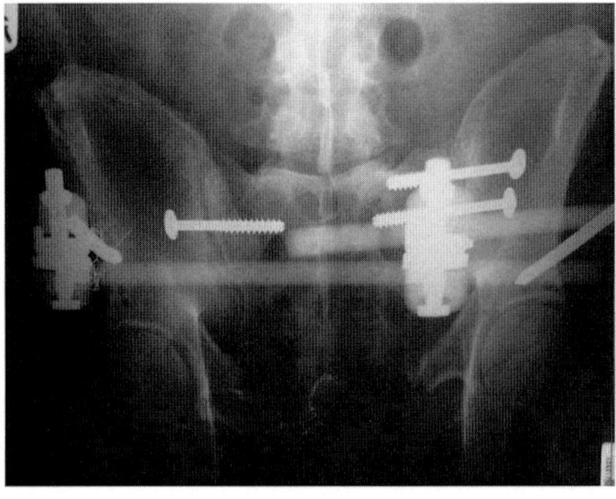

(B) (c)

Figure 6 (**B**) Staged surgical reconstruction in severe infection. Inadequate fecal diversion resulted in massive intrapelvic sepsis, with an abscess extending from the perineum into the subcutaneous tissue anterior to the diastasis. After referral for definitive care, the iliac-crest external fixator was swapped for an anterior construct, and colostomy and mucus fistula were performed. Aggressive local wound management was instituted. Once the infection was setting, posterior sacroiliac screw fixation was performed with close indirect reduction. Definitive fixation was performed three months after admission, with no infective complications. This was the last of 15 operative interventions.

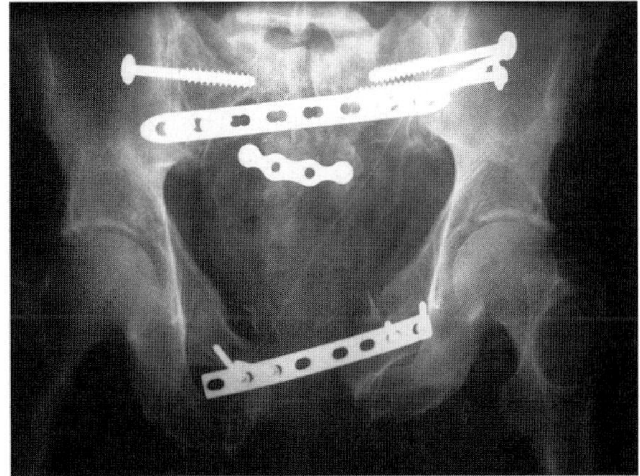

(d)

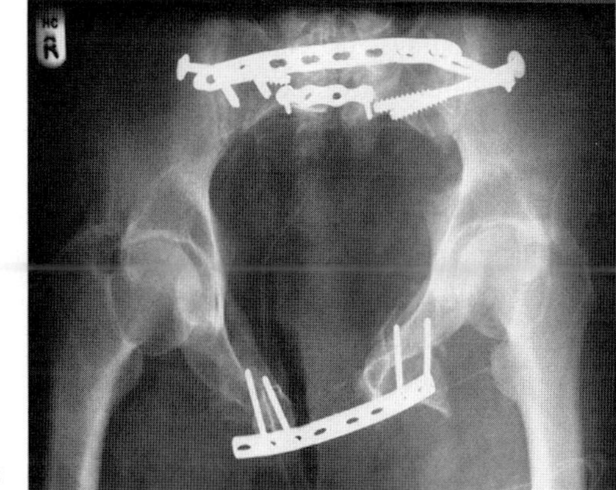

(e)

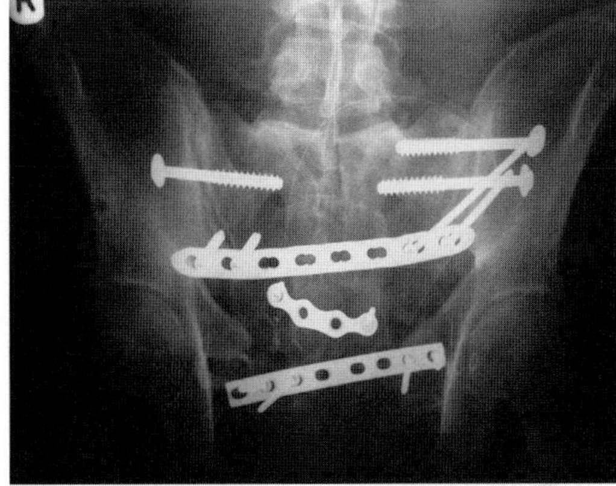

(B) (f)

Figure 6 *(Continued)*

be assured, although complete neurological recovery has not been documented (17,23). Nerve injuries associated with pelvic ring trauma are essentially injuries to peripheral nerves. Decompression of these nerves, by either direct or indirect reduction of fracture fragments, may well facilitate some recovery. This, however, cannot be guaranteed.

Other general arguments put forward to support the operative management of pelvic fractures include a more rapid reduction of pain and facilitation of nursing care and rehabilitation. However, such subjective criteria have not been reported in literature.

CIRCUMSTANCES WHERE EARLY PLANNED RECONSTRUCTION IS NOT FEASIBLE

Severe local problems, such as infection in neglected open pelvic fractures, open de-gloving injuries, or lack of access to modern health care, can present a surgeon with extremely difficult scenarios. Against expectations, patients can survive severe pelvic trauma in circumstances of austere health care. With time, despite nonunion and posterior instability, it is possible for them to make useful functional recoveries (Fig. 5).

Complex pelvic fractures associated with rectal injury can result in potentially lethal sepsis. Once established in the pelvis, standard operative fracture stabilization becomes unfeasible (Fig. 6). In such circumstances, adherence to the principles outlined above of reduction and stabilization of the posterior elements, aiming at healing, fusion, or ankylosis, hold the best chances of functional recovery. It may be necessary to achieve this in a sequential manner with minimally invasive methods, as illustrated.

SUMMARY

In the acute phase, in the presence of an unstable pelvic fracture with hypovolemic shock, damage-control management is essential, and application of a pelvic binder and, where necessary, full multidisciplinary surgical involvement are crucial.

Operative stabilization of displaced pelvic fractures must aim to restore not just pelvic symmetry but congruency and stability of the sacroiliac joints in particular. Vertical or anteroposterior displacement greater than 1 cm, diastasis of greater than 2.5 cm, or internal rotation of more than 15° are likely to be symptomatic (7).

When initial treatment is compromised by fulminant local infection or other comparable factors, the above principles may need to be applied with modified techniques. The goals, however, remain the same: posterior pelvic stability, avoidance of nerve injury, and restoration as far as possible of pelvic symmetry.

REFERENCES

1. Tile M. Pelvic ring fractures: should they be fixed? J Bone Joint Surg Br 1988; 70(1):1–12.
2. Henry SM, Tornetta P, 3rd, Scalea, TM. Damage control for devastating pelvic and extremity injuries. Surg Clin North Am 1997; 77(4):879–895.
3. Rommens PM, Hessmann MH. Staged reconstruction of pelvic ring disruption: differences in morbidity, mortality, radiologic results, and functional outcomes between B1, B2/B3, and C-type lesions. J Orthop Trauma 2002; 16(2):92–98.
4. Tornetta PrD, Matta JM. Outcome of rotationally unstable pelvic ring injuries treated operatively. Clin Orthop Relat Res 1996; 329:147–151.
5. Gautier ER, Matta JM. Late reconstruction after pelvic ring injuries. Injury 1996; 27(suppl 2):B39–B46.
6. Matta JMD, Markovich GD. Surgical treatment of pelvic nonunions and malunions. Clin Orthop Relat Res 1996; 329:199–206.
7. Mears DCV. Surgical reconstruction of late pelvic post-traumatic nonunion and malalignment. J Bone Joint Surg Br 2003; 85(1):21–30.
8. Vanderschot PD, Broos P. Surgical treatment of post-traumatic pelvic deformities. Injury 1998; 29(1):19–22.
9. Advanced Trauma Life Support for Doctors, 7th edition. American College of Surgeons. Chicago, 2005.
10. Biffl WLS, Moore WR, Gonzalez EE, et al. Evolution of a multidisciplinary clinical pathway for the management of unstable patients with pelvic fractures. Ann Surg 2001; 233(6):843–850.
11. Routt MLJF, Woodhouse A, Schildhauer E. Circumferential pelvic antishock sheeting: a temporary resuscitation aid. J Orthop Trauma 2002; 16(1):45–48.
12. Simpson TK, Heuer JC, Bottlang F. Stabilization of pelvic ring disruptions with a circumferential sheet. J Trauma 2002; 52(1):158–161.
13. Shank JRM, Smith SJ, Meyer WR. Bilateral peroneal nerve palsy following emergent stabilization of a pelvic ring injury. J Orthop Trauma 2003; 17(1):67–70.
14. Ertel WK, Eid M, Platz K, Trentz A. Control of severe hemorrhage using C-clamp and pelvic packing in multiply injured patients with pelvic ring disruption. J Orthop Trauma 2001; 15(7):468–474.
15. Dujardin FHH, Duparc M, Biga F, Thomine N. Long-term functional prognosis of posterior injuries in high-energy pelvic disruption. J Orthop Trauma 1998; 12(3):145–150.
16. Lindahl JH, Bostman E, Santavirta O. Failure of reduction with an external fixator in the management of injuries of the pelvic ring. Long-term evaluation of 110 patients. J Bone Joint Surg Br 1999; 81(6):955–962.
17. Majeed SA. Neurologic deficits in major pelvic injuries. Clin Orthop Relat Res 1992; 282:222–228.
18. Hanson PBM, Chapman JC. Open fractures of the pelvis. Review of 43 cases. J Bone Joint Surg Br 1991; 73(2):325–329.
19. Kottmeier SAW, Born SC, Hanks CT, Iannacone GA, DeLong WM. Surgical management of soft tissue lesions associated with pelvic ring injury. Clin Orthop Relat Res 1996; 329:46–53.
20. Copeland CEB, McCarthy MJ, MacKenzie ML, Guzinski EJ, Hash GM, Burgess CS. Effect of trauma and pelvic fracture on female genitourinary, sexual, and reproductive function. J Orthop Trauma 1997; 11(2):73–81.
21. Watnik NFC, Goldberger M. Urologic injuries in pelvic ring disruptions. Clin Orthop Relat Res 1996; 329:37–45.

22. Keating JFW, Blachut J, Broekhuyse P, Meek H, O'Brien RN. Early fixation of the vertically unstable pelvis: the role of iliosacral screw fixation of the posterior lesion. J Orthop Trauma 1999; 13(2):107–113.
23. Reilly MCZ, Matta DM. Neurologic injuries in pelvic ring fractures. Clin Orthop Relat Res 1996; 329:28–36.

5
Surgical Approaches for Pelvic Ring Injuries

Johannes K. M. Fakler
Department of Trauma and Reconstructive Surgery, Charité—University Medical School Berlin, Berlin, Germany

Ian Pallister
Department of Trauma and Orthopaedics, Morriston Hosptial, University of Wales Swansea, Morriston, Swansea, U.K.

Philip F. Stahel
Department of Orthopaedics, Denver Health Medical Center, University of Colorado School of Medicine, Denver, Colorado, U.S.A.

INTRODUCTION

Good outcome following surgery for pelvic ring injuries depends upon accurate reduction, stable internal fixation, and minimizing the risk of surgical complications. The pelvic ring injury must be fully understood before any surgical strategy is planned. Only by understanding the pattern of injury can the approach, reduction technique, and fixation be successfully achieved.

The pelvic ring links the axial skeleton to the lower limbs, anchors the major muscle groups of the anterior abdominal wall, lumbar spine and lower limbs, protects and provides routes of transit for the lumbosacral plexus, and finally, suspends the organs of the perineum. It is therefore hardly a surprise that surgical approaches to the pelvis are technically demanding, and carry a risk of iatrogenic injury. These may be due to intraoperative trauma to important neurovascular structures during exposure, reduction, or fixation, or related to wound breakdown.

Recent years have seen a great deal of interest in the development and application of minimally invasive and percutaneous fixation techniques in the hope of avoiding the morbidity associated with large surgical exposures. The success of these techniques when applied to injuries of the pelvic ring hinges upon the same considerations as elsewhere. The reduction (usually achieved by indirect means) must be accurate and the fixation sound. Image intensifier control of the highest quality is an essential requirement to ensure accurate and safe fixation.

The choice of an appropriate surgical approach represents the prerequisite for an adequate outcome after surgical fixation of unstable pelvic ring injuries. This is of particular importance due to the imminent risk of iatrogenic intraoperative damage of neurovascular structures or the bladder by anterior approaches, and of neurological sacral plexus injuries or wound healing problems by posterior approaches due to the thin dorsal soft tissue coverage of the sacrum and sacroiliac joint. Successful surgical exposures of the pelvic ring strictly depend on a correct preoperative positioning of the patient on the operating table. The use of bolsters, staples of sheets, or supports mounted to the operating table alleviate the approach and exposure of the fracture site. The use of a radiolucent operating table is strictly recommended in order to allow a multidimensional intraoperative fluoroscopy including inlet and outlet images of the pelvic ring. Before skin incision, anatomical landmarks should be identified and marked. A strict subperiostal dissection technique helps avoiding damage to neurovascular structures. Furthermore, the careful blunt detachment of musculature from the bone helps maintain the integrity of the muscle and protect neurovascular structures. An appropriate surgical approach contributes to minimal tissue trauma, offers good intraoperative exposure, enables short operating times, and minimizes the risk of iatrogenic tissue damage.

ANTERIOR APPROACH TO THE SYMPHYSIS AND PUBIC BONE

The anterior elements of the pelvic ring consist of the symphysis pubis and the superior pubic rami. Variations on the simple approach to these anterior structures can allow greater exposure for reduction and fixation of acetabular and posterior ring injuries.

For the simple anterior approach, the urogenital triangle is shaved following perurethral catheterization. This has often been performed beforehand during the resuscitation phase of the patient management. In cases of complete urethral transection, the placement of a suprapubic catheter may be required. Management of such urologic injuries remains controversial (1). Placement of the entry point of the catheter through the anterior abdominal wall, remote from the site of surgical incision, reduces the risk of infection.

The "Pfannenstiel" approach to the anterior pelvic ring represents a standard for open reduction and internal fixation of a ruptured pubic symphysis (Fig. 1). This approach can be extended laterally to expose the superior ramus of the pubic bone and anterior column of the acetabulum, if required. Retroperitoneal packing for urgent control of massive bleedings associated with pelvic ring disruption may also be performed through this approach. In cases of combined anterior pelvic ring and intra-abdominal injury, an

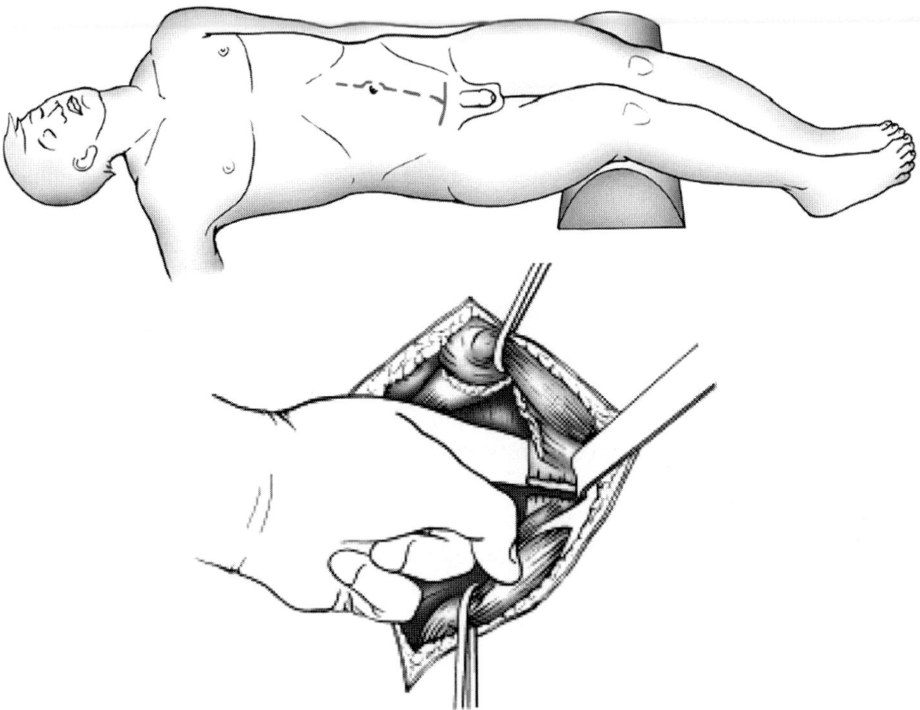

Figure 1 Anterior "Pfannenstiel" approach for fixation of a ruptured symphysis. The preoperative positioning in slight flexion and internal rotation of the hip and knees allows easier intraoperative reduction. Digital palpation of the Retzius' space allows an accurate control of reduction and protection of the bladder. An inferior median laparotomy can be chosen alternatively in cases with concomitant intra-abdominal injuries (*dashed line*). *Source*: Adapted from Ref. 14.

inferior median laparotomy is preferred to the "Pfannenstiel" approach for simultaneous access to the abdominal cavity (Fig. 1).

The incision is made approximately 3 cm proximal to the symphysis pubis. This is deepened to the anterior rectus sheath. Proximal dissection elevates the skin and all subcutaneous tissue halfway to the umbilicus. This dissection is extended distally about 2 cm distal to the upper border of the symphysis pubis.

The linea alba is identified and cutting diathermy used to incise precisely along the midline. The two bellies of the rectus abdominis are then separated. The thickness of the posterior rectus sheath is somewhat variable, but this should then be carefully incised for the whole length of the exposed sheath, keeping the dissection extraperitoneal. A number of large gauze swabs are then packed in the retropubic space to push the empty bladder posteriorly out of the operative field.

In some cases, avulsion of one or other rectus sheath may have occurred at the time of injury. In these circumstances, the exposure to the upper border of the body of the pubis is already performed. Transosseous repair of the avulsed rectus sheath often seems tenuous but usually heals very well.

In most injuries, the dissection can then be continued, with elevation of the rectus sheath from the anterior margin of the body of the pubis bilaterally, and sharp dissection onto the superior surface of the pubis, dividing the pectineal and lacunar ligaments. This plane is developed using a Cobb elevator, in the anterior, posterior, and lateral directions. Once the pubic tubercle is exposed, open anatomic reduction is easily performed by application of a reduction forceps.

Where the plating needs to extend more laterally to bridge associated ramus fractures, great care in dissection needs to be taken to identify, when present, the corona mortis vessels (2,3). These vessels communicate between the obturator and external iliac vessels, lying usually in a fairly lateral position, although there is considerable variability in the described location. Occasionally they are to be found more medially, adjacent to the lacunar ligament. Whether present as artery or vein, if injured inadvertently profuse bleeding occurs. Because of the location of the vessels, once they have been avulsed it is extremely difficult to locate the ends and gain bleeding control. With care, they can be identified and clipped, prior to division, without problem.

Once symphyseal diastasis, or overlapping, has been reduced and held, associated pubic ramus fractures may then require stabilization. The lateral window of the ilioinguinal approach may be used to allow the fracture to be bridged and secured to the sciatic buttress proximally (see below) (4,5). Alternatively, antegrade or retrograde anterior column screws may also be employed (see below).

This basic approach can be developed further to allow exposure of the pelvic brim, quadrilateral plate, and even the sacroiliac (SI) joints bilaterally. The modified Stoppa approach is described more fully in relation to acetabular fracture reduction and fixation (6). This has similarities to the approach described by Goris and Biert for unstable type C pelvic injuries (7). A midline skin incision is made extending from a few centimeters proximal to the umbilicus to a point a little distal to the symphysis. The linea alba is incised in the manner described above and then the rectus abdominis is mobilized from the posterior sheath. This is then incised as far lateral as possible, again taking care to stay extraperitoneal. The peritoneal sac is then pulled upwards and medially, allowing exposure of the inner surface of the pelvis. Identification of the femoral vessels, the psoas, the femoral nerve, and the spermatic cord allows these structures to be mobilized and protected using vascular slings in a manner similar to that used in the more familiar ilioinguinal approach. Both SI joints may be exposed and reconstruction begins posteriorly and continues anteriorly.

It is important to bear in mind the difference in orientation of the plate used to stabilize the pelvic ring via this approach. A straight plate contoured as a Roman arch will allow screw insertion through its most proximal holes. A standard plate "curved on the flat" has proximal holes, which are almost impossible to access via this approach. If this standard orientation is used, extreme difficulty will be encountered in drilling for screw holes in the region of the sciatic buttress, which may result in drill breakage and accidental vessel injury.

Upon closure, the retropubic space should be drained, and the rectus sheath repaired using strong, nonabsorbable sutures. Depending on the patient's build, a further drain may be required before closure of subcutaneous tissue and skin.

ANTEROLATERAL APPROACH TO THE ILIAC WING

The anterolateral Olerud approach, corresponding to the first window of the ilioinguinal Letournel approach (Fig. 2), allows exposure of the iliac wing and direct access to the anterior part of the SI joint. This approach is used for reduction and fixation of iliac wing fractures, transiliosacral "crescent" fractures, and disruptions of the SI joint. Apart from excellent direct visual control of these anatomical structures, optimal guidance of the drilling direction close to the SI joint is possible. Furthermore, reduction of fractures below the linea terminalis within the "true" pelvis can be performed under digital control. In contrast, sacral fractures cannot be adequately exposed and fixed through this approach.

The patient is placed supine on a radiolucent operating table. Stapled sheets are placed under the back to elevate the pelvis on the ipsilateral side. Free draping of the ipsilateral leg must be ensured to allow intraoperative reduction by axial traction. The opposite side of the pelvis should be braced by a support on the operating table in order to enable a safe intraoperative tilting to the contralateral side. A curved skin incision is made parallel to the iliac crest, beginning approximately 5 cm dorsal to the anterior superior iliac spine, and continuing for an additional 5 cm ventro-medially along the line of the inguinal ligament (Fig. 2). After deepening the skin incision through the subcutaneous fat, the aponeurosis of the oblique external abdominal muscle is exposed and detached from the iliac crest in a subperiostal fashion. At this time, the lateral cutaneous femoral nerve, which runs ventrally to the anterior superior iliac crest, has to be spared (Fig. 2). From the inner wall of the ilium, the iliacus muscle is detached by blunt subperiostal dissection with a periosteal elevator. Bleeding from nutrient vessels avulsed from the inner wall of the ilium can be controlled by bone wax. By retracting the iliacus and psoas muscles medially, the SI joint is exposed. Care has to be taken not

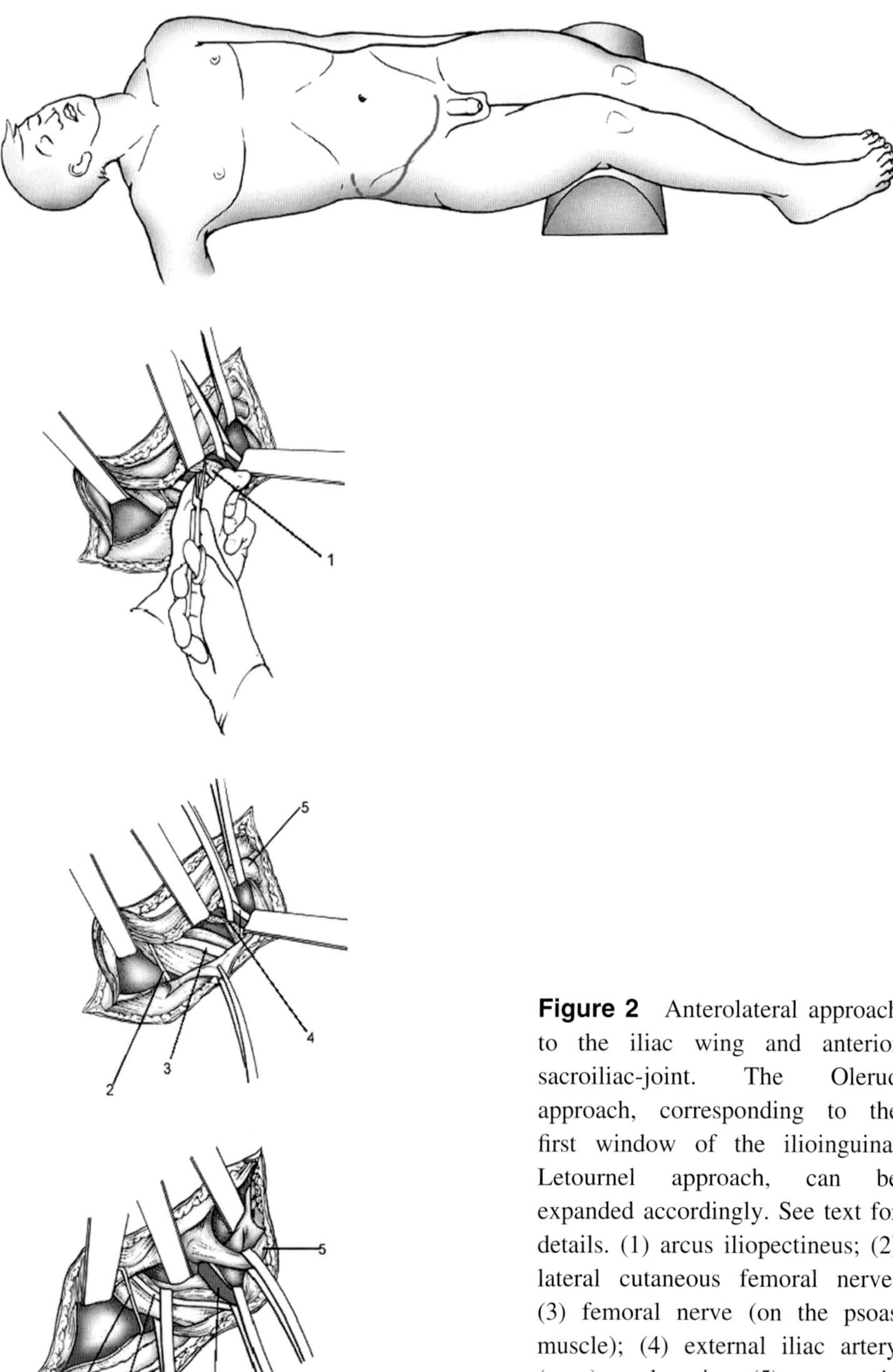

Figure 2 Anterolateral approach to the iliac wing and anterior sacroiliac-joint. The Olerud approach, corresponding to the first window of the ilioinguinal Letournel approach, can be expanded accordingly. See text for details. (1) arcus iliopectineus; (2) lateral cutaneous femoral nerve; (3) femoral nerve (on the psoas muscle); (4) external iliac artery (gray) and vein; (5) spermatic cord. *Source*: Adapted from Ref. 14.

to induce an indirect shearing injury to the plexus lumbosacralis by the use of Hohmann retractors.

The anterolateral Olerud approach can be extended anteriorly and medially through the "classical" three windows of the ilioinguinal Letournel approach (Fig. 2). The skin incision is extended in a curved manner caudally and medially towards the midline and about 1 to 2 cm above the pubic tuberosities. After deepening the incision through the subcutaneous fat, the aponeurosis of the oblique external abdominal muscle is incised distally towards the superficial inguinal ring in the line of its fibers. The spermatic cord is dissected, embraced, and retracted by a Penrose drain (Fig. 2). The posterior wall of the inguinal canal—consisting of the transversus abdominus and internal oblique abdominus muscle and fascia, respectively—is exposed and incised. Lateral to the deep inguinal ring, the deep abdominal muscles are detached from the inguinal ligament. The femoral vessels, the femoral nerve, and the iliopsoas muscle are exposed and retracted by a Penrose drain (Fig. 2). The arcus iliopectineous is partially incised with a scissor in the ventral dorsal direction in order to enable an easier mobilization of the iliopsoas muscle (Fig. 2). For access to the symphysis or the contralateral pubic bone the rectus abdominal muscle is incised transversely 1 to 2 cm proximally of its insertion. Blunt dissection of the Retziuś space separates the bladder from the symphysis, as described above for the "Pfannenstiel" approach.

POSTERIOR APPROACH TO THE SACRUM AND SI JOINT

The posterior approach allows an open reduction and internal fixation of fractures of the sacrum, posterior iliac wing, ruptures of the SI joint, and fixation of transiliosacral "crescent" fractures (Fig. 3). The approach is safe with regard to neurovascular structures since there is no true internervous plane. It has to be taken into account, however, that the prone positioning may not be adequate in acute cases for patients with concomitant severe intracerebral, intraabdominal, or thoracic injuries. The specific risks of posterior approaches are represented by the endangered soft tissue envelope and the possibility of inducing iatrogenic lesions to the sacral nerve roots by incorrect reduction or fixation techniques of the SI joint. The thin soft tissue coverage puts the posterior approach at risk for delayed or impaired wound healing and subsequent infections. The patient is placed prone on the operating table. The use of image intensifier is essential. Prior to skin preparation and draping, anteroposterior and 40° caudad and cephalad (inlet and outlet) views must be taken to ensure intraoperative views can be obtained. Bolsters should be placed under the lateral aspects of the chest and pelvis.

The open posterior approach to the sacrum and SI joint is employed to assure adequate reduction of the posterior ring in injuries with significant translational instability and also in fractures involving the sacral foramina and canal (8). Severe soft tissue injuries may well accompany these disruptions of the pelvic ring. In such circumstances, if the posterior approach must be used, it should be delayed until the soft tissue envelope has healed. Application of skeletal traction can be helpful in preventing further proximal displacement of the injured hemipelvis.

A straight skin incision is made beginning 1 to 2 cm proximal and lateral to the posterior superior iliac crest and extending vertically down to just distal to the level of

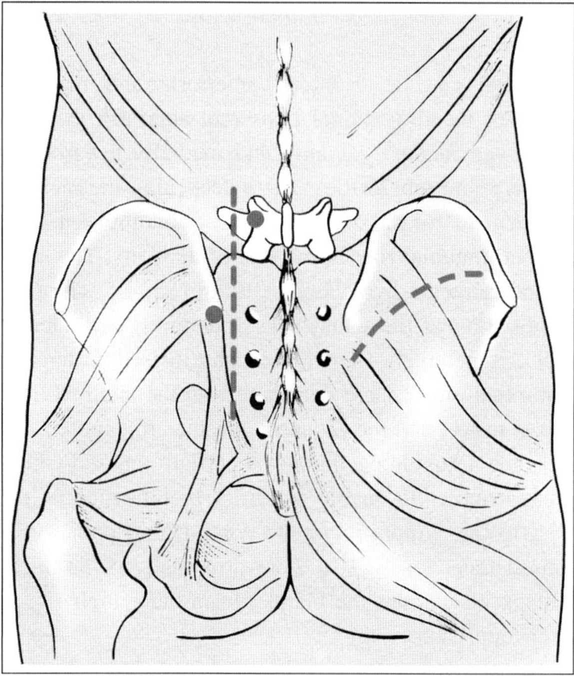

Figure 3 Posterior standard approaches to the sacrum and sacroiliac (SI) joint. A longitudinal skin incision is performed medial to the posterior superior iliac spine for fixation of the SI joint. The gray points mark the entry points for the pedicle screws for a distraction spondylodesis in unstable C-type "vertical shear" injuries (pedicle L5 to posterior iliac crest). For posterior fixation of the iliac wing, a curved incision is performed parallel to the posterior iliac crest. See text for details. *Source*: Adapted from Ref. 14.

the sciatic notch. Undermining of the skin edges must be avoided. The gluteus maximus is then identified and released from its origin on the iliac crest, sacrotuberous ligament, and also the muscle fibers, which are continuous with those of the erector spinae. The gluteus maximus is then reflected subperiosteally from the ilium, along with medius and minimus, as far as the iliac tubercle.

The dissection is then extended distally to expose the posterior inferior iliac spine and the inferior aspect of the SI joint. The superior gluteal artery is at risk as it exits the greater sciatic notch. Great care should be taken during this dissection to prevent injury to the artery and its accompanying nerve. Similarly, excessive retraction on the gluteal muscle mass must be avoided.

The piriformis muscle is then identified in the greater sciatic notch and mobilized to allow a finger to be inserted into the notch and allow palpation of the anterior aspect of the SI joint. Release of a portion of the sacrotuberous ligament may be necessary to allow adequate exposure. Further elevation of the erector spinae and multifidus muscles towards the midline allows the dorsal surface of the sacrum to be exposed if necessary.

Sufficient exposure is made to allow for the application of reduction clamps and the insertion of temporary screws as needed for their application. Once a reduction is performed, no further visualization of the fracture or dislocation is possible. It is important therefore to debride the fracture line or the SI joint before attempting a reduction. This is of particular importance in fractures involving the sacral canal or nerve root foramina. Hasty attempts at reduction of these fractures could clearly result in permanent neurological injury if the nerve roots are impaled upon displaced fragments of bone. A lamina spreader inserted into the fracture line can be used to gently distract the injury and facilitate debridement.

This approach is particularly useful for performing a distraction spondylodesis with polyaxial internal fixator from the pedicle of L5 to the posterior iliac crest (Fig. 3), for example, for indirect stabilization of "vertical shear" C-type injuries.

PERCUTANEOUS PROCEDURES FOR TRANSILIOSACRAL SCREW FIXATION

The percutaneous transiliosacral screw fixation is characterized by sparing the posterior soft-tissue envelope due to the minimal invasive procedure. The disadvantage is the requirement for exact fluoroscopic guidance in anteroposterior, inlet, and outlet views. This technique can be performed both in prone as well as in the supine position of the patient on a radiolucent table. While vertically undisplaced anterior-posterior compression (APC) II and APC III-type fractures may be fixed without requirement for reduction of the SI joint, the ipsilateral leg should be freely draped for all C-type ("vertical shear") injuries for allowing intraoperative reduction by axial traction. A small skin incision is performed dorsolaterally in projection to the first sacral vertebrae under fluoroscopic control. The exact corridor for the drill and the screw requires accurate fluoroscopic guidance in all views (anteroposterior, inlet, and outlet) in order to avoid a iatrogenic nerve root injury of the sacral plexus. Alternatively, this procedure can also be performed under computed tomography (CT) guidance in selected cases, even under local anesthesia. Technical details are described below.

TRANSPERITONEAL APPROACH FOR SACROILIAC RUPTURE

In cases of severe trauma with combined intra-abdominal and posterior pelvic ring injuries, the transperitoneal approach offers the possibility to stabilize the SI joint by internal fixation. After undermining the basis of the sigmoid mesenterium, the iliac vessels and the ureter are identified. These structures are carefully retracted medially. The lumbosacral plexus is also identified and carefully retracted to expose the SI joint safely for internal fixation. However, this time-consuming procedure should not be performed in highly unstable polytrauma patients who are candidates for a "damage control" procedure with early transfer to intensive care.

CONSIDERATIONS IN EMPLOYING SIMULTANEOUS OPEN AND PERCUTANEOUS TECHNIQUES

Percutaneous techniques offer the advantage that extensive approaches can be avoided. It is important to bear in mind, however, that the approach may represent the only effective way in which a satisfactory reduction can be achieved. If indirect reduction is possible, then percutaneous stabilization may be appropriate.

Stabilization of the SI joint using percutaneous screws is an exacting technique, as described above (10). In rotationally unstable injuries, SI screws may be used to achieve the final reduction, as well as stabilization. The patient is positioned supine on a radiolucent table. A liter bag of fluid swathed in gamgee can be placed posteriorly to allow the buttocks to hang a little, facilitating guidewire placement. A dry run with the image intensifier should be carried out, ensuring that anteroposterior (AP), inlet, and outlet views can be obtained. It is helpful to mark the floor of the operating room for the machine's position for the optimum views, as this speeds up intraoperative screening. After preparing the skin, the drapes should be applied and almost tucked under the patient's buttock to allow full access for the entry point.

A true lateral view of the sacrum should then be obtained and the entry point for the screw identified using the tip of a wire to point out the center of the sacral alar, proximal to the S1 level. This point is then incised and a wire introduced by hand and held against the bone using a Kocher. Once correct placement of the tip of the wire is confirmed, the AP, inlet, and outlet views are taken. The wire is then introduced slowly using power. As soon as the hard subchondral bone of the ilium at the SI joint is encountered, the trajectory must be rechecked in all three views. If the trajectory of the wire is unsatisfactory, it is helpful to leave the wire in place, allowing the surgeon to reference from it and also preventing the new wire from following the same path. The wire should cross the SI joint, head towards the center of the body of the sacrum on the inlet view, and be mid-way in the corridor proximal to the S1 nerve root foramen on the outlet view. Dense bone is encountered on the sacral side of the SI joint. The surgeon should be aware that further dense bone could represent the wire exiting the sacrum anteriorly, penetrating into a nerve root canal, or even into the sacral canal posteriorly. The guidewire should reach the middle of the sacral body, or just beyond. It is measured, subtracting 5 mm to allow for compression of the SI joint, and a washer is applied. A second screw can be inserted in the same manner. If the corridor between S1 and S2 is chosen, it must be remembered that this is considerably more narrow, and that any imperfection in reduction renders this more narrow still.

The anterior elements of the pelvic ring can, in some circumstances, be stabilized using the same technique described for percutaneous fixation of the anterior column of the acetabulum. Again, this is a method of stabilizing the fracture reduced by other, usually indirect means. An antegrade or retrograde screw may be inserted (11–13). In the dry run with the image intensifier, views must be obtained in a plane perpendicular to the superior pubic ramus. In order to ensure that penetration of the inner cortex is avoided, a clear inlet-iliac oblique must be seen. Correspondingly, to avoid penetration of the joint below or of the superior cortex in the region of the femoral vessels, the outlet-obturator oblique view must be seen.

For antegrade screw insertion, the patient is prepared and draped as for anterior stabilization and as if percutaneous SI screw fixation were to be performed. The line from the tip of the trochanter to the thickest part of the iliac crest is drawn out. This lies 4 to 5 cm posterior to the anterior superior iliac spine. A small stab wound is made a little proximal to the mid-point of the line and the guidewire introduced. Once the trajectory is confirmed the wire is advanced, with repeated screening throughout. Again, encountering dense bone warns of penetration of the joint, the inner, or the upper cortex. Leaving the unsatisfactory wire in place is usually helpful as with the SI screw technique.

Retrograde screw insertion is performed via a 3-cm anterior "mini-Pfannenstiel" incision and the entry point is just inferior to the pubic tubercle. Guidewire insertion proceeds in the same manner as above, initially aiming below and beyond the anterior inferior iliac spine.

As with all percutaneous techniques, the fact that a large exposure is avoided does not mean that the technique is easy. On the contrary, attention to detail must be absolute.

SUMMARY

Successful surgery for pelvic ring injuries is strictly dependent on the adequate surgical approach to the individual injury pattern. Furthermore, the general condition of the patient and the presence of concomitant extrapelvic injuries should guide the therapeutic protocol with regard to the choice of timing, modality of fixation, and the exact approach for stabilization of pelvic ring injuries. The accurate preoperative positioning, the knowledge of anatomical structures and landmarks, and the careful surgical dissection technique represent further prerequisites for the successful management of pelvic ring injuries.

ACKNOWLEDGMENTS

The figures were kindly drawn by Mrs. Marianne Peters, Charité University Medical Center, Campus Benjamin Franklin, Berlin, Germany.

REFERENCES

1. Watnik NFC, Goldberger M. Urologic injuries in pelvic ring disruptions. Clin Orthop 1996; 329:37–45.
2. Karakurt L, et al. Corona mortis: incidence and location. Arch Orthop Trauma Surg 2002; 122(3):163–164.
3. Tornetta P 3rd, Hochwald N, Levine R. Corona mortis. Incidence and location. Clin Orthop 1996; 329:97–101.
4. Hirvensalo E, Lindahl L, Bostman O. A new approach to the internal fixation of unstable pelvic fractures. Clin Orthop 1993; 297:28–32.
5. Letournel E. The treatment of acetabular fractures through the ilioinguinal approach. Clin Orthop 1993; 292:62–76.
6. Cole JD, Bolhofner BR. Acetabular fracture fixation via a modified Stoppa limited intrapelvic approach. Description of operative technique and preliminary treatment results. Clin Orthop 1994; 305:112–123.
7. Goris RJ, Biert J. A single, midline, extraperitoneal incision for internal fixation of type C unstable pelvic ring fractures. J Am Coll Surg, 1995; 181(1):81–82.
8. Moed BR, Karges DE. Techniques for reduction and fixation of pelvic ring disruptions through the posterior approach. Clin Orthop 1996; 329:102–114.
9. Leighton RK, Waddell JP. Techniques for reduction and posterior fixation through the anterior approach. Clin Orthop 1996; 329:115–120.
10. Routt ML, Jr. et al. Early results of percutaneous iliosacral screws placed with the patient in the supine position. J Orthop Trauma 1995; 9(3):207–214.
11. Routt ML Jr, Simonian PT, Grujic L. The retrograde medullary superior pubic ramus screw for the treatment of anterior pelvic ring disruptions: a new technique. J Orthop Trauma 1995; 9(1):35–44.
12. Starr AJ, Reinert CM, Jones AL. Percutaneous fixation of the columns of the acetabulum: a new technique. J Orthop Trauma 1998; 12(1):51–58.
13. Simonian PT, et al. Internal fixation of the unstable anterior pelvic ring: a biomechanical comparison of standard plating techniques and the retrograde medullary superior pubic ramus screw. J Orthop Trauma 1994; 8(6):476–482.
14. Stahel PF, Ertel W. Pelvic ring injuries. In: Rüter A, Trentz O, Wagner M, eds. Unfallchirurgie, 2nd ed. Munich: Urban & Fischer, 2004:907–934.

6
Reconstruction of the Injured Pelvis: Fixation Techniques

Deniz W. Baysal and Adam J. Starr
Department of Orthopaedic Surgery, University of Texas Southwestern Medical Center, Dallas, Texas, U.S.A.

INTRODUCTION

Less invasive methods of fracture stabilization are now more popular than ever. Today, surgeons realize that disturbance of the fracture environment, soft-tissue stripping, and removal of periosteal tissues will slow fracture healing and increase the risk of infection. New, minimally invasive techniques to approach and reduce bony fragments have been developed. The orthopedic industry has jumped on the bandwagon too. Better reduction tools and fixation devices now allow us to bring fractures to a correct position and hold them in place while they heal, with as little damage to surrounding tissues as possible. "Just enough dissection and stabilization" is the principle driving this revolution in fracture care.

The same revolution is taking place in pelvic fracture management. Open treatment of pelvic fractures predominated just a few years ago. Today, open methods are giving way to newer techniques of closed or limited open reduction, coupled with percutaneous stabilization. Percutaneous iliosacral screws are no longer a controversial novelty; percutaneous fixation of the superior pubic ramus is becoming more common, and percutaneous fixation of iliac wing fractures has been reported. Endoscopically assisted plate fixation of symphysis disruption has been described at several centers. Clearly, the push is to stabilize the pelvis with minimally invasive techniques.

Open techniques will always have a place in the trauma surgeon's armamentarium. In some cases, open approaches will yield better results than percutaneous methods. But, as long as minimally invasive techniques can yield adequate reductions, these methods will continue to grow in popularity; for the same reasons their popularity is on the rise elsewhere in the body. Less invasive surgery does less damage to the soft-tissue envelope, cuts down the risk of infection, leads to less scarring, and may hasten union.

This chapter reviews the methods of pelvic fracture stabilization. Methods of open reduction and stabilization are presented along with newer techniques of less invasive fixation.

POSTERIOR RING INJURIES

Sacroiliac Joint Injuries

The sacroiliac articulation is one of the most complex joints orthopedic surgeons deal with. The anatomy of the sacrum and surrounding structures make diagnosis and fixation difficult. Recognition of these injuries was difficult before the advent of roentgenograms. Until recent times, these injuries were treated conservatively, with no surgical intervention. Most pelvic injuries are stable, meaning they will not displace significantly when faced with physiologic loads (1). For the unstable injuries, conservative management results in deformity, leg length discrepancy, chronic pain, and occasionally nonunion (2). Attempts at closed reduction with traction and manipulation are often unsuccessful due to the strong deforming forces the posterior ring is subjected to. Early reports of persistent back pain and leg discomfort with conservative treatment led surgeons to become more aggressive with sacral injuries (3,4).

Early attempts with stabilization involved the use of external fixators. Although external fixation techniques are often successful in management of anterior pelvic injuries, posterior injuries are difficult to immobilize with frames, and loss of reduction with a posterior injury is common when anterior frames alone are used (2).

To avoid loss of reduction, surgeons turned to open stabilization. Early attempts at fixation involved an open posterior approach. Initial reports were promising. However, later studies showed that the soft-tissue complication rate was high. Kellam and associates reported a complication rate 25% of posterior injuries treated with open reduction and internal fixation (5). Goldstein and associates reported similar results, with an infection rate of 27% after open reduction and internal fixation of posterior pelvic injuries (6). Open reduction and internal fixation of posterior pelvic ring injuries

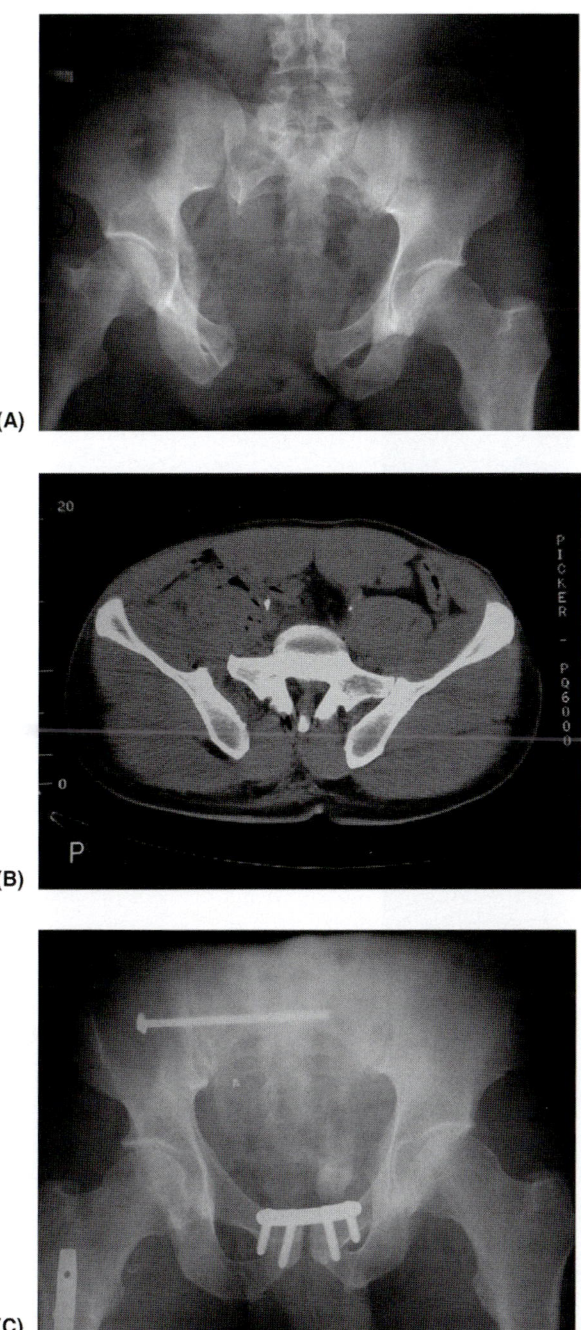

Figure 1 (**A**) Anteroposterior radiograph of a patient who sustained a right sacroiliac dislocation and widening of the symphysis pubis (APCIII). (**B**) Computed tomography of sacroiliac joint demonstrating disruption of anterior and posterior sacroiliac ligaments. Arterial hemorrhage "blush" is visible anterior to the right ala. (**C**) Postoperative anteroposterior radiograph demonstrates closure of sacroiliac joint with percutaneous iliosacral screw and plating of symphysis pubis with precontoured symphysis plate. (*Continued*)

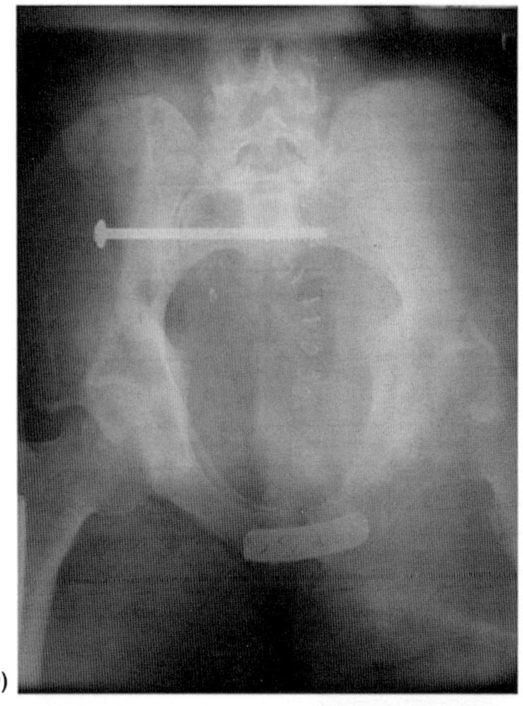

(D)

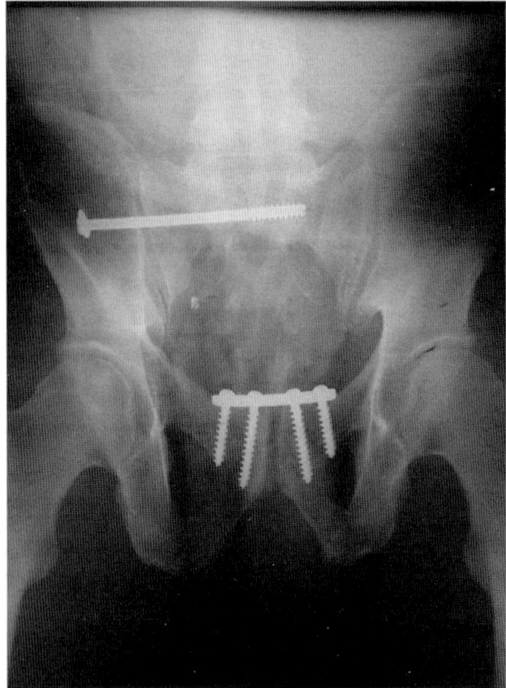

(E)

Figure 1 (*Continued*) (**D**) Postoperative inlet radiograph. Note the embolization coil anterior to the right ala. (**E**) Postoperative outlet radiograph.

is often lengthy surgery with significant blood loss. Additionally, many such patients are multiply injured and remain bedridden with trauma. Persistent bed rest may increase wound complications at the site of posterior pelvic incisions. Although operative treatment results in improved function and restoration of anatomy when compared to conservative treatment, it is clear that open approaches to the posterior ring carry significant risk of soft tissue complications.

In the early 1990s, Routt and associates reported the use of percutaneous fixation to stabilize posterior injuries involving the sacroiliac joint (7,8). With a large series of patients, Routt reported a low complication rate (8), with few screw-related problems, low operative time, and minimal blood loss. Most important, the rate of soft-tissue complication was dramatically minimized.

Despite the low complication rate, surgeons were slow to accept this technique. But, with improvements in intraoperative imaging and increased familiarity with percutaneous techniques, this method is now a common treatment for posterior pelvic injuries (Fig. 1A–E).

Open Posterior Approach

The open approach to the posterior pelvic ring requires that the patient be placed in a prone position on bolsters (9). This can make monitoring difficult, but prone position is usually well tolerated by patients and may actually be beneficial for pulmonary function. After identifying the posterior superior iliac spine, a longitudinal incision is made either medially or laterally to this landmark depending on whether the injury involves the sacrum or the sacroiliac joint. For fractures involving the iliac wing, the proximal extent of the incision can be curved laterally along the iliac crest. Due to the bony prominence of the sacral spine, an incision directly over the sacral midline is fraught with wound complications, especially in those patients who must remain supine in the intensive care for prolonged periods. The most commonly used skin incision is made just lateral to the sacral midline, extending from the level of the posterior superior iliac spine distally for 8 to 10 cm. The subcutaneous tissue is divided in line with the skin. The origin of the gluteus maximus is dissected off the ilium and sacrum and reflected downward and laterally. The erector spinae and multifidi muscles are elevated from the sacrum. With high-energy injuries, the dissection is often completed at the time of injury.

All components of anatomy should be identified, including the sacral neural foramina, the ala, and the superior aspect of the first sacral vertebra. The sacroiliac joint should be debrided and aligned anatomically. In case of sacroiliac joint disruption, bone reduction clamps are used to bring the ilium into correct alignment with the sacrum. Similarly, clamps can be used to align sacral fractures. Reduction is best judged with fluoroscopy and direct visualization. The anterior aspect of the sacrum is palpable through the greater sciatic notch, allowing the surgeon to assess the alignment of the disrupted joint.

Once the reduction is acceptable, several methods can be used to fix the injury. Matta described the use of iliosacral bars (10), a technique that avoids risk of damage to sacral nerve roots as the bar is placed through the posterior iliac wing, dorsal to the sacrum. This technique requires a second incision over the contralateral ilium in order to lock the bar, thus raising the risk of compromise of the soft tissues.

Mears and associates describe the use of a cobra plate along the posterior sacrum, reaching from one wing to the opposite (11). This method requires more dissection and may not be suitable for traumatized patients, especially when soft tissue coverage is compromised. Recent studies have described the use of smaller precontoured plates or small fragment plates to stabilize the posterior sacrum. These techniques require an open approach, but the implants are less bulky, while still preserving stability (12).

Open Anterior Approach

For anterior exposure of the sacroiliac joint, the patient is placed supine with the injured side tilted up with a roll for easier access and manipulation (13). The incision parallels the iliac wing, beginning at the anterior superior iliac spine, extending posteriorly. One must take care to protect the lateral femoral cutaneous nerve because injury to this nerve may cause a painful neuroma. The external oblique insertion on the ilium is lifted up, and the iliacus is elevated from the inner cortex of the iliac wing. As the dissection courses medially, the sacroiliac joint hump is reached. One to two centimeters medial to this joint lies the fifth sacral nerve root.

The limb is draped free so it may be manipulated into flexion to relax the iliopsoas muscle. In most dislocations, the ilium is displaced superiorly and posteriorly, so reduction requires that the hip be flexed and pulled with inline traction. A pelvic reduction clamp can be placed from the sacral ala to the ilium along the inner table. To help bring the ilium into place, a shanz pin placed in the ilium can be used to aid manipulation. The sacroiliac joint can be held in place temporarily with kirshner wires or a staple (14).

Once adequate reduction is obtained, permanent fixation is commonly achieved using one or two plates. Screw placement can be difficult due to both the tight confines of the approach and the anatomy of the sacrum. Examination of the field during fixation with fluoroscopy will make screw placement easier. One advantage of plate fixation is that the plate can be used as a reduction tool by over contouring. Either 3.5 or 4.5 mm plates can be used.

The major disadvantage of this technique is the amount of deep exposure required and the risk to large neurovascular structures. Authors report good ability to reduce the sacroiliac joint when using this approach. Ability to reduce the joint is reported to have 85% to 95% success if attempted within the first two weeks (13). The major disadvantage of this approach is the dissection required, with major neurovascular structures at risk.

The fifth lumbar-nerve root limits medial dissection and can be damaged by dissection or retraction. Reduction and visualization of the injured structures are limited by the confines of this approach. As noted previously, a problem with the anterior approach is the rate of lateral femoral cutaneous nerve injury. Up to 30% of patients are observed to have injury to this nerve, with 50% of them reporting pain or numbness at one year (13).

Percutaneous Iliosacral Screws

Percutaneous techniques were introduced with the aim of decreasing morbidity and mortality to the patient while maintaining a rigid and anatomic reduction. Intraoperative assessment of fracture reduction and percutaneous insertion of screws has become possible with improvements of imaging technology and an improved understanding of sacral anatomy. This technique was popularized by Routt and associates, who were the first to report on a large series of patients operated in the supine position (7).

With the patient in supine position, the entire lower abdomen is draped free from the nipple line distally, including the involved leg in case traction is required. A midline radiolucent bump is used to lift the buttock off the bed to achieve a better entry point. Prior to draping, fluoroscopy is used to ensure that adequate anteroposterior, inlet, and outlet views are visible. Preoperative images are assessed to ensure nothing is obscuring the sacral body or neural foraminae. Contrast in the abdomen or nitrous oxide inhalational anesthesia can obscure anatomic details and make the procedure more difficult. Nitrous oxide passes readily through the endothelial capillaries of the intestine and enters the bowel lumen. The resulting gas bubbles can mimic or obscure outlines of neuroforaminae; the procedure will have to be delayed by three to five days until the gas settles.

Under fluoroscopic guidance, the tip of the guidewire is passed through the gluteal skin and placed on the outer table of the ilium near the sacroiliac joint. The exact point of entry is determined by verifying the location of the guidewire tip on the inlet and outlet views. To approximate the entry point, one can view a direct lateral of the sacrum and, using a marking pen, trace out the dorsal and ventral aspects of the sacrum along with the superior endplate of S1 on the skin. This triangular shape demarcates the sacrum, the target for guidewire placement.

A cannulated bone spike helps maintain guidewire position on the ilium and also helps with reduction. Before inserting the guidewire, a maneuver may be required to reduce the sacroiliac joint. The lateral fracture fragment is usually displaced superiorly and posteriorly. The best way to reduce this is to apply mild traction while the hip is held in flexion. Depending on the mechanism of injury (either lateral compression or anterior–posterior compressions), the leg may need to be abducted or externally rotated to reverse the deforming forces with continuous traction. If the reduction is difficult, a shanz pin placed in the ilium can aid manipulation. This can be used as a joystick to maneuver the hemipelvis into a reduced position.

Lateral displacement of the ilium can be reduced with pressure from the cannulated bone spike. Usually the reduction is amenable to closed techniques or after open fixation of the anterior components, the sacroiliac joint falls into place.

Once reduction is obtained, the guidewire is inserted through the cannulated bone spike. The position is first checked on the outlet view to make sure the wire is aiming above the first sacral foramen. The inlet is then verified to ensure to wire is aimed toward the first sacral body. The position of the guidewire can also be checked by aiming the beam of the C-arm directly down the axis of the wire on a direct lateral view. The wire should lie caudal to the iliac cortical density and within the borders of the anterior and posterior bony margins of the sacrum. In general, the wire should be passed as far as safely possible, as this will increase screw purchase and hopefully decrease risk of failure. Once guidewire position is adequate, the length of the wire should be measured.

Large fragment cannulated screws of 6.5, 7.0, 7.3, 7.5, or 8.0 mm can be used. The choice of width is primarily up to surgeon preference. Fully threaded screws are used if no fracture compression is desired. Our practice is to use partially threaded screws for the majority of cases, with the amount of compression controlled by the surgeon. Washers are used only if greater compression is required. One screw is adequate for most sacroiliac injuries. For highly unstable patterns, two screws can be inserted. It is sometimes difficult to place two screws into the first sacral body. Therefore our practice is to place the second screw into the second sacral body.

Studies have shown that 30% of pelvises have a dysmorphic first sacral vertebrae (2). This makes insertion of screws unsafe and unpredictable due to decreased space available anteriorly and superiorly. The screw has an increased chance of exiting and damaging one of the nerve roots. In such cases, the screw entry point is dropped down to allow placement of the screw into the second sacral body.

Some authors advocate the use of somatosensory evoked potentials during fixation to guard against nerve injury (15). However, reports of percutaneous iliosacral screws placed with the use of somatosensory monitoring showed a low rate of nerve injury, bringing into question the need for monitoring (8). As the surgeon's experience improves, nerve injury becomes rare and evoked potential monitoring may become unnecessary.

The advantages of percutaneous sacroiliac screws in the trauma setting are numerous. Decreased soft tissue dissection, decreased blood loss, less operative time, cost-effectiveness, and less wound healing problems are obvious benefits. As the surgeon's proficiency rises, surgical risks decrease further. Modern series of posterior pelvic ring injuries show very low rates of malreduction, low operative time, and minimal blood loss. For example, Routt and associates reported on a series of 103 percutaneously placed sacroiliac screws (7). Their mean operative time was 29 minutes, with a mean blood loss of 10.2 mL. In this series, 17 complete SI joint dislocations required open reduction before insertion of iliosacral screws.

Postoperatively, there were 12 malreductions, most of which occurred in the Tile type C injuries. There were no reported nonunions or infections at 12 months.

Recent studies have also compared mechanical properties of percutaneous fixation versus traditional plating techniques. In a recent study, the stiffest construct in single limb stance simulation was created with two iliosacral screws (16). This was equivalent to two anterior sacroiliac plates, and superior to a posterior tension plate or even two posterior sacroiliac bars.

In the hands of an experienced surgeon, sacroiliac disruptions can be fixed using percutaneous techniques. At our center, open techniques are reserved for chronic nonunions and irreducible or locked sacroiliac joints. As knowledge of percutaneous techniques evolves, the technique will be applied to other areas of the pelvis, allowing patients to benefit. Orthopedic surgeons have only recently accepted the percutaneous technique to fix the posterior pelvis. It will only be a matter of time before more types of pelvic injuries are treated with percutaneous techniques.

Sacral Fractures

Sacral fractures are commonly associated with polytrauma and can be easily overlooked. Diagnosis begins in the emergency department with a detailed history and physical examination (17). Subtle signs include bruising along the lower lumbar vertebrae or buttock. It is important to document a detailed neurologic examination upon arrival in the emergency department. Any patient with disruption of the pelvic ring should be suspected of having sacral involvement until proven otherwise. Several large series have reported an incidence of sacral fractures in 30% of pelvic injuries (18). Spinal injury should also be suspected with these injuries since there is up to a 20% incidence of contiguous injury within the axial skeleton (6).

Radiographic evaluation should include the standard anteroposterior plain film of the pelvis along with inlet and outlet views. Subtle radiographic signs include asymmetric sacral foramen, lateral process fractures of the fifth lumbar vertebrae, and bony avulsions of sacral ligaments. Once diagnosed, further evaluation must be undertaken to determine the amount and direction of displacement. Computed tomography of the pelvis with fine cuts through the sacrum allows the surgeon to determine type of sacral injury (rotational vs. translational) along with the amount of displacement. Currently there are no guidelines to the usefulness of magnetic resonance imaging in this setting.

Classification systems have been created to help guide treatment and estimate prognosis. The most commonly used classification is that of Denis (18). He divides them into three injury patterns: those with fracture lines passing lateral to the foramina (transalar), through the foramina (transforaminal), and medial to the foramina (central). The Arbeitsgemeinschaft für Osteosynthesefragen (Association for the Study of Internal Fixation)/Orthopedic Trauma Association (AO/OTA) and the Hannover groups both have more complex classification systems, which include more complex injuries, including tranverse and bilateral injuries. These detailed systems are most useful in research settings. We will use the Denis system for further discussions in this chapter.

Denis showed that as the injury moves medial, the risk of neurologic injury increased (Type I 6% vs. Type III up to 60%) (18). Such injuries can result in motor and sensory deficits in the lower extremities as well as genitourinary and sexual dysfunction.

Treatment of sacral fractures is based primarily on the amount of displacement and stability. Complete sacral fractures with displacement are usually best served with surgical stabilization. Other indications for fixation include unremitting pain and polytraumatized patients unable to mobilize. Stabilization can lessen pain and permit mobility in some cases.

Open reduction and internal fixation of sacral fractures carries inherent risks. As with sacroiliac disruptions, open approaches to sacral fractures can be complicated by soft tissue complications. The overlying soft tissue is often injured by the force of trauma, and wound dehiscence and infection have been reported with open procedures (5,6). These risks, coupled with advances in imaging technology and minimally invasive surgical techniques, have driven an increase in use of percutaneous techniques (Fig. 2A–F). Both open and percutaneous techniques will be discussed here.

Open Treatment

Our current indications for open reduction and internal fixation of sacral fractures include patients whose fractures cannot be reduced using closed means, fractures that have gone on to malunion or nonunion, or fractures associated with lower lumbar spine

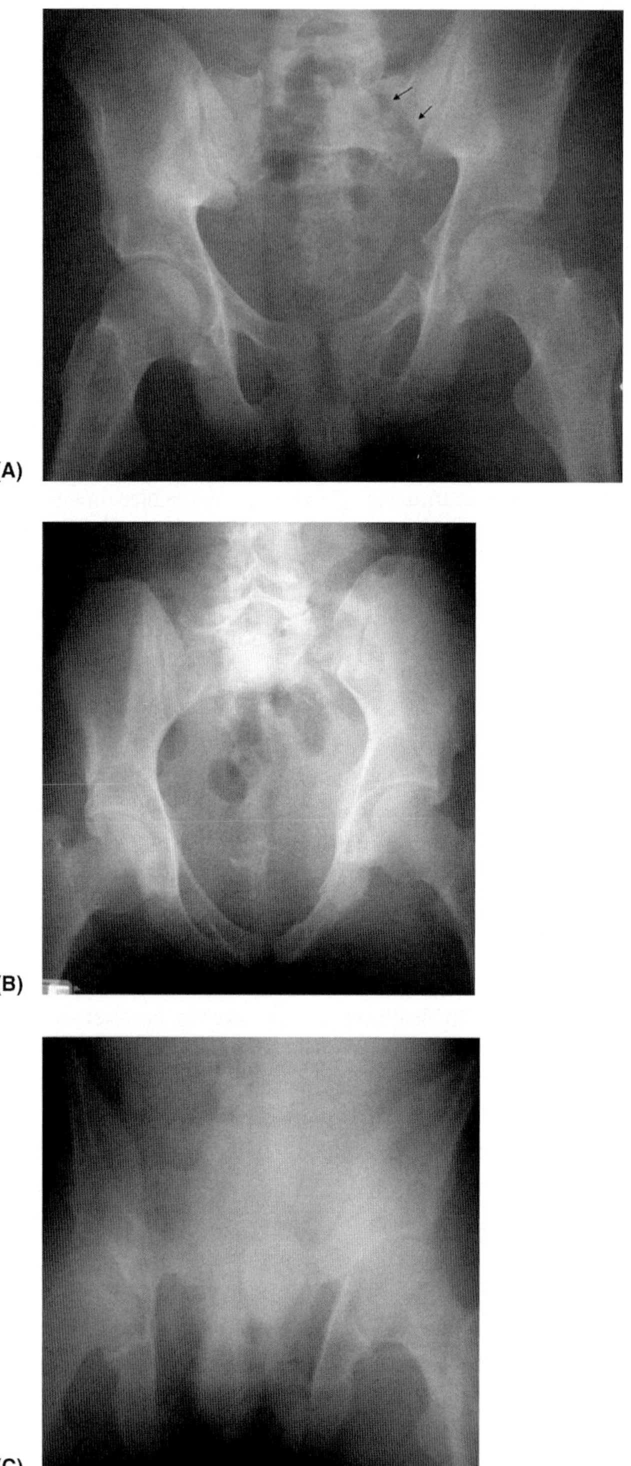

Figure 2 (**A**) Anteroposterior radiograph of a patient who sustained a fall. *Arrows* demonstrate a left sacral fracture (Denis I) and anterior rami fractures. (**B**) Inlet view showing posterior displacement of left hemipelvis. (**C**) Outlet view revealing minimal superior displacement. (*Continued*)

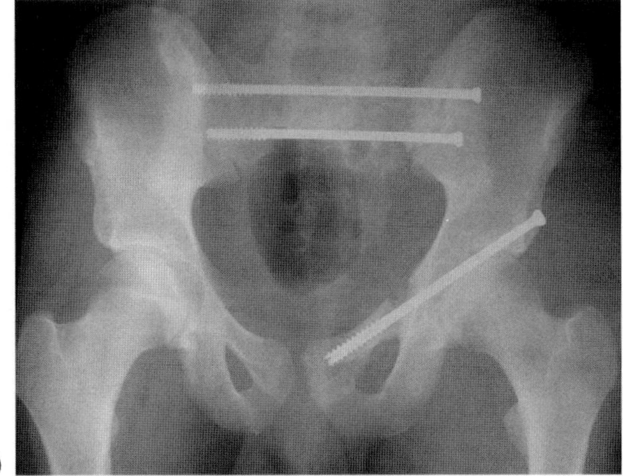
(D)

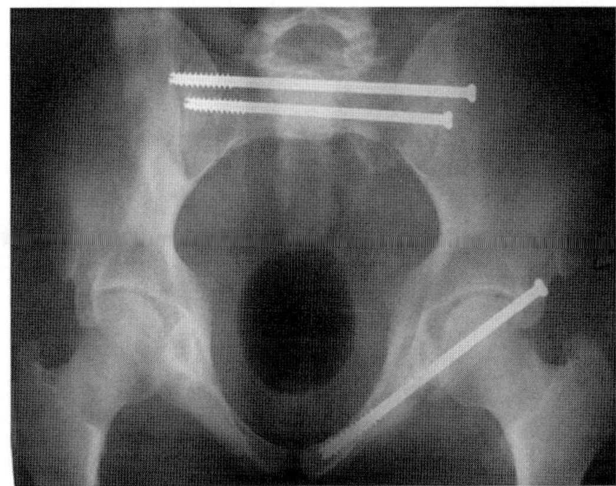
(E)

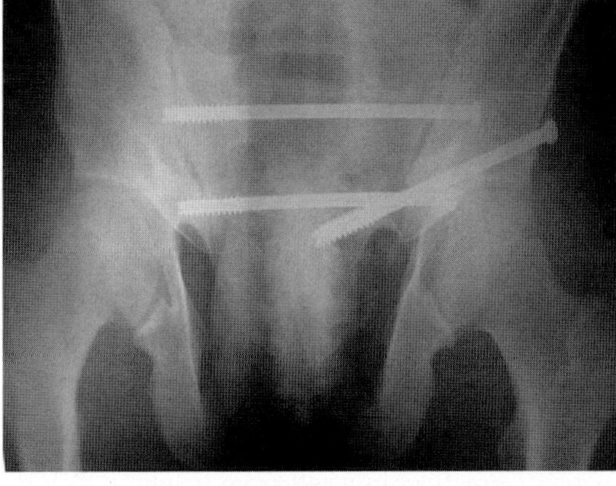
(F)

Figure 2 (*Continued*) (**D**) Postoperative anteroposterior radiograph demonstrates two iliosacral screws engaging the opposite cortex for stability. Antegrade superior ramus screw was used for increased stability. (**E**) Inlet radiograph shows the posterior displacement has been reduced. Fracture comminution anterior to the left ala is clearly visible. (**F**) Outlet radiograph. Screws have been placed in both S1 and S2 to increase stability. Comminution at the superior aspect of the left ala is visible.

fractures. The surgery is done with the patient in prone position on a radiolucent table. Preoperative inlet and outlet views must be assessed prior to the incision. The entire back is draped from mid-thorax to below the sacrum with the involved leg free limbed in case manipulation is required. For bilateral sacral fractures, it may be necessary to include both legs. For Denis type I and II injury patterns, a longitudinal paramedial incision is made between the iliac crests. The thoracolumbar fascia is incised in line with the skin incision, exposing the underlying erector spinae muscle. The muscle is elevated from midline and moved laterally, exposing the posterior cortex of the sacrum. The neural foramina are visualized and the nerve roots exposed. For Denis III fractures, occasionally a midline incision directly over the spinous process can be used. In such a case, elevation of the erector spinae from both sides of the sacrum may be needed to expose the fracture. Bony fragments within the canal are removed; a small laminectomy may be required to decompress the nerve roots.

Once exposed, the fracture is cleaned and then reduced with a pelvic reduction clamp. A posterior external frame distractor can also be used by placing pins in the posterior superior iliac spines. Distraction of the fracture may assist in fracture debridement, but great care must be taken to avoid damage to anterior vessels or nerve roots. Traction may be required on the legs to reduce a vertical shear component. The injuries are similar to sacroiliac disruptions in that the lateral fragment can be displaced superiorly and posteriorly.

Once a reduction is obtained, the surgeon has the option of placing hardware directly onto the posterior sacrum or using fluoroscopy to place percutaneous screws. For Denis type I injuries, a plate can be placed over the fracture extending from the intact medial ala to the lateral alar fragment or even the ilium if necessary. Screws in this plate are placed medially into the first sacral pedicle below the lumbosacral facet. Fluoroscopic guidance is useful in guiding screw placement. Special H-shaped plates can be used for this injury pattern, or acetabular reconstruction plates can be contoured to extend across the injury. Fixation should be obtained from lateral to medial at the first sacral level and one level below, usually the third or fourth sacral level, with two screws lateral to the fracture and at least one medial at each level. For Denis type II injuries, a similar technique is used, with reconstruction plates crossing the fracture at two levels.

Denis type III injuries or bilateral sacral fractures require two reconstruction plates at the first and third sacral levels to achieve fixation. These should extend laterally over good bone in the ala across to the opposite side since the canal is directly midline.

Special patterns of injury, such as the H-shaped sacral fracture that involve bilateral sacral fractures with a horizontal component, require special attention. Roy-Camille described three types of H-shaped fracture patterns based on extension or flexion of the proximal fragment (19). These are strongly associated with sacral plexus injuries (19). These fractures are often found in patients involved in a fall from height, which results in traumatic spondylolisthesis of the first sacral level over the remaining sacrum, along with bilateral sacral fractures.

Initial treatment of H-shaped fractures starts with reduction of the fracture with the patient in prone position and hyperextension of both legs. This maneuver is not always successful. The need for reduction is controversial. Some authors recommend percutaneous fixation in situ, others suggest open reduction and internal fixation. Open treatment involves a direct midline incision over the spine beginning at the third lumbar vertebrae and extending distally over the sacrum. The paraspinal muscles are elevated subperiosteally and the pedicles of the fourth and fifth lumbar vertebrae are isolated. Pedicle screws are inserted into the spine, usually 5.5 mm in diameter. The posterior iliac spines are also isolated and large pedicle screws (6.5 mm) approximately 80 to 90 mm in length are inserted. These are directed anteriorly toward the anterior inferior iliac spine, directly above the acetabulum. A finger palpating the greater sciatic notch can help direct these screws anteriorly. The position of these screws should be verified on iliac and obturator oblique views of the posterior sacrum as well as a perpendicular view of the ilium to ensure the screw does not exit the inner or outer table. The fluoroscopic beam can also be aimed directly down the shaft of the screw and a teardrop outline of the supra-acetabular region will be seen, with the screw directly in the middle. These screws are connected to the lumbar pedicle screws with connector bars similar to those used in posterior instrumentation for lumbar decompression and fusion.

As previously discussed, placing hardware directly onto the sacrum can create problems with wound healing, damage to nerve roots, and other neurovascular structures. The bony anatomy of the sacrum in certain areas is thin and oblique; screw placement can be difficult. One can also place iliosacral bars, but as previously discussed with sacroiliac joint disruptions, these require a fairly large dissection and leave prominent hardware. In a recent series of 11 patients with H-shaped sacral fractures treated with open reduction and internal fixation, three developed infection, two developed seromas, and one had a secondary neurologic deficit (20). Open treatment of the sacrum should not be taken lightly, especially with the advancements of percutaneous screw fixation.

Percutaneous Fixation

At our institution, sacral fractures are treated with closed reduction and percutaneous screw fixation. Even markedly displaced fractures can be reduced early and stabilized with percutaneously placed iliosacral screws. Closed reduction is difficult. It requires multiple assistants, traction, and compression of the ilium to reduce the fracture. The technique of screw placement is similar to that used in sacroiliac joint disruptions. If the pelvis is widened anteriorly, it is recommended that the symphysis diastasis be addressed first (see section on "Anterior Pelvic Injuries"). The percutaneous method of posterior fixation preserves all soft tissues, and is less risky for nerve roots, if done properly under fluoroscopy by an experienced surgeon.

There are some subtle differences for percutaneous fixation for sacral fractures when compared to sacroiliac disruptions. The preoperative setup and reduction techniques are similar; however the direction of screw placement is slightly different. The guidewire should be placed directly across the fracture, with a more anterior starting point on the outer table. The wire is directed perpendicular to the fracture, not the sacroiliac joint, and if possible should be advanced all the way across the sacral body into the opposite iliac wing to improve fixation.

Large fragment cannulated screws should be used. The partial versus fully threaded screw question is controversial. At our center, partially threaded screws are used for virtually every case. The surgeon controls compression and care must be taken to avoid overcompressing the fracture. Some authors advocate the use of somatosensory evoked potentials to prevent nerve injury during fixation, but this is controversial (15). Two screws are placed to prevent rotational instability and provide enough fixation to allow the patient to mobilize early (Fig. 2D). A recent study showed that, following percutaneous iliosacral screw fixation, injuries involving vertical shear patterns have a higher risk of fixation failure with surgery than sacroiliac joint dislocations (21). These sacral fractures differ from sacroiliac dislocations or fracture dislocations involving the ala because there is no cortical bone available for screw purchase. On either side of the sacral fracture, the screw is surrounded by comminuted cancellous bone, unlike the sacroiliac disruption, where the screw is able to purchase into cortical bone in the ilium and ala. For this reason, it is recommended that, for sacral fractures, the sacroiliac screw cross as far as possible across the fracture into the opposite sacroiliac joint if possible for bony cortical purchase (Fig. 2D).

With reduction and stabilization, patients with sacral fractures can mobilize early. At our center we allow "foot flat" weight bearing for three months. Thus complications of bed rest are avoided.

Crescent Fractures

When the posterior pelvic disruption passes through the lower portion of the sacroiliac joint and exits through the ilium, this is known as a "crescent fracture." A portion of the iliac wing remains attached to the sacrum by means of the sacro-iliac ligaments. The piece of bone fractured from the iliac wing resembles a crescentic moon, hence the term (Fig. 3A–H). The most common mechanism of injury is lateral compression, resulting in the wing being impinged against the dense sacral bone (22). These fractures are rotationally unstable, and are classified as lateral compression type II in the Young–Burgess classification system (23).

Traditionally, these fractures have been stabilized with open reduction and internal fixation. They can be approached anteriorly, via an iliac fossa approach, or posteriorly, by elevating the gluteus maximus to expose the posterior ilium. These open approaches are beneficial in that they allow direct manipulation of bone fragments. As noted by Routt, the posterior approach allows for debridement of devitalized muscle tissue disrupted by the injury (11). Reports of open reduction and internal fixation of crescent fractures have shown uniformly good results. But, as with other open procedures, open reduction of crescent fractures carries a moderate risk of soft tissue complication. Due to the risk, percutaneous methods have been attempted for this injury pattern.

Percutaneous Technique

The patient is placed on a radiolucent table in supine position, and the entire pelvis from the base of the penis up to the nipple line is prepped and draped, including the entire iliac crest and as far as posteriorly and laterally over the gluteus maximus. The ipsilateral leg is draped into the surgical field. Intraoperative imaging is checked preoperatively to ensure that proper views are obtainable and that there are no obstructions to the fluoroscopy such as nitrous oxide gas or abdominal contrast. The surgeon must be able to visualize inlet and outlet views as well as obturator views of the pelvis.

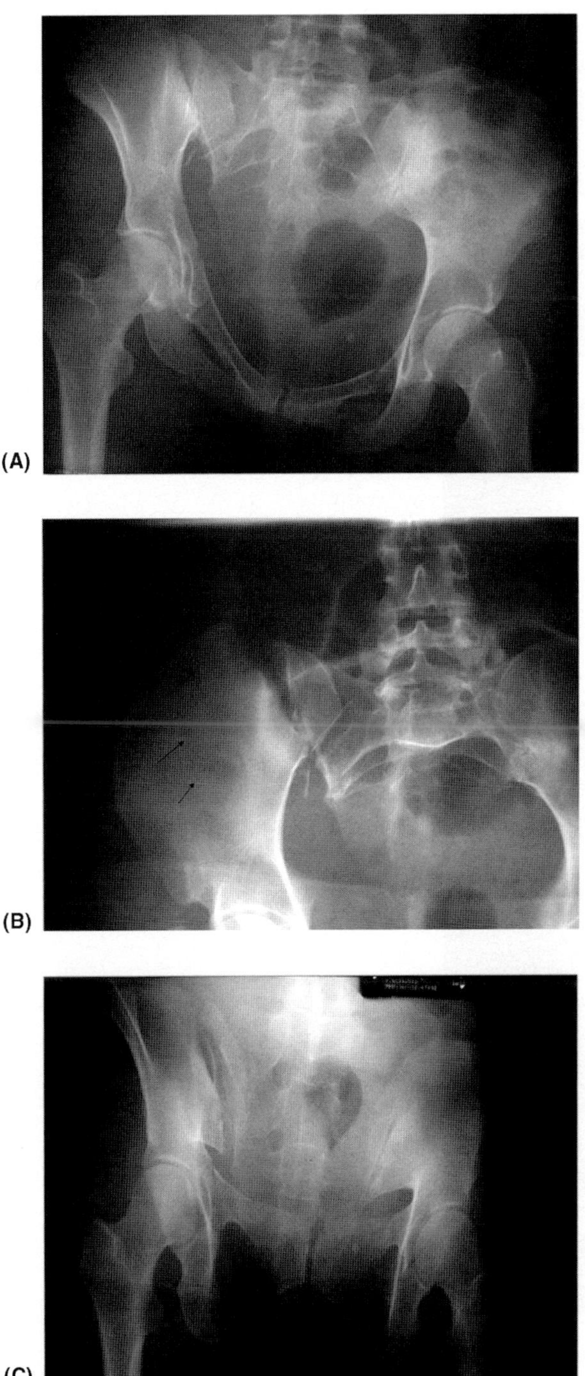

Figure 3 (**A**) Anteroposterior radiograph reveals a fracture through the right sacroiliac joint and right ilium, demonstrating the "crescent fragment." (**B**) Close-up inlet radiograph shows the crescent fragment (*arrows*) still attached to the sacrum. The iliac wing has displaced superiorly and posteriorly. (**C**) Injury outlet radiograph. The patient's S1 is dysmorphic. (*Continued*)

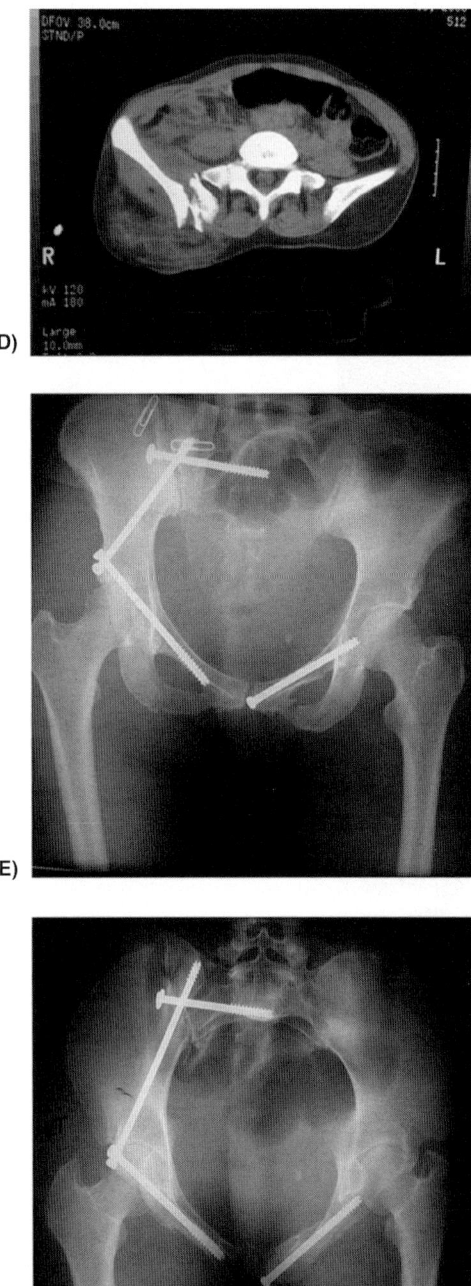

Figure 3 (*Continued*) (**D**) Computed tomography demonstrates the "crescent fragment" still attached to the sacrum. The iliac wing fragment is clearly displaced posteriorly and laterally. (**E**) Postoperative anteroposterior radiograph. Traction, to reduce superior and posterior translation, coupled with a ball spike pusher placed through a stab incision to reduce lateral translation of the ilium, provided adequate reduction. The iliac wing fracture was stabilized using an LC 2 screw. Then, the SI joint disruption was stabilized using an iliosacral screw placed in S2. Finally, both superior ramus fractures were stabilized using percutaneous screws. (**F**) Postoperative inlet radiograph. This view reveals residual slight internal rotation deformity of the right ilium. The pathway of the LC2 screw is clearly visible. (*Continued*)

(G)
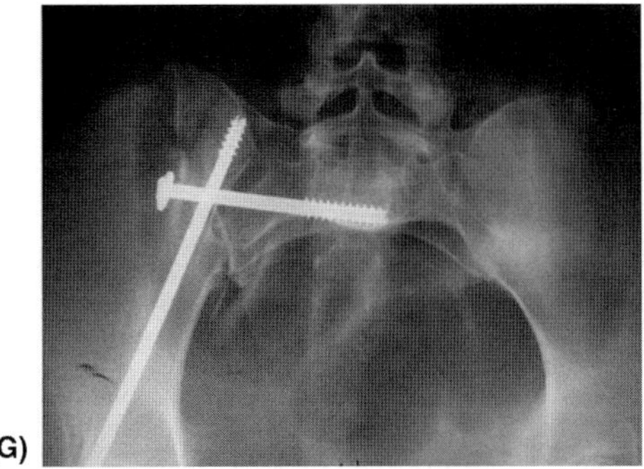

(H)
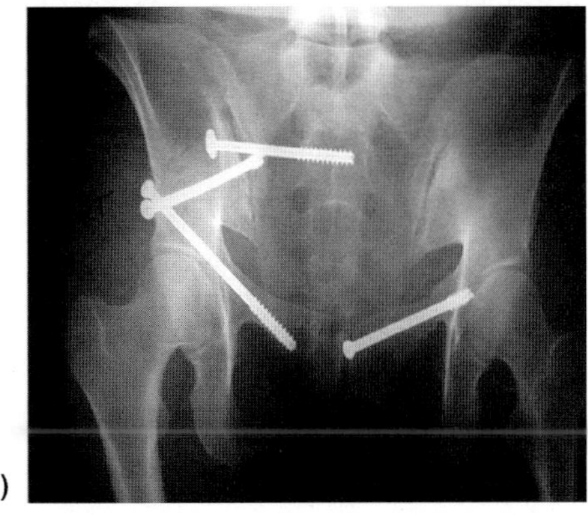

Figure 3 (*Continued*) (**G**) This closeup inlet view reveals the reduction of the ilium to the crescent fragment. The reduction is not anatomic. The threads of the LC 2 screw are visible in the crescent fragment. (**H**) Postoperative outlet view reveals reduction of the lateral and superior displacement of the ilium.

If attempts at percutaneous reduction are not successful, the anterior approach is used to access the injury; for this reason, it is important to drape the area large enough to allow access through the front. The injury mechanism is often a lateral compression, which results in internal rotation of the hemipelvis. External rotation and abduction of the hip often serve to correct the deformity. Occasionally, the iliac wing will be translated laterally away from the crescent fragment at the fracture site. This can usually be corrected by using a bone spike introduced through a stab incision passing through the abductor muscles. A shanz pin can be inserted into the iliac crest just proximal to the anterior superior iliac spine is also useful in gaining reduction. In conjunction with traction and manipulation of the hip, crescent fractures can usually be adequately aligned.

Once the fracture is visualized and can be reduced, the bony landmarks are identified for guidewire insertion. The direction of the screw is directly in line from the anterior inferior iliac spine to the posterior inferior iliac spine. This allows the screw to pass above the acetabulum through the thickest portion of the ilium and provides good purchase in the posterior iliac wing. Under fluoroscopic guidance, the entry point for the guidewire is identified directly over the anterior inferior iliac spine and a small elevator is used to clear the soft tissue. At this point, a cannulated bone spike is placed over the entry point and the guidewire inserted into the bone.

The direction of the guidewire is assessed with several fluoroscopic views. The view to demonstrate the correct starting point—the "Teepee view"—aims directly down the axis from the anterior inferior iliac spine to the posterior inferior iliac spine and is obtained by directing the fluoroscopy machine towards an obturator oblique position. Adjustment of the fluoroscopy will reveal a teepee shape just above the acetabulum. This shape represents the cortical confines of the thick column of bone that passes from the anterior inferior iliac spine to the posterior inferior iliac spine. If the cannulated bone spike is placed correctly, the surgeon should be able to see directly down its center, with the spike in the middle of the teepee shape.

Once the guidewire is started in the center of the "Teepee," its direction is checked on an iliac oblique. This ensures that the wire proceeds superior to the sciatic notch. Moving the fluoroscope to an inlet view, then rolling the C-arm over the injured side, a third view looking down the iliac wing is obtained. This "top-down" view of the iliac wing is used to ensure that the wire does not penetrate the inner or outer cortices of the iliac wing, as it moves posteriorly. Reduction is assessed continuously as the wire crosses the fracture and enters the crescent fragment itself (Fig. 4).

Once correct guidewire position is determined, the guidewire is measured and an appropriate length large fragment cannulated screw is placed. Reduction maneuvers should be continued during screw placement to ensure that no loss of alignment occurs. No washer is necessary, unless the bone is of very poor quality. Screw position is verified using multiplanar fluoroscopy. A second screw can be inserted above the first, as long as enough room remains superiorly on the "Teepee" view.

These fractures can be associated with sacroiliac disruptions. If so, an iliosacral screw can be placed to stabilize the sacroiliac joint.

Postoperatively, the patient is allowed to mobilize with "foot flat" weight bearing for three months.

Results from percutaneous treatment of these injuries result in less soft tissue dissection and blood loss without compromising reduction and stability to the fracture (22). This is a viable treatment option for these injuries, provided the indications are appropriate and the surgeon is confident in his ability to perform an adequate reduction using minimally invasive techniques.

ANTERIOR RING INJURIES

Ramus Fractures

Fractures of the anterior aspect of the pelvis can occur due to a lateral compression mechanism or from an anteroposterior compression mechanism. Lateral compression type injuries typically produce horizontal fracture planes, where the bone cracks and the fragments slide past each other. Anteroposterior compression (APC) type injuries produce vertical fracture planes as the bone is pulled apart, separating the two fragments. In practice, truly horizontal or vertical fracture alignment is rare, but examination of ramus fracture anatomy can provide some clue as to the force that produced the fracture.

Indications for stabilizing pubic ramus fractures are controversial. If left untreated, most ramus fractures will heal uneventfully. Conservative treatment is often an acceptable course of management. However, surgical stabilization of the rami can yield some benefit to the patient. Fixation can help provide added stability to pelvic

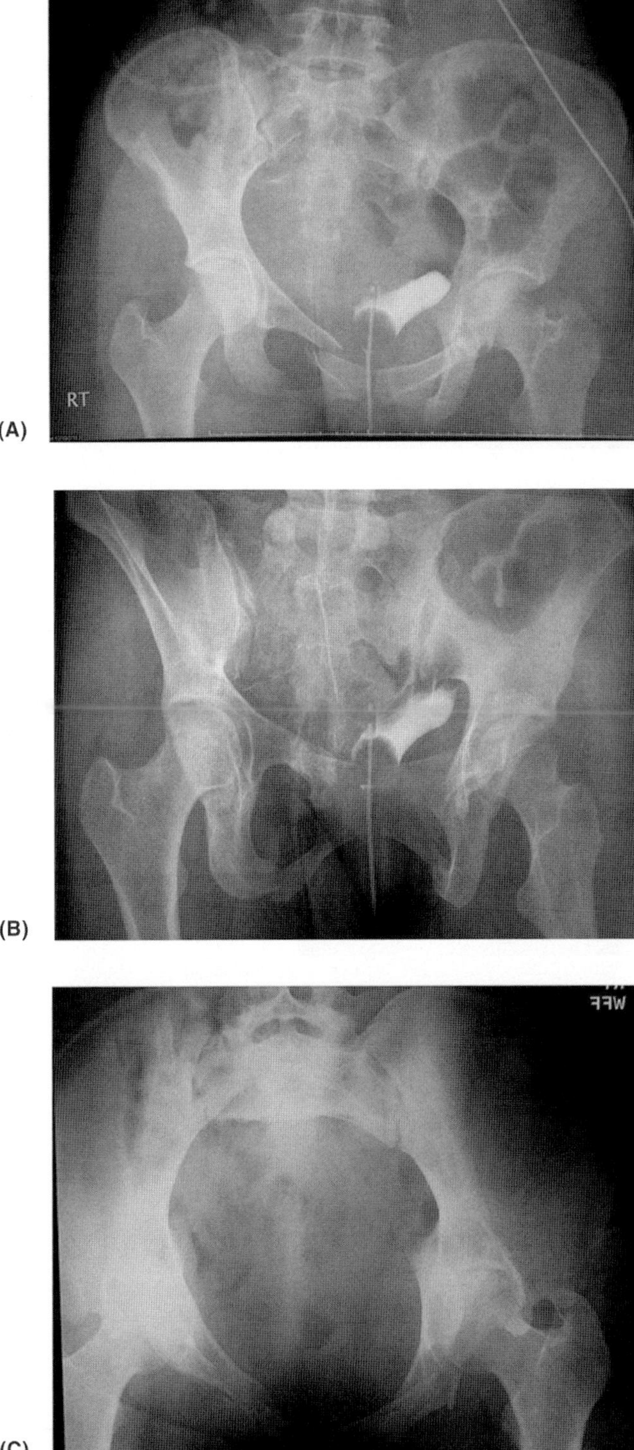

Figure 4 (**A**) Anteroposterior radiograph of a 22-year old female involved in a motor vehicle collision, sustaining a sacral fracture and bilateral rami fractures. (**B**) Outlet view. (**C**) Inlet view. Severe right sacral alar comminution is seen. (*Continued*)

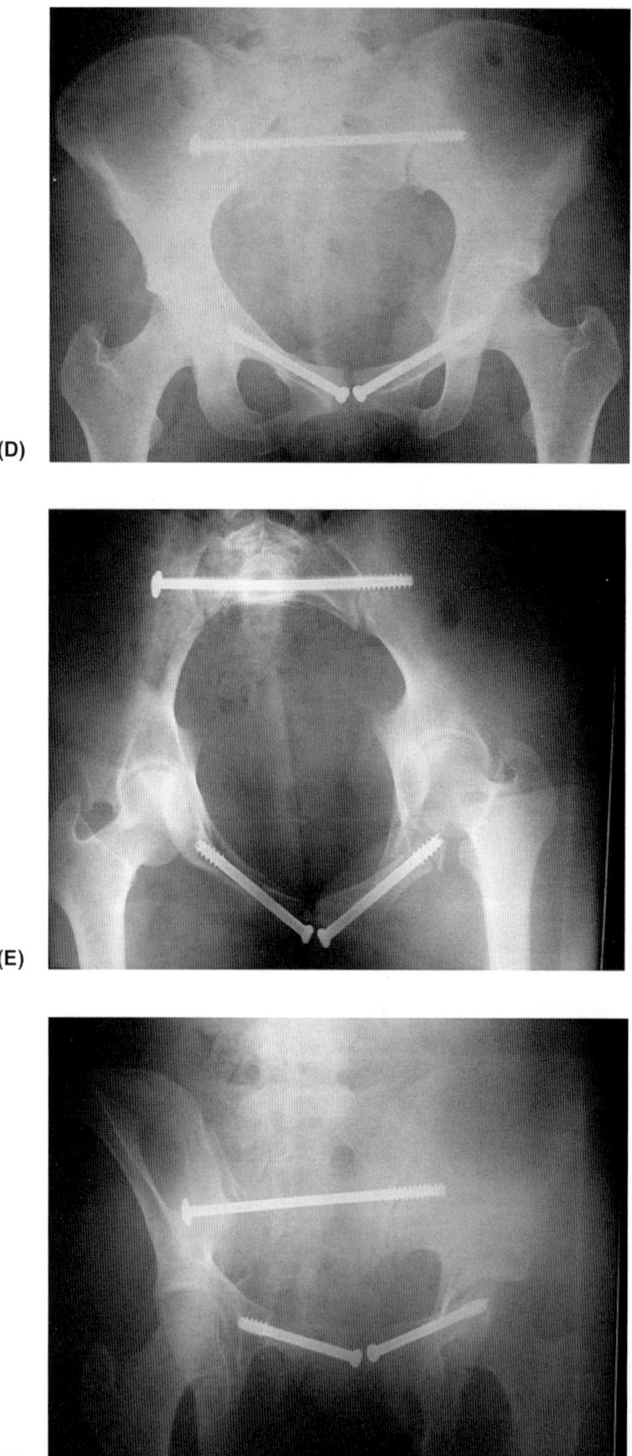

Figure 4 (*Continued*) (**D**) Postoperative radiograph, showing bilateral retrograde ramus screws. This patient was up sitting in a chair on postoperative day one, with minimal discomfort. (**E**) Inlet view. (**F**) Outlet view.

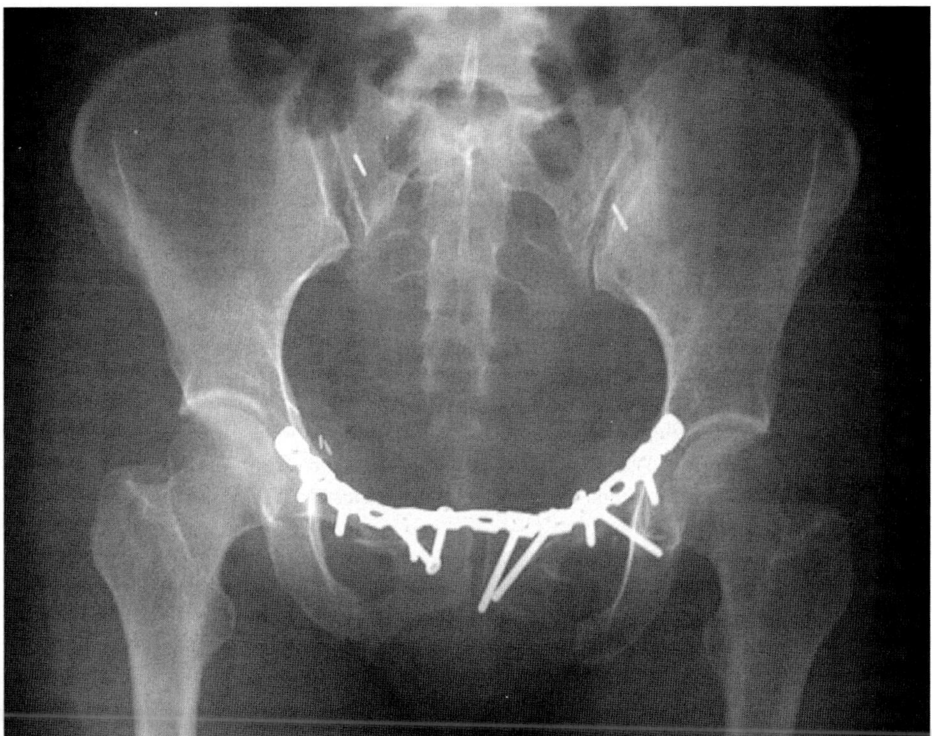

Figure 5 Bilateral superior ramus fractures treated with open reduction and internal fixation using a 3.5 mm reconstruction plate.

ring. The reduction and stabilization can restore anatomy and can prevent problems such as dyspareunia in females with impingement on the vagina from displaced ramus fractures. Additionally, stabilization of ramus fractures alleviates pain, and this can be a marked benefit for patients who sustain pelvic ring fractures. Pain may prevent patients from mobilizing early and expose them to further risks involved with these injuries such as thromboembolic disease or deconditioning (Fig. 5).

The surgeon must weigh the risks involved with an operative procedure versus the morbidity of the fracture. In the past, anterior stabilization required external fixation, which can be uncomfortable for the patient, or open reduction and internal fixation. Open reduction and internal fixation of the rami can involve extensive dissection and frequently requires mobilization of the femoral neurovascular bundle and spermatic cord. The advent of percutaneous techniques have made anterior fixation more attractive (Fig. 5).

External Fixation

The traditional anterior pelvic external fixator is placed along the iliac wing with three pins aiming directly down from the iliac ridge centrally, towards the thin portion of the wing. These pins often exit the inner or outer table thus compromising the fixation and strength of the fixator. An alternative fixation construct employs one pin in each anterior inferior iliac spine, aimed toward the thick bone above the sciatic notch. A skin incision is made directly over the anterior inferior iliac spine and the soft tissue is cleared using a small elevator. The fluoroscope is aimed directly down the axis from the anterior inferior iliac spine towards the posterior superior iliac spine. The inner and outer tables of the iliac wing are visible as the sides of a "teepee" shape, with the floor made up of the acetabular roof. The starting point of the pin should be in the center. Once the pin penetrates the cortex, an iliac oblique view is obtained to make sure the pin is directed towards the bone above the sciatic notch; it is not necessary to advance it all the way to the notch. A third view can be obtained by looking directly down the wing with fluoroscopy to ensure the pin is not exiting the inner or outer cortex. Once the pins are in the appropriate position, they are connected with one bar between them.

The pins can be used to manipulate the pelvic ring and may allow indirect reduction of the ramus fractures. The reduction should be judged using multiplanar fluoroscopy. Once acceptable reduction is obtained, the external fixator pin clamps are tightened to maintain the reduction. This type of frame uses two versus six pins and, after surgery, allows the patient to sit up with the frame on while allowing access to both the abdomen and the pelvis.

Open Anterior Approach

The pubic rami can be approached through a pfannensteil incision. This exposure allows easy access to the medial portion of both superior rami. More lateral portions of the rami can be accessed by retracting the rectus abdominus muscles laterally. However, ramus fractures lateral to the mid-ramus are difficult to access through the Pfannensteil incision, especially if an open reduction and internal fixation is planned (24). For complete open exposure of the superior ramus, the ilioinguinal approach is the workhorse approach. The ilioinguinal allows complete access to the superior ramus up to the iliac wing and is useful in open reduction and internal fixation of ramus fractures, especially those that involve the "root" of the ramus. Once exposed, open reduction and internal fixation can proceed with reduction and stabilization using a 3.5 mm pelvic reconstruction plate contoured to fit the ramus (Fig. 6).

Percutaneous Techniques

The advantages of percutaneous fixation include avoidance of complications associated with open procedures including damage to the femoral nerve, artery, or vein, damage of the spermatic cord/round ligament, infection, hernias, lymphadema, and heterotopic ossification (23,25). Percutaneous fixation also allows maintenance of fracture hematoma, which should hasten union. Percutaneous screw fixation of superior ramus fractures is akin to internal fixation of the femur or tibia; the goal is maintenance of length and alignment while maintaining healing potential. Anatomic reduction is not required. Screws can be placed either retrograde or anterograde depending on fracture location and patient factors.

The surgeon must be sure before surgery that there is no contrast material in the patient's gastrointestinal tract because it will obscure bony detail when using fluoroscopy. The surgery is done under a general anesthetic. Nitrous oxide should not be used because the gas can enter the intestinal tract and can obscure detail. Two grams of cefazolin are given 30 minutes before surgery.

The patient is placed on a radiolucent table. With the fluoroscopy machine on the opposite side of the involved ramus, the surgeon must make sure that anteroposterior, inlet, outlet, and oblique views of the pelvis are clearly visible. The patient's skin is then circumferentially prepared and draped to a level 5 cm above the iliac wing, so that the entire affected hemipelvis and leg are free. The perineum is draped out of the surgical field. It is important to include the symphysis pubis, anterior-superior iliac spine, and ischial tuberosity in the field.

Antegrade Superior Ramus Screw. The superior ramus screw can be placed in either an antegrade or retrograde direction. Retrograde screw placement can be difficult if the patient is obese because the contralateral thigh may block the drill or guidewire. In slender patients, however, retrograde screw placement is usually technically easier than antegrade placement.

The starting point for antegrade placement of the anterior column screw is determined by a line drawn between the tip of the greater trochanter and the thick part of the iliac crest (usually 4–5 cm back from the anterior superior iliac spine). In thin patients, the skin stab wound for the guidewire is made just above the midpoint of this line. In heavy patients, the stab wound must be made closer to the iliac crest. We prefer to make the initial stab wound with the guidewire rather than with a knife. After a "ballpark" skin starting point is determined, a 1-cm skin incision can be made to allow use of a drill guide to better position and direct the guidewire. The wire is then passed

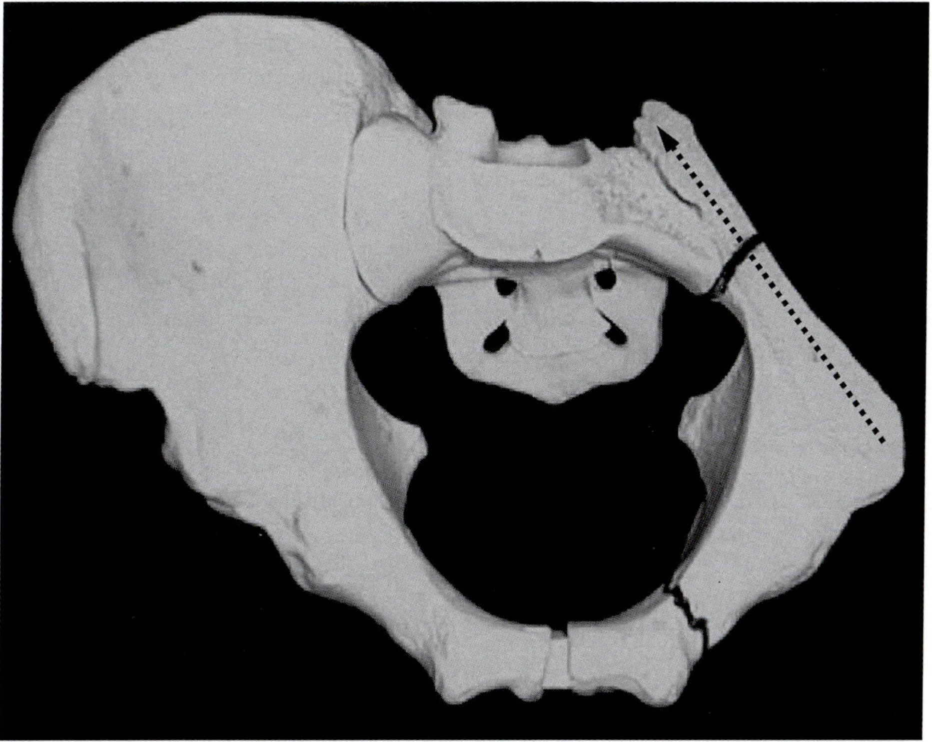

Figure 6 LC 2 screw pathway. The dotted arrow reveals the path from the anterior inferior iliac spine to the posterior inferior iliac spine.

down the superior pubic ramus toward the symphysis pubis. Outlet-obturator oblique and inlet-iliac oblique views are used to guidewire placement.

After the anterior column guidewire is inserted, the wire depth is measured and the screw hole is drilled, tapped, and filled with a partially threaded 7.3 mm cannulated screw. The small stab wound incisions are irrigated and closed with sutures (Figs. 2D–F, 3F, and 3G).

If the guidewire does not pass easily due to displacement, a minimal open reduction can be performed. A stab incision near the medial end of the superior ramus allows placement of a joker to manipulate the ramus, while the assistant provides manipulation of the iliac wing or limb. A large shanz pin in the iliac wing can be used as a joystick to rotate the hemipelvis, while the joker or bone spike provides pressure on the ramus. The surgeon must be aware of the risk of injury to the spermatic cord in males or ovarian ligament in females, along with the external iliac artery as they pass under the inguinal ligament.

For cases of severe impaction of the ramus, a femoral distractor can be placed across the anterior pelvis. This will assist with reduction and maintain distraction during screw placement.

Retrograde Superior Ramus Screw. This technique is used when the fracture is more medial, and closer to the symphysis pubis. This technique also works very well in thin people. It becomes very difficult and almost relatively contraindicated in the very obese or in those males with a large base of the penis.

For retrograde placement, the guide pin is placed against the ipsilateral pubic tubercle through a 3-cm minipfannensteil incision. It is aimed just posterior and inferior to the anterior inferior iliac spine. The wire is then passed up the superior pubic ramus using the inlet-iliac oblique and outlet-obturator oblique to ensure that the guidewire does not cut out of the inner cortex of the pubic ramus or iliac wing or enter the hip joint. A large fragment cannulated screw is used, similar to the antegrade technique. For displaced fractures, reduction techniques as previously described can be used (Fig. 5).

Postoperatively, the patients are kept on subcutaneous heparin, 5000 units three times a day, coupled with foot pumps. Physical therapy is begun as soon as possible, usually by the first postoperative day. The patients are instructed to bear weight "foot-flat" with a walker. They are kept from bearing full weight for three months. The patients are discharged home when they are using the walker independently. No anticoagulation and no formal therapy are used after discharge.

Symphysis Pubis Injuries

Most pubic diastasis injuries arise from an anteroposterior compression mechanism. The Young-Burgess classification system provides an elegant mechanistic approach to describing these injuries (23). The system promotes an understanding of the pathoanatomy and guides our treatment. The classification describes three types of anteroposterior compressions. Type 1 involves diastasis of the symphysis pubis of less than 2.5 cm, with no disruption of the posterior pelvic structures (APC I). Type 1 is both rotationally and vertically stable. Type 2 involves tearing of the anterior sacroiliac ligaments with diastasis of the symphysis pubis of greater than 2.5 cm (APC II). These are rotationally unstable. The hemipelvis rotates externally while the posterior sacroiliac ligaments act as a hinge. Type 3 involves tearing of both the anterior and posterior sacroiliac ligaments as well as widening of the symphysis pubis (APC III). Type 3 results in instability of the injured hemipelvis rotationally and vertically.

Treatment of these patterns is based on injury type. Type I injuries can be treated symptomatically, since the posterior ligaments are in tact and rotational instability is minimal. These patients may weight bear as tolerated; however, it is wise to obtain postambulatory films (anterior posterior, inlet, and outlet) to ensure that these injuries truly are type I.

Type II injuries can usually be treated with anterior pubic fixation alone. By doing so, the anterior sacroiliac joint is reduced; rotational stability is regained and the pelvic integrity restored. Reduction should be verified intraoperatively with inlet and outlet fluoroscopy views. APC type III injuries are unstable posteriorly and anteriorly and should be fixed at the sacroiliac joint as well as the anterior pubis.

Method of Fixation

There is little controversy regarding the treatment of symphysis diastasis. Most pelvic fracture surgeons employ open reduction and internal fixation with plates. Certain injuries, such as contaminated, open fractures or hemodynamically unstable patients, can be treated using an anterior external fixator. This is not ideal treatment because the posterior elements are not addressed appropriately and this construct is cumbersome and often does not allow as perfect a reduction as can be obtained with open techniques.

Most symphysis disruptions are treated using plates. Most orthopedic surgeons agree with this method of treatment; the controversy lies in the type and number of plates. Some authors recommend one plate superiorly for APC type II injuries, with two plates for more unstable APC III type injuries (23). Studies show that the strongest construct is biplanar type fixation either with one plate superiorly and one anteriorly, or a specially designed biplanar box plate (26). However, our experience has been that the anterior structures do not require biplanar fixation. A single plate seems to provide adequate stability. At our institution, we use a specially designed four-hole, large-fragment plate that is precontoured to fit on the superior aspect of the symphysis pubis. The holes in the plate are redesigned to allow increased angulation of 6.5 mm cancellous screws without impinging on the plate (Smith & Nephew, Memphis, Tennessee) (Fig. 1C–E).

Therefore it is always advisable to communicate with the surgical team or urologist prior to any incisions or percutaneous placement of urinary catheters directly in the field of the incision. The vertical incision usually made during a celiotomy is far enough superior that it will not interfere, or can easily be incorporated into the orthopedic approach. If a diverting urinary catheter or diverting colostomy is to be placed, then it should be done away from the incision.

The patient is placed on a radiolucent table in the supine position. The abdomen is prepped and draped from the nipple line down to the base of the penis and the hair overlying the symphysis pubis is shaved. A foley catheter and nasogastric tube is inserted prior to commencement in order to decompress the abdomen. Under general anesthetic, a pfannensteil incision is used to expose the symphysis pubis. After incising through the subcutaneous fat, the fascia overlying the rectus abdominus is identified and swept clean using a sponge. The fibers of the linea alba are identified directly in line with the umbilicus. A vertical incision is made through the linea in this location using a number 15 blade. Care must be taken not to damage the underlying bladder. The surgeon's finger is used to develop the space between the rectus and bladder. The injury hematoma is evacuated.

The space of Retzius is entered by retracting the rectus abdominus muscle on either side. The muscle is sometimes torn off the superior aspect of the pubis in high-energy injuries. The superior pubis is exposed using a cobb elevator while protecting the bladder. Care must be taken during lateral dissection in order to avoid injury to the spermatic cord in males or ovarian ligament in females.

Once the superior rami are exposed, the diastasis is reduced using a large reduction clamp. The clamp tines can be seated on the pubic tubercles, or in the obturator foramina. Once reduced, alignment is verified on both inlet and outlet radiographs. The surgeon should strive for perfect alignment—rotational displacement may lead to leg length discrepancy and pain.

After anatomic reduction, the plate is placed on the superior aspect of the rami and screws are inserted to affix it to the bone. If reduction is difficult, the plate can be affixed to one side with a single screw. Then one tine of the reduction clamp is placed on the side opposite the plate, and the second tine placed in a hole in the plate. This provides a better anchoring point and cuts down the risk of dislodging the clamp. Once reduction is obtained, a second screw is inserted into the hole most proximal to the symphysis pubis on the remaining side. Once in place, the reduction is checked under fluoroscopy. Once satisfied with the position, the final two screws should be placed into position (Fig. 1C–E).

After final radiographs are taken, any injury to the rectus abdominus muscle is repaired. The split in the linea alba is repaired and the subcutaneous tissues and skin are closed. No drain is necessary. The patient is to remain foot-flat weight bearing on the side with the involved sacroiliac joint for three months.

Other techniques used to stabilize the symphysis pubis have been described. Endoscopically assisted fixation has been described for symphysis disruptions (27,28). Endoscopic techniques have been successful during gynecologic, urologic, and general surgical procedures in this region, and this method of fixation will undoubtedly see greater use in the future.

REFERENCES

1. Bucholz R, Heckman J. Rockwood and Greens: Fractures in Adults, 5th ed. Baltimore: Lippincott Williams & Wilkins, 2001.
2. Tile M, Helfet DL, Kellam J. Fractures of the Pelvis and Acetabulum, 3rd ed. Philadelphia: Lippincott Williams & Wilkins, 2003.
3. Raf L. Double vertical fractures of the pelvis. Acta Care Scand 1965; 131:298–305.
4. Semba R, Yasukawa K, Gustilo R. Critical analysis of results of fifty-three Malgaigne fractures of the pelvis. J Trauma 1983; 23:535–537.
5. Kellam J, McMurtry R, Paley D, Tile M. The unstable pelvic fracture: operative treatment. Orthop Clin North Am 1987; 18:25–41.
6. Goldstein A, Phillips T, Sclafani SJ, et al. Early open reduction and internal fixation of the disrupted pelvic ring. J Trauma 1986; 26:325–333.
7. Routt M, Kregor P, Simonian P, Mayo K. Early results of percutaneous iliosacral screws placed with the patient in the supine position. J Orthop Trauma 1995; 5:207–214.
8. Routt M, Simonian P, Mills WJ. Iliosacral screw fixation: early complications of the percutaneous technique. J Orthop Trauma 1997; 11:584–589.
9. Ruedi T, von Hoechstetter A, Schlumpf R. Surgical Approaches for Internal Fixation. Berlin: Springer-Verlag, 1984.
10. Matta J, Saucedo T. Internal fixation of pelvic ring fractures. Clin Orthop 1989; 242:83–97.
11. Mears DC, Capito CP, Deleeuw H. Posterior pelvic disruptions managed by the use of the double cobra plate. In: Bassett FH III, ed. Instructional Course Lectures XXXVII. Park Ridge IL: American Academy of Orthopaedic Surgeons, 1988:143–150.
12. Pohlemann T, Tscherne H. Fixation of sacral fractures. Tech Orthop 1995; 9:315.
13. Leighton R, Waddell J. Techniques for reduction and posterior fixation through the anterior approach. Clin Orthop 1996; 329:115–120.
14. Leighton R, Waddell J. Open reduction and internal fixation of vertical fractures of the pelvis using the sacroiliac joint plate. J Orthop Trauma 1991; 5:225.
15. Helfet DL, Koval KJ, Hissa EA, et al. Intraoperative somatosensory evoked potential monitoring during acute pelvic fracture surgery. J Orthop Trauma 1995; 9:28–34.
16. Yinger K, Scalise J, Olson SA, et al. Biomechanical comparison of posterior pelvic ring fixation. J Orthop Trauma 2003; 7:481–487.
17. McCormick JP, Morgan SJ, Smith WR. Clinical effectiveness of physical examination in diagnosis of posterior pelvic ring injuries. J Orthop Trauma 2003; 4:257–261.
18. Denis F, Steven D, Comfort T. Sacral fractures: an important problem, retrospective analysis of 236 cases. Clin Orthop 1988; 227:67–81.
19. Roy-Camille R, et al. Transverse fracture of the upper sacrum: suicidal jumper's fracture. Spine 1985; 10(9):838–845.
20. Gansslen A, et al. Suicidal Jumper's Fractures. Analysis of Treatment in 17 cases. Louisville, KY: Orthopaedic Trauma Association, 1999.
21. Griffin DR, Starr AJ, Reinert CM, Jones AL, Whitlock S. Vertically unstable pelvic fractures fixed with percutaneous iliosacral screws: does posterior injury pattern predict fixation failure? J Orthop Trauma 2003; 17:399–405.
22. Starr AJ, Walker JC, Harris RW, et al. Percutaneous screw fixation of the iliac wing and fracture-dislocations of the sacro-iliac joint (OTA types 61-B2.2 and 61-B2.3, or Young–Burgess lateral compression type II pelvic fractures). J Orthop Trauma 2002; 2:116–123.
23. Young JWR, Burgess AR. Radiologic Management of Pelvic Ring Fractures. Baltimore: Urban and Schwarzenberg, 1987:45.
24. Letournel E, Judet R. Fractures of the Acetabulum, 2nd ed. Berlin: Springer-Verlag, 1993.

25. Routt M, Meier M, Kregor P. Percutaneous iliosacral screws with the patient supine technique. Oper Tech Orthop 1993; 3:35–45.
26. Simonian PT, Schwappach JR, Routt ML Jr, et al. Evaluation of new plate designs for symphysis pubis internal fixation. J Trauma 1996; 41(3):498–502.
27. Rubel IF, Seligson D, Mudd L, et al. Technical tricks: endoscopy for anterior pelvis fixation. J Orhop Trauma 2002; 16(7):507–514.
28. Zobrist R, Messmer P, Levin LS, et al. Endoscopic-assisted, minimally invasive anterior pelvic ring stabilization: a new technique and case report. J Orthop Trauma 2002; 16(7): 515–519.

7
Diagnosis and Treatment of Acetabular Fractures: Historic Review

Steven A. Olson
Division of Orthopaedic Surgery, Duke University Medical Center, Durham, North Carolina, U.S.A.

INTRODUCTION

In 2007, displaced fractures of the acetabulum are generally considered an indication for surgical reduction and fixation unless strict criteria for nonoperative treatment or contraindications for operative treatment exist. Left untreated, a displaced acetabular fracture can be a source of significant long-term morbidity. The techniques and methods used for diagnosis, classification, surgical exposure, and operative reduction and fixation have been developed over the past 50 years. However, only in the past two decades has this body of knowledge been widely disseminated.

THE NONOPERATIVE ERA

Displaced fractures of the acetabulum are the result of significant skeletal trauma. Historically, this was a relatively uncommon injury. The anatomic location of the acetabulum, as well as the three-dimensional structure of the bone elements, make the treatment of these injuries extremely challenging. The severity of these injuries is demonstrated by the fact that early descriptions of acetabular fractures are the result of autopsy findings of patients who had sustained significant trauma (1). Callisen in 1788 is said to have reported the case of an acetabular fracture, but without significant detail in his description (1). In 1821, Cooper reported the first detailed description of an acetabular fracture. This case described autopsy findings in a patient with an associated central dislocation of the femoral head into the pelvis (2). In 1909, Schroeder reported a detailed compendium of the first 49 cases reported in the literature (1). The majority of these are reports of autopsy findings in patients who died of complications related to hemorrhagic shock or the late onset of intra-abdominal sepsis.

Early diagnosis of the injury was made by noting the physical findings of the lack of prominence of the greater trochanter, limitation of range of motion of the hip, shortening of the limb, and a bony protuberance medially into the pelvic cavity noted on rectal examination (1,3,4). Early terminology to described these injuries include central dislocation of the hip, stove-in hip, and fractura acetabuli perforans. In 1911, Skillern reported an additional four cases of fracture of the "floor" of the acetabulum (5). Early literature refers to fractures through the area of the cotyloid or acetabular fossa below the roof, either anteriorly or posterioly, as fractures of the floor of the acetabulum. Throughout most of the 20th Century, there was little uniformity in terminology, classification and description, and treatment of these injuries. Whitman in 1920 recognized that the medialization of the proximal femur led to a loss of abduction secondary to impingement of the greater trochanter on the ilium and superior acetabular rim (4). He advocated manipulation of the lower limb to reestablish a normal abduction arc as a treatment method. In 1921, Palmer, in reporting on central dislocation of the hip, noted that the majority of medical textbooks of the day did not mention diagnosis or treatment of acetabular fractures (3). In 1926, MacGuire described the lateral traction and treatment via a percutaneously placed threaded pin into the proximal femur (6). Approximately three months of immobilization was recommended at that time.

Bergmann in 1931 and Dyes in 1932 were the first to report avascular necrosis of the femoral head following traumatic dislocation of the hip (7,8). In 1934, Phemister reported on four cases of avascular necrosis following traumatic hip dislocation and recommended prolonged weight-bearing in the recovery period to prevent collapse of the femoral head (9). Campbell reported on the treatment of posterior dislocation of the hip with acetabular fractures in 1936 (10). He noted that fracture of the acetabulum was relatively common with dislocation of the hip. This work also points out the necessity for a prompt diagnosis and reduction of the hip to prevent irreparable damage to the hip joint.

BEGINNINGS OF OPERATIVE MANAGEMENT

In the early 1940s, Levine reported the early successful results of open reduction and internal fixation of a central fracture of the acetabulum (11). Review of his case reports revealed a both-column acetabular fracture, which at the time was treated through a Smith-Peterson approach with a plate on the internal iliac fossa. Although his report had relatively short follow-up, it was one of the first to advocate a more aggressive treatment.

Prior to the 1940s, acetabular fractures were relatively uncommon injuries. World War II, however, brought an increase in the number of these injuries. Young servicemen traveling at relatively high speeds in military jeeps and other vehicles accounted for relatively large numbers of these types of injuries. Two reports are particularly notable from this era. Armstrong et al. reported on the experience of the Royal Air Force (12). The classification used in his report consisted of four types of injuries:

1. A simple dislocation
2. Dislocation with acetabular rim fracture
3. Dislocation with acetabular floor fracture
4. Dislocation with femoral head fracture

The authors recommended that central and posterior dislocations be managed with arthrodesis of the hip. They also observed that sciatic nerve palsies were associated with displaced bony fragments. They recommended exploration of these cases and that the fragments be repositioned away from the nerve as part of the treatment. Urist et al. reported on a treatment of U.S. military personnel (13). In 27 cases of posterior fracture dislocation of the hip he reported successful treatment of the posterior wall fracture dislocation with operative repair. He stated that "in matched cases of fractures, treated conservatively and by open reduction, good function and little or no disability were shown when the hip joint surfaces were restored as perfectly as possible, but this could be accomplished only by open reduction."

In the 1950s, Thompson and Epstein published their classification of hip dislocation and fracture dislocation, modifying the original classification of Armstrong into five categories (14). They separated dislocation with posterior rim fracture into two categories—those with a single large posterior piece and those with a comminuted posterior rim. They noted that dislocation with a minor rim fracture (Type I) or one large fragment (Type II) did better than those with a comminuted rim fracture, acetabular floor fracture, or an associated femoral head fracture (Types III–V). They advocated open reduction to remove loose osteochondral fragments as a routine practice. Stewart and Milford reported on experience treating over 100 patients with acetabular fractures (15). They reported 52% good-to-excellent clinical results with nonoperative treatment of posterior fracture dislocation compared with 30% reduction result with operative treatment in contrast to Urist's findings (13,15). Similarly, they reported 100% good-to-excellent result with nonoperative treatment of ventral fracture dislocations as compared with 25% good-to-excellent results with operative treatment. This report reinforced the commonly held view of acetabular fractures held by many surgeons at that time that nonoperative management was the preferred method of treatment. Eichenholtz echoed these findings and advocated attempts at open reduction and internal fixation only in those patients without medical comorbidities (16).

Despite this overall dim view of surgical treatment, several authors persisted in attempts to improve operative management of these injuries. Elliott was one of the first to report on attempts at open reduction in four cases of open reduction and pin fixation (17). Knight and Smith described operative reduction of "central dislocation of the acetabulum" (18). These authors proposed the use of forceps (reduction clamps) to manipulate the bone fragments to obtain a reduction. They advocated the use of radiographs to better understand the fracture pattern. These authors described fractures as vertical (i.e., column-type fracture) or horizontal (i.e., transverse-type fracture pattern). Knight and Smith advocated restoration of the "weight-bearing vault" of the acetabulum. They also advocated an anterior (iliofemoral) approach for horizontal fractures and a posterior approach for the vertical fracture types, which in their series were largely posterior column injuries (18).

There was even a brief trial of femoral head mold arthroplasty as a treatment for displaced acetabular fractures. This method typically used fractures with central displacement of the femoral head and consisted of a surgical dislocation of the hip with placement of a vitalian cup arthroplasty over the native femoral head. The theory behind this treatment was that the vitalian coating on the femoral head would effectively "mold" the acetabulum into an appropriately shaped socket on healing in this displaced position. Although short-lived, this demonstrates that many surgeons were not satisfied with the hip function of patients in which these injuries were left untreated.

In the early 1960s, Pearson et al. (19) reproduced injury mechanisms that would result in acetabular fractures. Using a weighted pendulum that struck the greater trochanter of a cadaver, they were able to recreate fractures of the acetabular floor. The review of the article suggests that, in terminology of Letournel, the fractures that they actually created included an anterior wall with a posterior hemitransverse component, a transverse fracture, and low anterior-column injuries (20).

In 1962, Brav described a series of 523 patients with hip dislocations and fracture dislocations with follow-up on 264 of these patients in two years. He made the following treatment recommendations (21):

1. Early recognition and closed reduction were not under force when it was possible.
2. Anterior–posterior (AP) and lateral radiographs after reduction.
3. Open reduction when closed reduction was unsuccessful or when there was an incarcerated bone fragment.
4. He recommended that all anterior dislocation and simple dislocations without fractures should be kept in skin traction for three weeks and then mobilized after that with non–weight-bearing in the involved hip. He recommended beginning weight-bearing at 12 weeks postinjury. For all other posterior fracture dislocations he recommended skeletal traction for six weeks, with weight-bearing permitted no earlier than 12 to 16 weeks.

In 1961, Rowe and Lowell published their landmark article entitled "Prognosis of Fractures of the Acetabulum" (22). This is a retrospective study of 93 acetabular fractures in 90 patients, all with a minimum of one-year follow-up. This was the first study that attempted to look at injury-related factors and correlate them with long-term clinical outcome. Some of the fractures had been treated operatively but the majority was treated nonoperatively. The authors reported on four aspects of the fracture anatomy and/or characteristics of the hip joint that appeared to play a role in the long-term outcome. The factors that appear to be important in the maintenance of a normal appearing hip joint long-term outcome are:

1. An intact superior acetabulum, which was referred to as the weight-bearing dome.
2. The maintenance of a normal relationship between the femoral head and the superior acetabulum (the description referring to the maintenance of a congruent relationship of the femoral head to the acetabulum).
3. An intact femoral head, as the fractures resulting in impaction or fractures of the femoral head were shown to result in progressive arthrosis.
4. The maintenance of a stable hip joint, as those fractures that went on to late instability or subluxation of the femoral head invariably resulted in post-traumatic arthrosis.

In addition, Rowe and Lowell also described the first oblique view of the pelvis. They described a view with the patient placed prone, with the uninjured hip rotated to 60° to evaluate for a posterior acetabular fracture.

THE CONTRIBUTIONS OF LETOURNEL

In 1964, Judet et al. published their now classic article entitled "Fractures of the Acetabulum, Classification and Surgical Approaches for Open Reduction" (23). This manuscript describes the use of the AP and two 45° oblique views of the pelvis to evaluate the acetabular fractures. These radiographic views, now known as "Judet" views, named after the author, include the AP pelvis, the obturator view, and the iliac oblique view. These are now the standard radiographic films used for evaluation of acetabular fractures. This article represented a substantial step forward in the understanding of acetabular anatomy and fracture classifications. The principles put forth in this article, which represent major advances, included (23):

1. The recommendation of careful study of the radiographic lines of the acetabulum on all three plain radiographic views (Figs. 1 and 2).
2. The establishment of the basic terms of surgical anatomy of the acetabulum including the anterior column and the posterior column.
3. The understanding of the morphology or pattern of the fracture was important preoperatively to select the appropriate surgical approach to be able to perform a surgical reduction.
4. The beginnings of the establishment of an anatomic classification of acetabular fractures.
5. Similar to the recommendations of Urist, the authors strongly advocated for the anatomic restoration of the articular surface (they stated "in our experience, the unsatisfactory results of nonoperative treatment of fractures of the acetabulum displacement are usually not due to failure to reduce the dislocation of the femoral head but, rather, to the inability to produce the acetabular fractures").
6. The first description of impaction of the articular surface is marginal impaction.

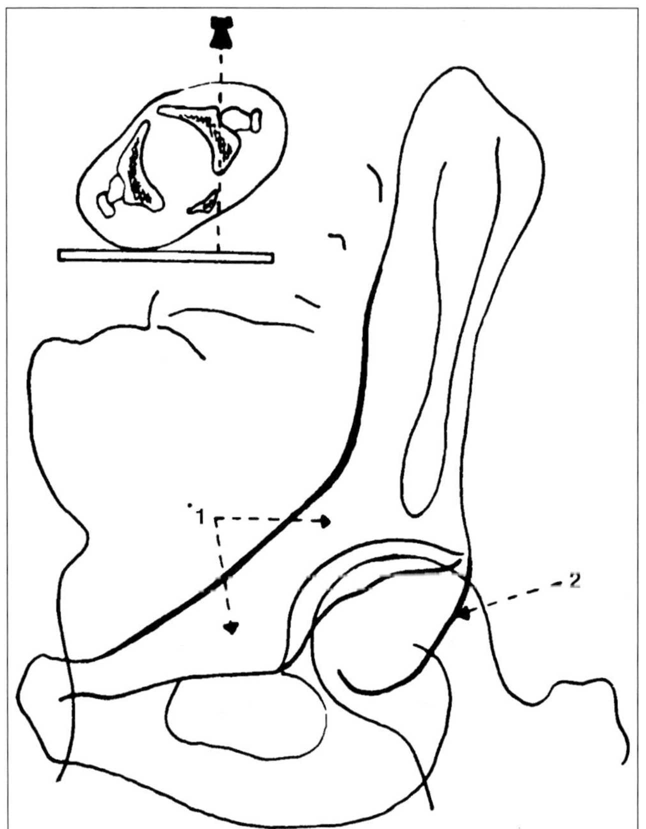

Figure 1 Recognition of significant acetabular landmarks on the obdurator oblique X-ray image. (**1**) crosses the iliopectineal line and points to the anterior column, (**2**) points to the line corresponding to the posterior wall of the acetabulum.

This 1964 article is often quoted as the source of the modern Judet and Letournel fracture classification. However, the student of acetabular fractures will find substantial differences in some of the terminology and classification used in the 1964 article compared with the modern version of the Letournel system (Fig. 3). In the original 1964 article, the term "superior channel" was used for the radiographic landmark, which is now commonly referred to at the iliopectineal line. The original description of the anterior column extended from the pubic symphysis only to the area of the iliopectineal eminence on the anterior wall of the acetabulum (Fig. 1). The 1964 article fracture classification scheme included the following terminology: (*i*) posterior lip fractures, (*ii*) fracture of the ilioischial column (posterior column), transverse fractures, transverse fractures with a posterior lip fracture, T-shaped fractures, fracture of the iliopubic column (anterior column), anterior ridge fracture (anterior wall), and associated fracture of both columns (23). The modern version of the Letournel fracture classification was initially published in French (24). It was not widely adapted in North American literature until after the 1981 English translation of Letournel's text (20). This is evidenced by the literature in the area of acetabular fractures published

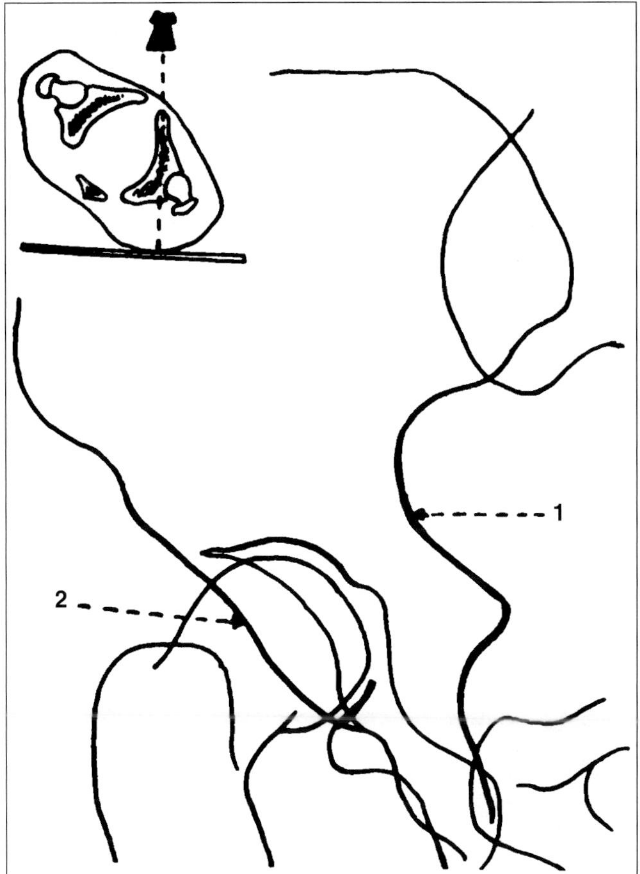

Figure 2 Recognition of acetabular landmarks on the iliac oblique xray image. (**1**) points to the ilioischial line, which represents the edge of the posterior column, (**2**) points to the line corresponding to the anterior wall of the acetabulum.

in North America in the 1970s. The majority of these authors used fracture classification schemes and terminology from the works of Knight and Smith and Rowe and Lowell (25–29).

Throughout the 1970s, the North American literature reflected a skepticism toward open reduction internal fixation of acetabular fractures. In 1973, Neurubay et al. reported results of treatment of 111 acetabular fractures (28). They reconfirmed the findings of Rowe and Lowell and emphasized the poor characteristics of the fracture needed for good outcome as originally outlined in 1961. Barnes and Stewart advocated nonoperative treatment of central fractures of the acetabulum with closed reduction and traction for three months as the recommended management (25). Carnesale et al. continued to recommend nonoperative treatment, and they noted "thus, the treatment of fracture-dislocations with the weight-bearing dome intact probably should be by closed methods, while the proper treatment of disrupted acetabular remains uncertain" (26). Rogers et al. incorporated the use of Letournel's definitions of anterior and posterior columns in their work (29). They also independently verified the need for oblique

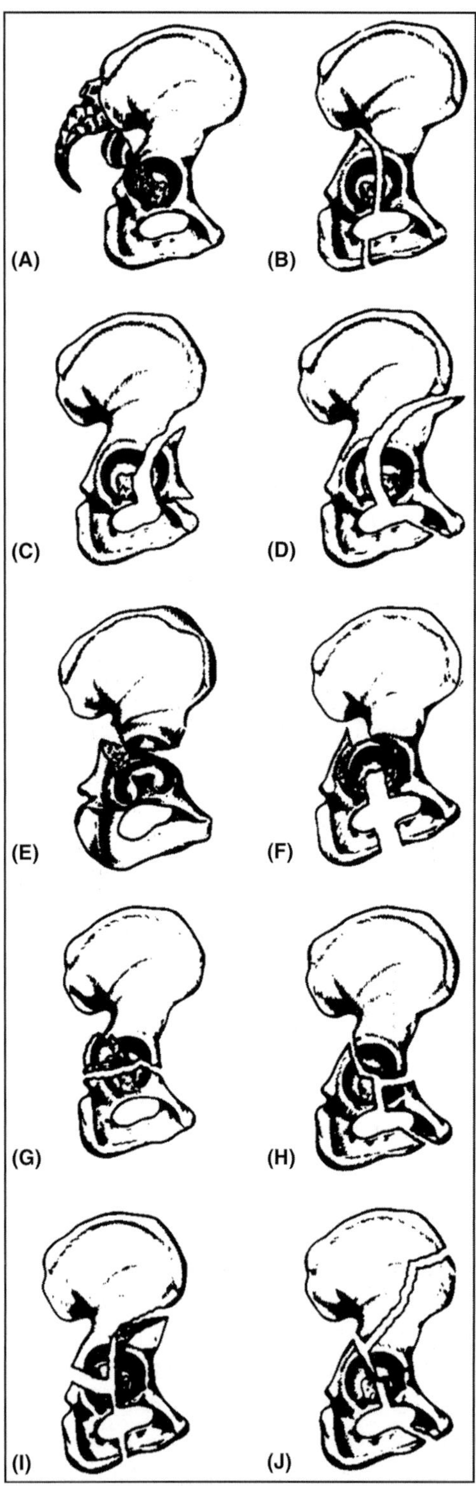

Figure 3 Schematic representation of the Judet classification of acetabular fractures. (**A–E**) are the elemental patterns. (**F–J**) are the associated patterns.

views of the pelvis as they reported there were four cases in which the fracture was not seen on the AP view. Epstein presented his long-term follow-up from posterior fracture dislocation to the hip in 1974 (30). He continued to advocate for open reduction of fracture dislocation to the hip. However, only in cases where a single large posterior fragment could be reduced and fixed stably resulted in superior outcomes.

The 1980s saw substantial developments in the treatment of acetabular fractures. The advancement of fracture care in North America was influenced by the contributions of several individuals.

By far the greatest influence was that of Emile Letournel. In 1980, Letournel came to the University of Southern California as a visiting professor (J.M. Matta, personal communication, 2002). From then on, several North American surgeons subsequently studied with Letournel and brought his teachings back to North America. In 1984, Letournel held his first international course on treatment of fractures of the pelvis and acetabulum in Paris. In 1988, the first such course was held in North America in Los Angeles, California.

In 1986, Matta published two articles that helped establish the modern basis of nonoperative treatment of acetabular fractures (31,32). Matta used the work of Rowe and Lowell and Neurobay as the basis of his investigation. Both of these authors had identified having the "weight-bearing dome" of the acetabulum intact was important. However, neither author had attempted to quantify what portion of the superior acetabulum was actually that critical portion. Using the AP and the 45° oblique Judet views of the pelvis, Matta developed the concept of a "roof arc measurement." Using the measurements of the roof arc, he was able to estimate the amounts of the superior acetabulum left intact after fracture (Fig. 4). He thereby came up with roof arc criteria for a nonoperative management. These were further clarified in the 1988 publication where a roof arc measurement of 45° or greater on all three radiographic views, a maintenance of a congruent relationship between the femoral head and the acetabulum out of traction, and no associated posterior wall fracture that might lead to instability were considered criteria for nonoperative treatment (33).

THE MODERN ERA

The 1980s saw a substantial increase in the overall knowledge base of orthopedic surgery throughout the world with regard to treatment of acetabular fractures. The majority of these developments can be tied to Letournel's publication of the English translation of his text in 1981 (20). These advancements include: (*i*) the formal description of the plain radiography of the pelvis and acetabulum; (*ii*) the completion of the current-day Letournel classification system of acetabular fractures; (*iii*) the dissemination of Letournel's work on the development of the ilioinguinal exposure, the extended iliofemoral exposure, and Letournel's refinements on the points of dissection of the Kocher–Langenbeck approach; (*iv*) the modern concept of the anterior column, which is now seen as extending from the anterior part of the iliac crest to the pubic symphysis, as well as the concept of the acetabulum, which sits at the base of the arms of an inverted "Y" formed by the junction of the anterior and posterior columns (Fig. 2) (the columns themselves are linked by the articular surface of the sacroiliac joint that Letournel termed "sciatic buttress"); (*v*) the need to flex the knee and extend the hip

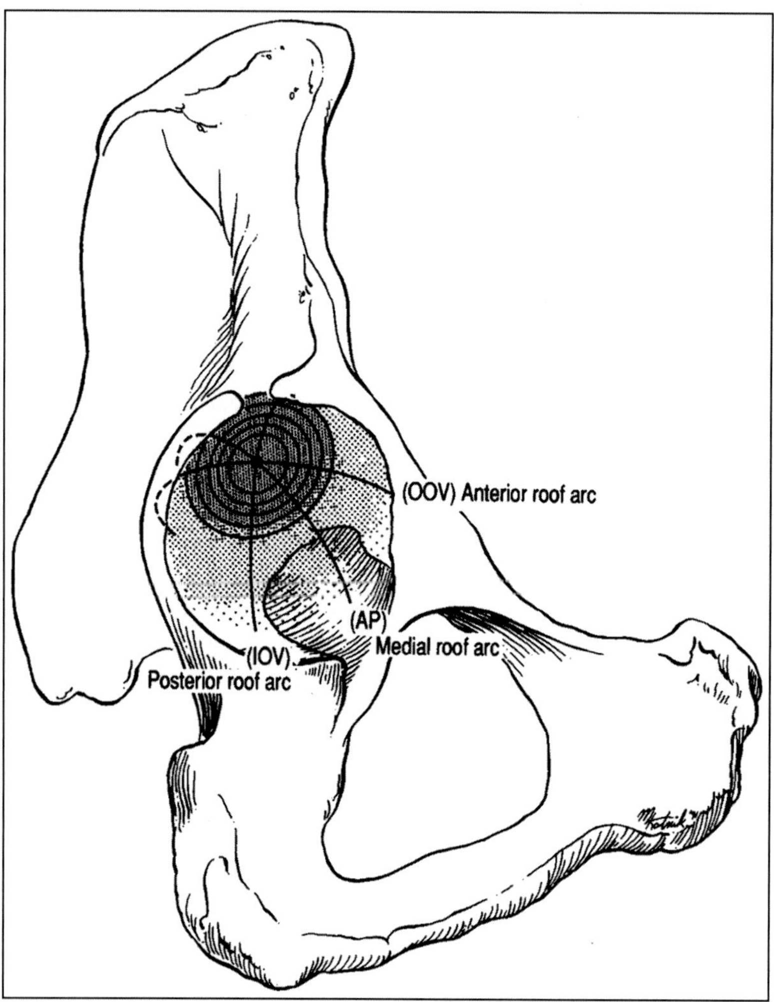

Figure 4 Representation of the anterior, medial and posterior roof arc concept.

during the posterior approaches to protect the sciatic nerve; (*vi*) the use of the fracture table to facilitate surgical approach and reduction of the fractures; and (*vii*) the first comprehensive collection of long-term clinical outcome data regarding open reduction and internal fixation of acetabular fractures.

Computed tomography was introduced in the 1980s and was widely championed by Mears and others (34–36). Tile continued to build on the work of his mentor George Pennal (37). He made significant contributions to the field of pelvic and acetabular surgery (38).

Over the past 20 years, a variety of authors have contributed widely to the field of acetabular fracture surgery. The multiple authors have described these procedures as trochanteric osteotomy or variations of extensile surgical exposures for acetabular fractures (39–41). The prevention of treatment-related complications, neuropalsy, pulmonary embolism, heterotopic ossification, and so on, have also been described (42–44). These subjects are covered in later chapters in this book and will not be described here in detail.

Roof arc measurements were further defined with the development of the computed tomography subchondral arc (45). This measurement describes the use of the normal bony anatomy of the superior acetabulum as visualized in computed tomography to provide an equivalent measure of the roof arcs. As such the study determined that the superior 10 mm of the acetabulum represents the equivalent area of a roof arc of 45° (Fig. 5). The current treatment recommendation for nonoperative management would include: (*i*) that the superior 10 mm of the CT subchondral arc are intact; (*ii*) that the femoral head remains congruent with the acetabulum on the AP and two 45° oblique views of the pelvis taken out of traction; (*iii*) there is no low associated posterior wall fracture of substantial size (greater than 40–50% of the wall); and (*iv*) that intraoperative stress views demonstrate no evidence of femoral head subluxation (45,46).

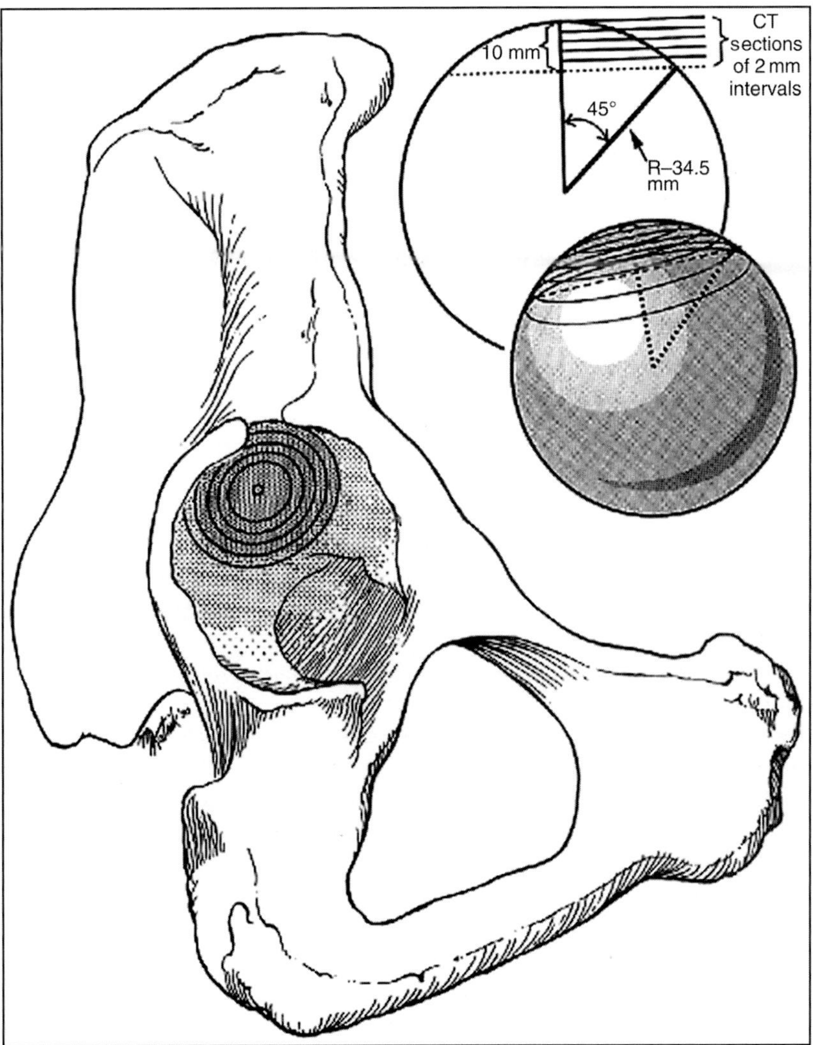

Figure 5 Representation of the roof arc concept with CT measurement to define the subchondral ring.

Letournel advocated an approach or protocol to treatment of acetabular fractures that includes extensive study of the X-rays to understand the anatomy of the fracture pattern and subsequent correct classification followed by appropriate operative positioning of the patient whenever possible to operate the fracture through a single surgical approach. Emphasis has been placed on obtaining an anatomic reduction of the articular surface. Long-term clinical outcome data suggest that the more accurate the articular reduction, the greater the likelihood for an improved clinical outcome of the patient's hip joint (47–50). Other authors have advocated protocols with multiple approaches, either simultaneously or consecutively, as a routine approach for certain types of acetabular fractures (51–53), while others have advocated the use of manipulative closed reduction with percutaneous fixation techniques for certain types of acetabular fractures. The published data of clinical outcomes from surgeons who follow Letournel's protocol remain the most consistently successful.

REFERENCES

1. Schroeder WE. Fracture of the acetabulum with displacement of the femoral head into the pelvic cavity (Central Dislocation of Femur). Bulletin of the Northwestern Medical School 1909; 9–42.
2. Cooper SA. Surgical essays 1818; Part I(Second Ed.):51.
3. Palmer DW. Central dislocation of the hip—with report of three cases. Am J Surg 1921; 35(5):118–121.
4. Whitman R. The treatment of central luxation of the femur. Ann Surg 1920; 71:62–65.
5. Skillern PG, Pancoast HK. Fracture of the floor of the acetabulum. In Philadelphia Academy of Surgery. Edited, Philadelphia, October 2, 1911.
6. MacGuire CJ. Fracture of the acetabulum. Ann Surg 1926; 83(718–1926).
7. Bergmann E. Uber kielherde im huftkopf. Deutsche Zeitschr Chir 1931; 233:252–261.
8. Dyes O. Huft kopfnekrosen nach traumatise huftgelenk sluxccrium. Arch f Klin Chirg 1932; 172:339–359.
9. Phemister DB. Fractures of neck of femur, dislocations of hip and obscure vascular disturbances producing aseptic necrosis of head of femur. Surg Gyn and Obstet 1934; 59:415–440.
10. Campbell WC. Posterior dislocation of the hip with fracture of the acetabulum. J Bone Joint Surg 1936; 18(4):842–850.
11. Levine MA. A treatment of central fractures of the acetabulum. J Bone Joint Surg 1943; 25(4):902–906.
12. Armstrong JR. Traumatic dislocation of the hip joint. JBUS 30B:430–445.
13. Urist MR. Fracture dislocation of the hip joint. J Bone Joint Surg 1948; 30A:699–727.
14. Thompson VP, Epstein HC. Traumatic dislocation of the hip. JBJS 1951; 33A:746–777.
15. Stewart MJ, Milford LW. Fracture dislocation of the hip. J Bone Joint Surg 1954; 36A:315–342.
16. Eichenholtz SN, Stark RM. Central acetabular fracture. J Bone Joint Surg 1964; 46A: 695–713.
17. Elliott RB. Central Fracture of the Acetabulum—Described 4 cases of central dislocation, open reduction, pin fixation. Clin Orthop and Related Res 1956; 7:189–201.
18. Knight RA, Smith H. Central fracture of the acetabulum. J Bone Joint Surg 1958; 40A: 1–16.
19. Pearson JR, Hergaden EJ. Fractures of the pelvis involving the floor of the acetabulum. J Bone Joint Surg 1962; 44B:550–561.

20. Letournel E, Judet R. Fractures of the acetabulum, 1st ed. Berlin: Springer-Verlag, 1981.
21. Brav EA. Traumatic dislocation of the hip. J Bone Joint Surg 1962; 44-A(6):1115–1134.
22. Rowe CR, Lowell JD. Prognosis of fractures of the acetabulum. J Bone Joint Surg 1961; 43-A:30–59.
23. Judet R, Judet J, Letournel E. Fractures of the acetabulum: classification and surgical approaches for open reduction. J Bone Joint Surg 1964; 46A(8):1615–1646.
24. Letournel E, Judet R. Les fractures du cotyle masson et cie. 1974.
25. Barnes SN, Stewart MJ. Central fracture of the acetabulum. Clin Orthop 1976; 114: 276–281.
26. Carnesale PG, Stewart MJ, Barnes SN. Acetabular disruption and central fracture dislocation of the hip. J Bone Joint Surg 1975; 57-A:1054–1059.
27. Guthlin G, Hindmarsh J. Central dislocation of the hip. Acta Orthop Scandinav 1970; 41:476–487.
28. Nerubay J, Glancz G, Katznelson A. Fractures of the acetabulum. J Trauma 1973; 13(12):1050–1062.
29. Rogers CF, Novy SB, Harnis NF. Occult central fracture of the acetabulum. Am J Roentgenol 1975; 124:96–101.
30. Epstein HC. Posterior fracture dislocation of the hip. J Bone Joint Surg 1974; 56A(1103–1127).
31. Matta JM, Anderson LM, Epstein HC, Hendricks P. Fractures of the acetabulum. A retrospective analysis. Clin Orthop and Related Res 1986; 205:230–240.
32. Matta JM, Mehne DK, Roffi R. Fractures of the acetabulum. Early results of a prospective study. Clin Orthop and Related Res 1986; 205(241–250).
33. Matta JM, Merritt PO. Displaced acetabular fractures. Clin Orthop and Related Res 1988; 230:83–97.
34. Burk DL, Mears DC, Cooperstein LA, Herman GT, Udupa JK. Actabular fractures: three-dimensional computer tomographic imaging and interactive surgical planning. Journal of Computed Tomography 1986; 10(1):1–10.
35. Harley JD, Mack LA, Winquist RA. CT of acetabular fractures: comparison with conventional radiography. Am J Roentgenol 1982; 138(3):413–417.
36. Mears DC, Rubash HE. Pelvic and acetabular fractures. Edited, Thorofare, NJ, Slack, 1988.
37. Tile M. Fractures of the pelvis and acetabulum. Edited by Tile M. Baltimore, Williams & Wilkins, 1995.
38. Olson SA, Tile M. Acute management. In Fractures of the Pelvis and Acetabulum. Edited.
39. Bray TJ, Esser M, Fulkerson L. Osteotomy of the trochanter in open reduction and internal fixation of acetabular fractures. J Bone Joint Surg 1987; 69(5):711–717.
40. Reinert CM, Bosse MJ, Poka A, Schacherer T, Brumback RJ, Burgess AR. A modified extensile exposure for the treatment of complex or malunited acetabular fractures. J Bone Joint Surg Am 1988; 70(3):329–337.
41. Senegas J, Liorzou G, Yates M. Complex acetabular fractures: a transtrochanteric lateral surgical approach. Clin Orthop 1980; 151:107–114.
42. Bosse MJ, Poka A, Reinert CM, Ellwanger F, Slawson R, McDevitt ER. Heterotopic ossification as a complication of acetabular fracture. Prophylaxis with low-dose irradiation. J Bone Joint Surg Am 1988; 70(8):1231–1237.
43. Fishmann AJ, Greeno RA, Brooks LR, Matta JM. Prevention of deep vein thrombosis and pulmonary embolism in acetabular and pelvic fracture surgery. Clin Orthop 1994; 305:133–137.
44. Helfet DL, Hissa EA, Sergay S, Mast JW. Somatosensory evoked potential monitoring in the surgical management of acute acetabular fractures. J Orthop Trauma 1991; 5(2): 161–166.

45. Olson SA, Matta JM. The computerized tomography subchondral arc: a new method of assessing acetabular articular continuity after fracture (a preliminary report). J Orthop Trauma 1993; 7(5):402–413.
46. Tornetta P, III: Non-operative management of acetabular fractures. The use of dynamic stress views. J Bone Joint Surg Br 1999; 8(1):67–70.
47. Letournel E, Judet R. Fractures of the acetabulum. Springer-Verlag, Berlin, 2nd ed. 1992.
48. Matta JM. Fractures of the acetabulum: accuracy of reduction and clinical results in patients managed operatively within three weeks after the injury. J Bone Joint Surg 1996; 78-A(11): 1632–1645.
49. Mayo KA. Open reduction and internal fixation of fractures of the acetabulum, Results in 163 fractures. Clin Orthop 1994; 305:31–37.
50. Ruesch PD, Holdener H, Ciaramitaro M, Mast JW. A prospective study of surgically treated acetabular fractures. Clin Orthopand Related Res 1994; 305:38–46.
51. Routt ML, Swiontkowski MF. Operative treatment of complex acetabular fractures. Combined anterior and posterior exposures during the same procedure. J Bone Joint Surg 1990; 72A:897–904.
52. Wright R, Barrett K, Christie MJ, Johnson KD. Acetabular fractures: long-term followup of open reduction and internal fixation. J Orthop Trauma 1994; 8(5):397–403,
53. Ylinen P, Santavirta S, Slatis P. Outcome of acetabular fractures: a 7-year follow-up. Journal of Trauma-Injury Infection & Critical Care 1989; 29(1):19–24.

8
Classification of Acetabular Fractures

Scott A. Adams and David J. Hak
Department of Orthopaedics, Denver Health Medical Center, University of Colorado School of Medicine, Denver, Colorado, U.S.A.

Treatment should not be commenced until a full understanding of the fracture is achieved
Emile Letournel

INTRODUCTION

Classification of acetabular fractures is a key element in understanding the injury and is the first stage of surgical planning. Decisions concerning the choice of approach and the alternative fixation techniques available require full appreciation of the fracture anatomy. The complex three-dimensional structure of the acetabulum with its supporting columns, in combination with the numerous fracture patterns, makes categorizing these injuries an involved task. The two most frequently used and interrelated classification systems are both based on the anatomy of the fracture.

Letournel and Judet's (1) anatomical classification is divided into two groups: elementary and associated fractures, with five patterns in each. Good intra- and interobserver agreement has been reported, and it is the most widely accepted system among surgeons today. Tile (2) described a modification of Letournel's classification. This modification enables these complex fracture patterns to be categorized into the A, B, and C types of the comprehensive classification of fractures developed by the Arbeitsgemeinschaft Für Osteosynthesefragen

(AO)/Association for the Study of Internal Fixation (ASIF) group and adopted by the Orthopaedic Trauma Association (OTA) (3). The goal of this modification is to "allow surgeons to speak the same language" and to aid in determining prognosis. An important additional aspect of the Tile classification is the correlation between the category and surgical approach and fracture reduction tactics.

Complementing a comprehensive history and physical examination, adequate radiographic imaging of the patient is required in order to classify acetabular injuries. In addition to the anteroposterior (AP) pelvis film taken as part of the trauma series, Judet views (iliac and obturator oblique) should be acquired once the patient is stable. Inlet and outlet projections of the pelvis are not required for isolated acetabular fractures but are indicated in combined acetabular and pelvic ring injuries. Computed tomography (CT) scanning of the pelvis provides additional information on the degree of displacement and impaction of the acetabular fracture as well as identifies any intra-articular fragments. The gold standard in terms of accurate classification of acetabular fractures remains, however, the AP and oblique radiographic views.

LETOURNEL AND JUDET CLASSIFICATION

The Letournel and Judet classification system has weathered the test of time and has remained essentially unchanged since 1965. This system is an anatomical classification with fractures divided into two groups (Fig. 1) with five subtypes in each group. The first group, elementary fractures, consists of injuries with one major fracture line. The associated fracture group is also made up of five fracture patterns, each with two or more major fracture lines. The importance of these distinct and separate patterns is well illustrated in the comprehensive text published by Letournel and Judet (1). They note that the surgical approach correlates with the fracture classification.

Elementary Fractures

Posterior wall fractures (Fig. 2) often associated with hip dislocation involve varying extents of the posterior articular surface. The fragment size, degree of wall displacement, and impaction can be seen on the AP and obturator oblique view; the ilioischial line will, however, remain intact. The Gull-Wing sign (4) has been described where the posterior wall fragment hinges supero-medially, giving the appearance of a wing on the AP view. The stability of the hip following these injuries is dependent on the size of

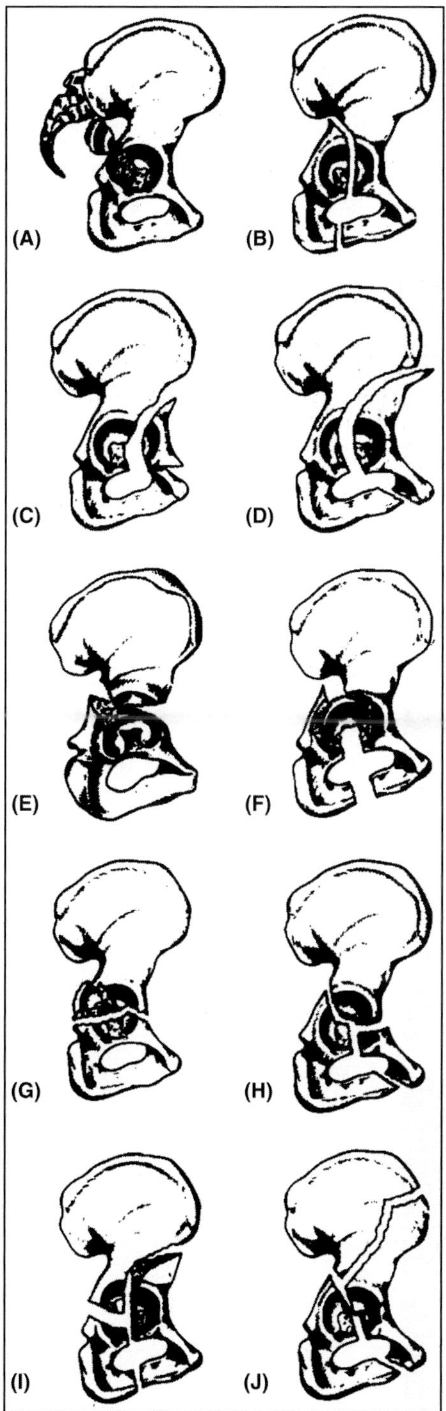

Figure 1 Letournel and Judet's classification of acetabular fractures. Elementary fractures; (**A**) posterior wall fracture, (**B**) posterior column fracture, (**C**) anterior wall fracture, (**D**) anterior column fracture, (**E**) transverse fracture. Associated fractures; (**F**) posterior wall with posterior column fracture, (**G**) transverse with posterior wall fracture, (**H**) T-shaped fracture, (**I**) anterior column with posterior hemitransverse fracture, (**J**) both column fracture.

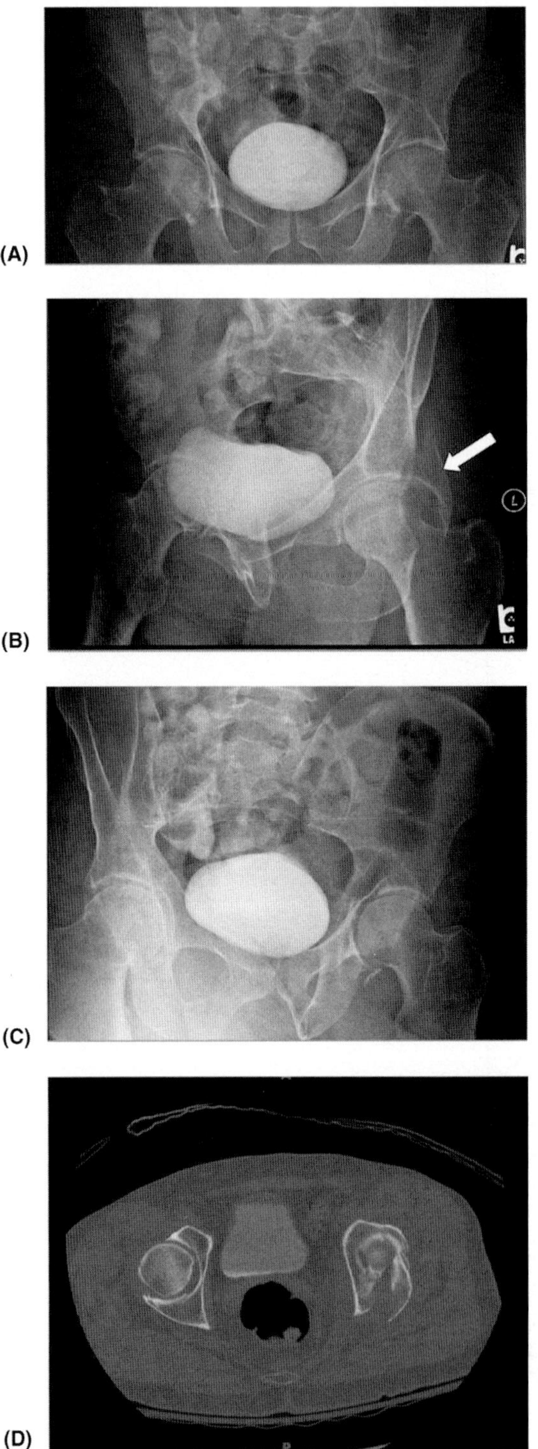

Figure 2 (**A**) Anteroposterior radiograph of a posterior wall fracture, (**B**) obturator oblique view radiograph of a posterior wall fracture, showing the Gull-Wing sign (*arrow*), (**C**) iliac oblique view radiograph of a posterior wall fracture, (**D**) computed tomography of a posterior wall fracture.

the fragments as well as their position relative to the weight-bearing area. The fragments can be described as pure posterior—the most common in Letournel's series—posterosuperior, or postero-inferior. Posterosuperior fragments are particularly important due to the involvement of the weight-bearing acetabular roof. Fragment size, comminution, and extent of marginal impaction have an influence on hip stability and degree of potential degenerative arthritis and will therefore have an impact on operative decision-making. The greater the involvement of the weight-bearing area and higher degree of marginal impaction or comminution, the more guarded the prognosis.

Posterior column fractures involve a breach of the ilioischial line on the AP and iliac oblique views. Posterior column fractures are rare—just over 3% of acetabular fractures in Letournel's series. They are important to recognize, however, since the typical fracture pattern detaches the entire posterior column, extending from the greater sciatic notch, through the acetabulum, and into the inferior pubic rami. Varieties of this pattern include extended posterior column fractures, in which the pelvic tear drop (corresponding to the floor of the cotyloid fossa) is attached to the column piece, producing a large joint fragment, and minimally displaced fractures with varying degrees of articular involvement.

Anterior wall injuries demonstrate a break in the iliopectineal line and anterior wall but do not extend into the superior pubic ramus, and therefore only involve the central portion of the anterior column. These rare injuries are usually associated with an anterior dislocation of the hip caused by abduction and external rotation.

Anterior column (Fig. 3) injuries involve variable extents of the segment of bone running from the midpoint of the iliac crest through the anterior acetabulum to the superior and inferior pubic rami. Four main categories have been described; (*i*) very low or distal fractures involve just the anterior horn of the articular surface and may be considered a high ramus pelvic ring injury, (*ii*) low fractures exit superiorly at the psoas gutter; the femoral head tends to remain subluxed anteriorly with the detached fragment, (*iii*) intermediate types exit superiorly between the anterior iliac spines, and femoral head positioning is similar to the low variety, and (*iv*) the fracture may extend though the iliac crest, resulting in a massive anterior segment. This large column piece is often minimally displaced because of extensive soft tissue attachments along its length and breadth.

Transverse fractures (Fig. 4) split the acetabulum horizontally and therefore break the anterior rim, iliopectineal, and ilioischial lines and often the posterior wall. Though these fractures involve both columns, there is a single fracture line and the columns themselves are not separated from each other. Therefore transverse fractures are not classified as acetabular both-column fractures and belong in the elementary fracture group. The fracture line can cross the acetabulum at various levels; transtectal, at the level of the roof; juxtatectal, at the junction of the roof and cotyloid fossa; and infratectal, below the weight-bearing dome. The obturator foramen is intact in transverse fractures. Not only can the fracture obliquity vary from horizontal through to almost vertical, but the fracture line may run from the postero-inferior aspect of the acetabulum exiting superiorly in the anterior column or vice versa. The degree of displacement of the femoral head can differ considerably from minimal to complete central dislocation. In osteoporotic bone transverse fractures often involve central dislocations because of

(*Text continues on page 149.*)

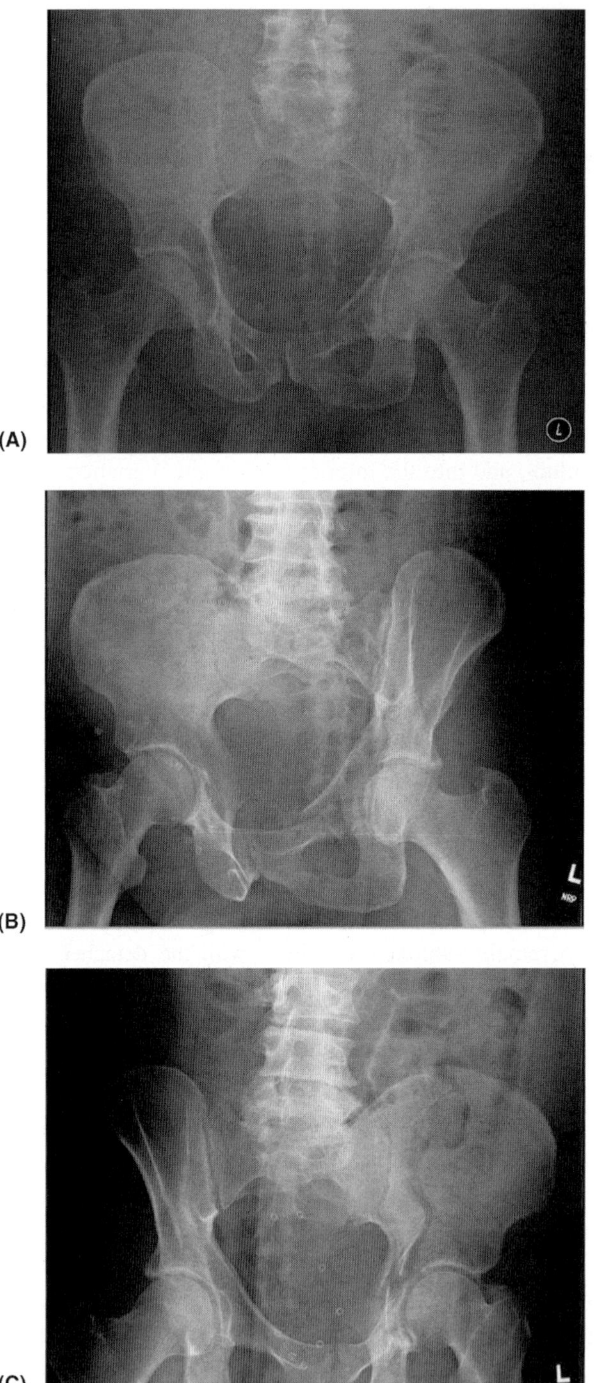

Figure 3 (**A**) Anteroposterior radiograph of an anterior column fracture, (**B**) obturator oblique view radiograph of an anterior column fracture, (**C**) iliac oblique view radiograph of an anterior column fracture. (*Continued*)

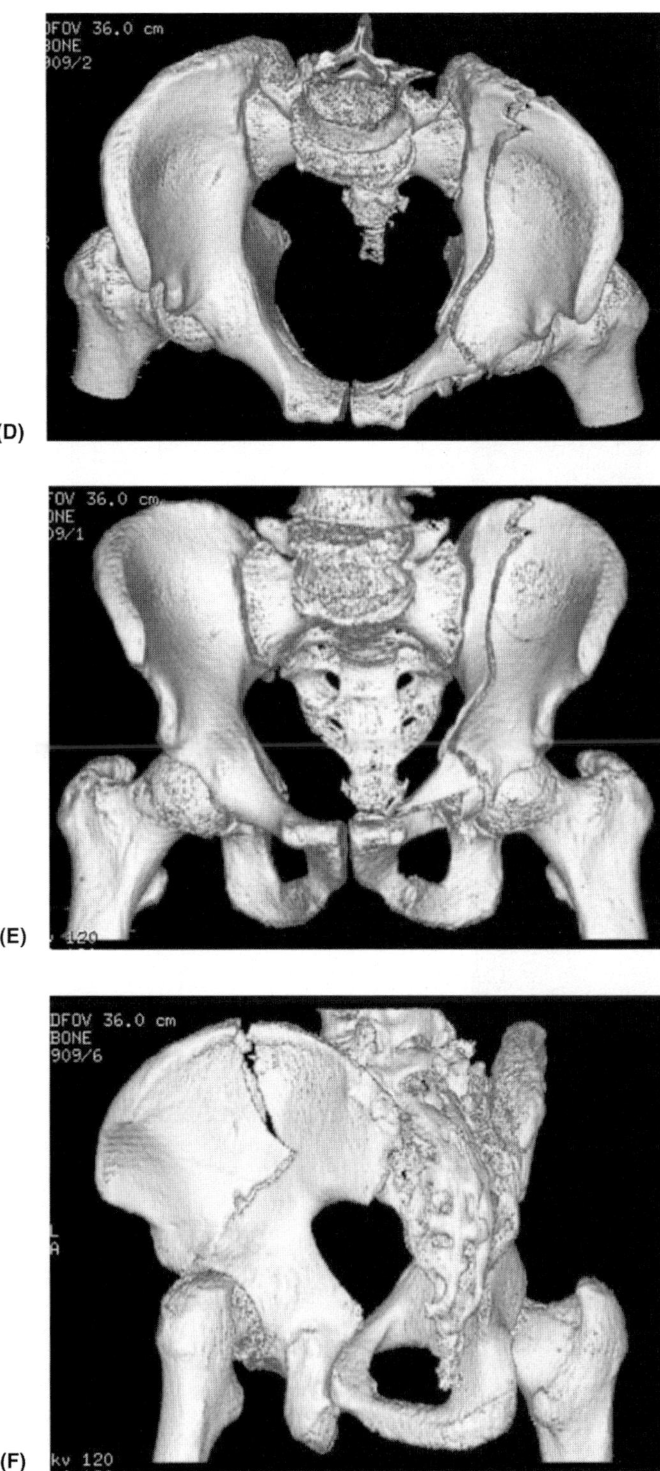

Figure 3 (*Continued*) (**D**) Computed tomography (CT) reconstruction of an anterior column fracture, (**E**) CT reconstruction of an anterior column fracture, (**F**) CT reconstruction of an anterior column fracture.

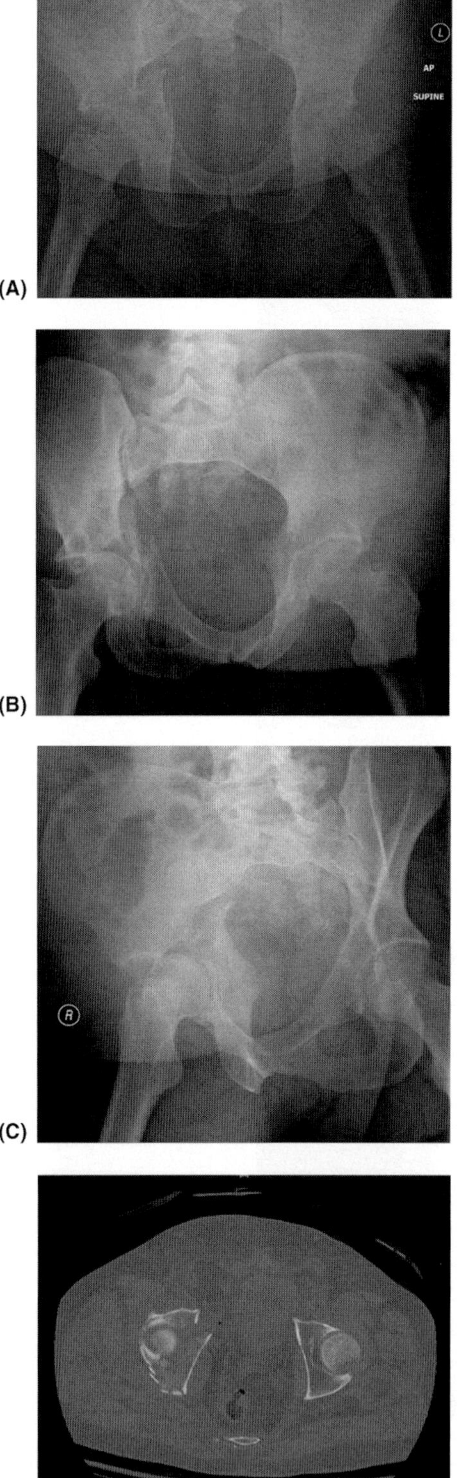

Figure 4 (**A**) Anteroposterior radiograph of a transverse fracture, (**B**) obturator oblique view radiograph of a transverse fracture, (**C**) iliac oblique view radiograph of a transverse fracture, (**D**) CT of a transverse fracture. *Abbreviation*: CT, computed tomography.

comminution of the quadrilateral plate. The extent of the displacement has considerable prognostic significance, particularly in high-energy injuries.

Associated Fractures

In associated posterior column with posterior wall fractures, the anatomy of the wall fracture and of the posterior column injury must each be considered. Similar to isolated posterior wall fractures, the size, number of fragments, degree of marginal impaction, and site of the wall fragment determine the instability of the hip and potential for post-traumatic arthritis. The column fracture may often be minimally displaced and incomplete. In some, however, there can be significant comminution and displacement. Therefore, careful analysis of both the wall and column fractures is required prior to decision-making regarding the techniques of fracture reduction and the method of fixation.

Transverse with posterior wall fractures is a frequent combination (Fig. 5). In these injuries there is segmental disruption of the posterior rim of the acetabulum, with involvement of the iliopectineal and ilioischial lines, and usually an intact obturator foramen. These injuries are caused by high-energy mechanisms, and a high rate of complications is common. Sciatic nerve injury and avascular necrosis of the femoral head can be devastating and can cause irreversible secondary injuries. The transverse fracture component may appear undisplaced on initial radiographs. There is a significant risk of secondary displacement if this fracture is not fixed concomitant with the posterior wall fixation.

The T-shaped fracture (Fig. 6) is a transverse fracture associated with a vertical split that enters the obturator foramina. The transverse fracture component can divide the acetabulum at any level and in the variety of orientations possible with the isolated pattern. The vertical fracture divides the anterior and posterior columns and enters the inferior pubic ramus. The split usually runs through the central portion of the acetabulum but can exit more obliquely either anteriorly or posteriorly. Letournel includes associated posterior column and anterior hemitransverse fractures within this group, as radiographically and surgically they require a similar approach. These fracture combinations may be associated with a central dislocation of the femoral head, particularly with high-energy mechanisms or osteoporotic bone.

The anterior column or wall with posterior hemitransverse fracture (Fig. 7) is described as a variant of the T-shaped pattern by Tile. Letournel states that the differences are subtle and often require CT scanning to determine the classification. In the T-shaped fracture, the anterior fracture runs vertically on the CT scan, disrupting the anterior rim. While in the associated anterior column or wall with posterior hemitransverse fracture the anterior breach exits higher with either a horizontal (column fracture) or a 45° oblique fracture plane (wall fracture). The posterior column fracture behaves similarly to the transverse pattern and can exit at the same levels as described above.

Both-column fractures (Fig. 8) are unique among the other associated patterns that involve the anterior and posterior columns. In both-column fractures, the articular surface is completely separated from the posterior ilium, which remains attached to the axial skeleton. It is this intact posterior segment of the innominate bone that produces the spur sign on the obturator oblique view as the articular elements are displaced medially. The both-column fracture can be regarded as a floating acetabulum or complete

(Text continues on page 155.)

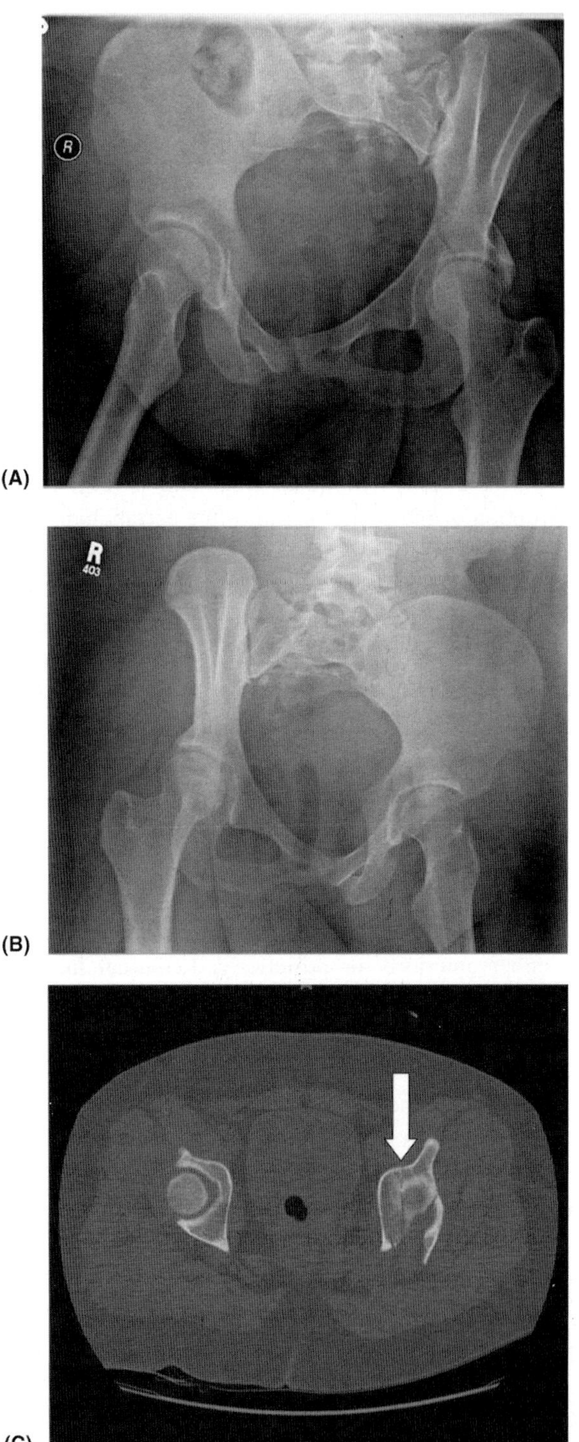

Figure 5 (**A**) Obturator oblique view radiograph of a transverse with posterior wall fracture, (**B**) iliac oblique view radiograph of a transverse with posterior wall fracture, (**C**) computed tomography of a transverse with posterior wall fracture, (*arrow*) shows transverse element.

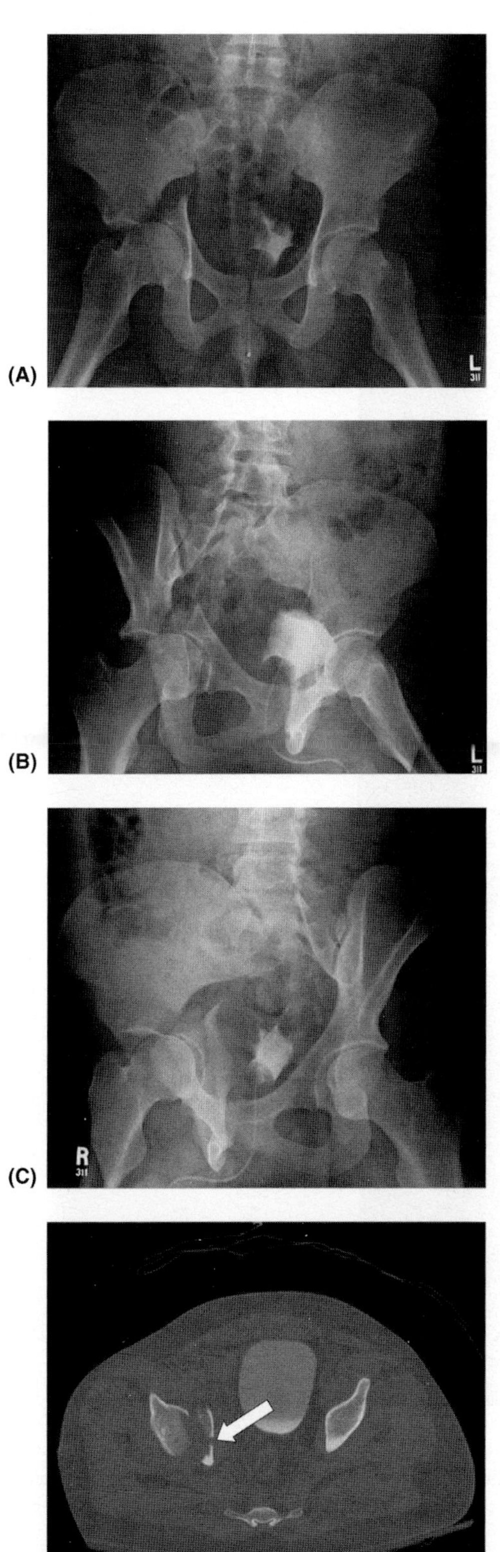

Figure 6 (**A**) Anteroposterior radiograph of a T-shaped fracture, (**B**) obturator oblique view radiograph of a T-shaped fracture, (**C**) iliac oblique view radiograph of a T-shaped fracture, (**D**) computed tomography of a T-shaped fracture, (*arrow*) shows vertical split.

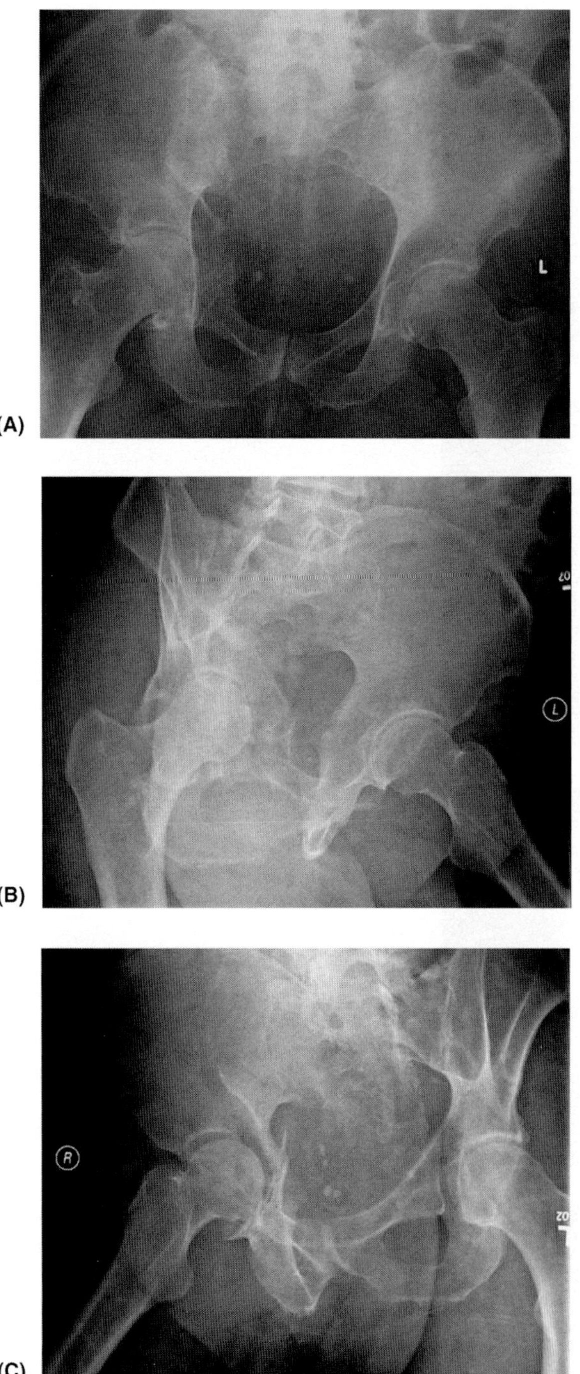

Figure 7 (**A**) Anteroposterior radiograph of an anterior column with posterior hemitransverse fracture, (**B**) obturator oblique view radiograph of an anterior column with posterior hemitransverse fracture, (**C**) iliac oblique view radiograph of an anterior column with posterior hemitransverse fracture. (*Continued*)

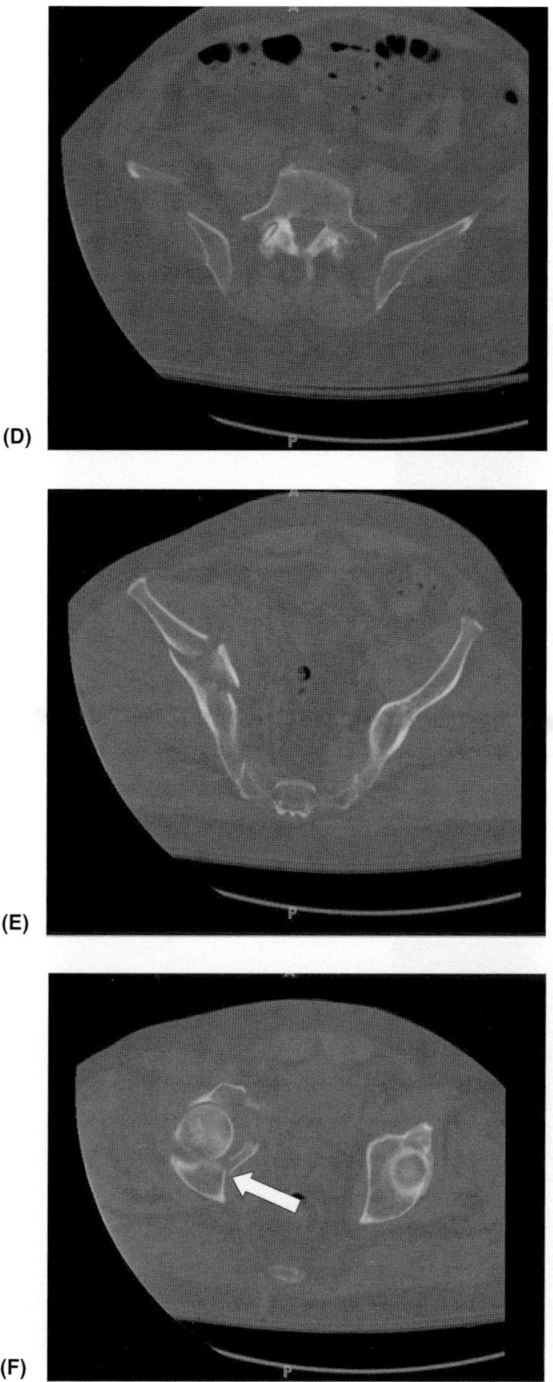

Figure 7 (*Continued*) (**D**) Computed tomography of an anterior column with posterior hemitransverse fracture, showing anterior column fracture line, (**E**) CT of an anterior column with posterior hemitransverse fracture, (**F**) CT of an anterior column with posterior hemitransverse fracture, (*arrow*) shows posterior split.

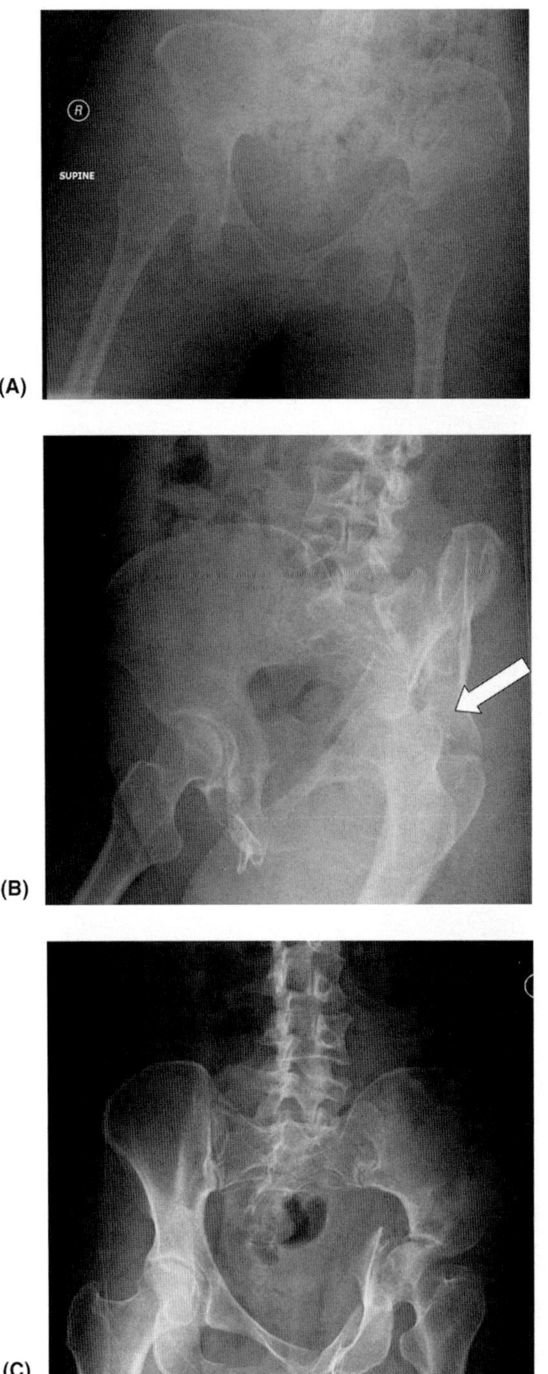

Figure 8 (**A**) Anteroposterior radiograph of a both-column fracture, (**B**) obturator oblique view radiograph of a both-column fracture, showing spur sign (*arrow*), (**C**) iliac oblique view radiograph of a both-column fracture.

articular dissociation. In some cases, the anterior and posterior columns reduce to the femoral head, producing secondary congruence. There are several varieties of the both-column pattern characterized by the exit level of the ilial fracture; low, high, or involving the sacro-iliac joint.

COMPREHENSIVE CLASSIFICATION

Tile's AO modification of Letournel's classification attempts to fit the various fracture patterns into the nomenclature of a comprehensive classification. The three types, Type A, fractures of one column or wall, Type B, fractures involving both columns but leaving part of the articular surface attached to the axial skeleton, and Type C, fractures involving both columns with complete articular separation, can each be subdivided into groups 1, 2, and 3 (Table 1) and further into subgroups and qualifiers (3). In the AO comprehensive classification system, fractures are assigned an alpha numerical code depending on the anatomical position of the fracture and its morphology. The numerical code of an acetabulum fracture is 62. Each fracture can therefore be assigned a unique identifier, which allows for easy data entry and classification recollection. For example, a posterior column fracture through the obturator ring involving the tear drop is a 62-A2.22.

MECHANISM AND INJURY MODIFIERS

In addition to the anatomical type of the fracture, there are several factors that also influence the type of the injury. The degree and vector of energy transfer and the position of the femur in relation to the acetabulum at the time of injury all have a bearing on the fracture pattern and associated injuries. The surgical approach, reduction, and fixation technique, as well as the predicted prognosis, will all be influenced by these variables.

When classifying the individual injury, it is necessary to appreciate the amount and direction of fragment comminution and displacement, whether the joint is subluxed or dislocated, and any associated femoral or knee fracture. The condition of the joint

Table 1 Comprehensive Classification: Acetabular Fractures

Type A: Partial articular fractures, one column	
A1	Posterior wall fracture
A2	Posterior column fracture
A3	Anterior wall or anterior column fracture
Type B: Partial articular fractures, transverse	
B1	Transverse fracture
B2	T-shaped fracture
B3	Anterior column and posterior hemitransverse fracture
Type C: Complete articular fractures, both columns	
C1	High
C2	Low
C3	Involving sacroiliac joint

Table 2 Comprehensive Classification: Articular Surface Modifiers

α: Femoral head subluxation	
α^1	Femoral head subluxation, anterior
α^2	Femoral head subluxation, medial
α^3	Femoral head subluxation, posterior
§: Femoral head dislocation	
$§^1$	Femoral head dislocation, anterior
$§^2$	Femoral head dislocation, medial
$§^3$	Femoral head dislocation, posterior
χ: Acetabular surface	
χ^1	Acetabular surface, chondral lesion
χ^2	Acetabular surface, impacted
δ: Femoral head surface	
δ^1	Femoral head surface, chondral lesion
δ^2	Femoral head surface, impacted
δ^3	Femoral head surface, osteochondral fracture
ϵ^1	Intra-articular fragment requiring surgical removal
$\emptyset^1$	Nondisplaced fracture of the acetabulum

surface needs to be assessed and the presence of any intra-articular fragments identified. The degrees of marginal impaction and osteochondral fracture have significant effect on the prognosis. Associated closed degloving soft tissue injuries such as a Morel Lavallee lesion (5) may influence the choice of approach; the extent of capsular injury will influence the risk of avascular necosis of the femoral head; and sciatic nerve involvement will necessitate emergent reduction of any dislocation. Tile's modification of the comprehensive classification attempts to describe some of these modifiers (Table 2).

Tile also emphasizes the direction of displacement as an aid to further classification and therefore surgical decision making. He notes that posterior acetabular injuries—posterior wall, posterior column, transverse, and T-shaped fractures with displacement—result frequently from the knee hitting the dashboard during road traffic accidents. In this mechanism, knee injuries are common and posterior hip instability is associated with wall fractures, necessitating open reduction and stabilization via a posterior approach. Anterior rotation of a transverse fracture with minimal displacement posteriorly will demand an alternative approach.

CONCLUSION

The care of patients who have sustained acetabular trauma begins with the management of any associated hemodynamic instability or limb-threatening injury. Once stabilized, further clinical examination and imaging will provide addition information to allow the surgeon to understand the acetabular injury. Classification of the fracture pattern and its reproduction on dry bones will allow individualized surgical planning that takes into account the type of the injury. Accurate understanding of the fracture classification and associated variables is the first critical step toward successful treatment.

REFERENCES

1. Letournel E, ed. Fractures of the Acetabulum, 2nd ed. New York: Springer-Verlag, 1993.
2. Tile M, ed. Fractures of the Pelvis and Acetabulum, 2nd ed. Baltimore: Williams & Wilkins, 1995.
3. Fracture and Dislocation Compendium. Orthopaedic Trauma Association Committee for Coding and Classification. J Orthop Trauma 1996; 10(suppl 1):v-ix, 1–154.
4. Berkebile RD, Fischer DL, Albrecht LF. The full wing sign value of the lateral view of the pelvis in fracture-dislocation of the acetabular and posterior dislocation of the femoral head. Radiology 1965; 84:937–939.
5. Morel-Lavallee. Decollements traumatiques de la peau et des couches sous-jacentes. Arch Gen Med 1863; 1:20–38, 172–200, 300–332.

9

Initial Management and Surgical Indications for Acetabular Fracture Reconstruction

Steven J Morgan and Patrick M. Osborn

Department of Orthopaedics, Denver Health Medical Center, University of Colorado School of Medicine, Denver, Colorado, U.S.A.

INTRODUCTION

Acetabular fractures resulting from high-energy trauma generally occur in a younger adult population (1). The long-term ramifications of this intra-articular injury are severe if improperly diagnosed and mistreated. Late reconstructive options in this population are generally inferior to preservation and acute reconstruction of the native hip joint. Early diagnosis and selection of the appropriate treatment option or prompt referral to a surgeon comfortable with the care of acetabular fractures is paramount for achieving acceptable long-term functional outcomes.

EPIDEMIOLOGY

Motor vehicle accidents are the primary cause of most acetabular fractures (2,3). The type of fracture produced by the trauma is dependent on the direction of force and the orientation of the femoral head in the acetabulum at the time of impact. The force required to create an acetabular fracture can be applied at four sites: the greater trochanter, the knee with the hip in the flexed position, the foot with the knee and hip in extension, and the posterior aspect of the pelvis (2). The rate of load application and the muscular response at the time of injury play a role in determining the initial degree of fracture displacement.

INITIAL DIAGNOSIS AND EVALUATION

The initial management of any trauma patient should follow the Advanced Trauma Life Support (ATLS) guidelines (4). The presence of an acetabular fracture is usually heralded by pain in the hip or groin area. The injured extremity may present similar to a dislocated hip, appearing shortened and externally rotated. In the obtunded patient or patients without obvious clinical deformity, the majority of acetabular fractures will be visualized on the anterior–posterior (AP) pelvis radiograph obtained during the initial trauma radiographic survey.

Though life-threatening hemorrhage is rare in acetabular fractures without a simultaneous pelvic ring injury, any hemodynamically unstable patient must be investigated and treated aggressively under the ATLS guidelines. There is no indication for emergent mechanical stabilization of the acetabular fracture with external fixation for hemorrhage control or maintenance of fracture reduction in these patients. While arterial injury is rare, there have been case reports to suggest that injury to arterial structures is possible. Damage to the hypogastric artery has been reported with displaced associated both-column fractures (5). Injury to the femoral vein (6) and the iliofemoral artery (7) can be the result of a traction injury caused by an anterior column fracture. Those fractures traversing the greater sciatic notch are at higher risk for arterial injury (8–10). It has been shown in at least one study that signs of contrast extravasation on computed tomography (CT) scan are highly predictive of the need for angiography (11). In cases of ongoing blood loss without another identifiable source of hemorrhage, arteriography should be considered as a treatment modality to identify and selectively embolize arterial sources of blood loss. Nonselective embolization should be avoided since occlusion of certain arteries may compromise the blood supply vital for soft tissue survival in some surgical exposures. The superior gluteal artery (SGA) is the primary supply to the hip abductors. Extensile approaches in the presence of SGA lesions may result in devascularization of the abductor flap. The collateral flow to the abductor mass arises from the ascending branch of the lateral femoral circumflex and the deep iliac circumflex arteries. If an arterial injury is suspected, or if nonselective embolization has been performed, some authors suggest that preoperative angiography be performed on patients prior to performing extensile approaches to the acetabulum (9,12).

A thorough neurologic examination should be performed, as the incidence of nerve palsy in patients who have sustained acetabular fractures is between 12% and 25%. The sciatic nerve is the most commonly injured nerve with a reported incidence of 3% to 12.2% (2,13,14). This is caused by displaced fracture fragments or a dislocated femoral head. The peroneal branch is more commonly injured than the tibial portion of the sciatic nerve. Function of ankle dorsiflexion and plantarflexion, ankle inversion, and eversion and toe extension and flexion should be well documented when the patient is able to comply with an examination. The femoral nerve is also at risk by entrapment though less likely as it is protected by the iliopsoas muscle. Again a thorough neurologic examination ensuring function of the quadriceps must be recorded (15). Obturator nerve palsy is infrequent risk with a reported incidence of 1% to 2% (16,17). It has been theorized that the obturator nerve is at greater risk with an anterior wall or column fracture. If possible, adductor function should be evaluated at the time of admission to determine the status of the obturator nerve.

Inspection of the skin for open wounds or the presence of a subcutaneous degloving injury (Morel–Lavalle lesion) may alter management of the acetabular fracture. A Morel–Lavalle injury represents a traumatic separation of skin and subcutaneous tissue from the fascia. Letournel and Judet reported the incidence of degloving injury to be 8.3% in patients who sustained a blow to the greater trochanter (2). It can be recognized by the hallmark finding of an area of fluctuance (18); this area is often large and when present is frequently apparent on CT scan (19). Decreased skin sensation or skin hyper-mobility may also be present (20,21). Obvious signs of trauma such as tire marks or ecchymosis should raise suspicion for this injury. This injury can also account for significant blood loss in the absence of associated injuries and has been reported to have a high incidence of bacterial colonization and subsequent infection if not debrided early. Bacterial colonization of these lesions is not uncommon (18). Current recommendations suggest that when the Morel lesion is in the operative field, it should be debrided either preoperatively or at the time of operative intervention for the acetabular fracture. In either case, at the time of surgical wound closure only the fascia should be closed and the Morel lesion should be left open to be closed in a delayed fashion once the soft tissue injury has stabilized (18,22,23). Morel lesions not involved with the surgical approach can be observed and will often resolve spontaneously; however, vigilance must be maintained for infection. Aspiration of the lesion and evaluation of the fluid as part of a fever work up is mandatory in the perioperative period if sepsis is suspected.

Genitourinary lesions are seen in 6% to 16% of pelvic and acetabular fractures (3,24,25). These lesions can be detected by a thorough genital and rectal examination as well as routine urinalysis. Urethral injury is indicated by perineal ecchymosis and edema, a high-riding or ballotable prostate on rectal examination, or difficulty passing a urinary catheter. There should be a low threshold for obtaining a retrograde urethrogram or CT cystogram. An anuric patient must also be aggressively investigated. Though likely caused by insufficient hemodynamic resuscitation, there have been reports of a pelvic compartment syndrome causing anuria in some patients (26). This phenomenon is analogous to the abdominal compartment syndrome and causes postrenal failure from compression of the ureters. These cases have been seen in patients with concomitant acetabular and severe pelvic injuries.

Ultimately the force required to fracture the acetabulum is often transmitted from the knee or foot to the femur and proximally to the acetabulum. Associated injuries of the ipsilateral extremity are not uncommon and frequently include the femur, patella, and tibia. Therefore a search for associated fractures in the ipsilateral extremity is mandatory and radiographs should be ordered when clinically appropriate (3).

INITIAL MANAGEMENT

Management of the acetabular fracture in the emergency department includes reduction of a dislocated femoral head and occasional application of skeletal traction. Letournel and Judet eschewed the use of skeletal traction going so far to say that their first step in "treatment is to remove the traction pin" (2); however, this remains controversial. In the case of posterior hip dislocation associated with an acetabular fracture, emergent reduction is mandatory to potentially reduce the severity of sciatic nerve injury (27–29). The reduction usually remains stable when hip and knee flexion is avoided, which is easily accomplished with application of a knee immobilizer. When significant joint incongruity is absent, traction is not necessary. Significant fracture displacement and associated major subluxation of the joint probably warrant skeletal traction via a femoral or tibial traction pin to relieve the pressure on the articular surface of the femoral head. Decisions regarding definitive care of the fractured acetabulum should be made on radiographs obtained out of traction (2,30,31).

In the preoperative period, patients will be largely immobilized and non-weight bearing on the affected extremity. Initial and continued fracture displacement is also felt to be a cause of endothelial damage and venous stasis, respectively, further increasing the risk of deep venous thrombosis (DVT). The risk of DVT is as high as 60%, while the incidence of pulmonary embolus (PE) is reported to be relatively low at 2% (32–40). While the level of evidence supporting preoperative DVT prophylaxis is poor, it is reasonable and prudent to offer those awaiting acetabular fracture surgery preoperative prophylactic measures, such as external compression devices, chemical prophylaxis that is easily reversible (heparin or low-molecular-weight heparin), or a combination of mechanical and chemical prophylaxis. The most effective pre- and postoperative prophylaxis regimen is unclear in the literature. Preliminary studies have shown that there may be some advantage to low molecular weight heparin compared to low-dose heparin, but this continues as a subject of debate (40–42). The associated risks of inferior vena cava (IVC) filter placement and the unknown long-term effects if retention is required of such an implant exclude its use as a routine prophylactic measure. Temporary IVC filters, which can be later removed, should be considered in the very high-risk patient with contraindications to traditional chemical and mechanical prophylaxis (43).

In the case when treatment has been delayed or no preoperative prophylaxis has been performed, the patient should be screened for DVT. The most common methods for preoperative DVT screening are duplex ultrasonography and magnetic resonance venography (MRV) (44–49). Ultrasound however is notoriously poor at detecting deep thigh and pelvic thromboses, and while MRV has been shown to be highly sensitive for DVT, its specificity has been questioned. There is no "gold standard" in regards to when and how to perform preoperative DVT screening.

INDICATIONS FOR NONOPERATIVE MANAGEMENT

Nonoperative management of acetabular fractures may be considered for non-displaced fractures or minimally displaced fractures (<2 mm displacement), fractures that do not involve the weight-bearing dome of the acetabulum as determined on CT or by roof-arc angles, and in cases of secondary congruence (31). The hip must remain congruently reduced without evidence of subluxation on radiographs and CT scans obtained with the patient out of traction. For displaced fractures, an adequate weight-bearing dome is rarely present (5%), and the presence of secondary congruence is a more common indication for nonoperative treatment (31).

The stability of nondisplaced fractures and fractures below the weight-bearing dome has been questioned. Though controversial, some reports indicate a possible role for stress radiographs obtained in the operating suite to determine fracture stability. Surgery is recommended for fractures not involving the weight-bearing dome or non-displaced fractures that demonstrate fracture instability or joint subluxation under fluoroscopic examination (50–53).

Controversy continues to exist surrounding the appropriate management of the posterior wall acetabular fracture with or without associated hip dislocation. Nonoperative treatment can be considered for a concentrically reduced joint in the absence of marginal articular impaction or incarcerated articular fragments. Proponents of nonoperative therapy mantain that the hip remains stable through a full range of motion when the degree of articular involvement is less than a third of the joint surface based on CT evaluation (51,52,54). Proponents of operative intervention suggest that even small fractures of the posterior wall involving less than a third of the joint surface will alter joint contact forces leading to early arthrosis and advocate anatomic reduction of all wall segments (3,55,56). There is general agreement that operative intervention should be undertaken in cases of instability, incarcerated fragments, marginal impaction, and large articular surface involvement (56,57).

Elderly patients with severe osteopenia or patients suffering from metabolic bone disease with inadequate bone stock for internal fixation should be considered for initial nonoperative therapy (30). Advanced age alone is not an indication for nonoperative management. Several articles suggest that acetabular fractures in the elderly demonstrate good functional outcomes following open reduction and internal fixation (2,3,56,57). Reduction and fixation of acetabular fractures through nonextensile exposures, particularly posterior wall fractures, result in an easier total joint reconstruction at a delayed time point if one is required at all.

The decision to treat a patient nonoperatively generally requires that the patient undergo a period of bed rest and, occasionally, use of skeletal traction. Skeletal traction is not used to reduce the fracture but to allow gentle motion with the joint mildly distracted, particularly in cases of displaced fractures with secondary congruence (30). In some cases, early mobilization with crutches or transfers to a wheel chair may be warranted (58). In either case, close radiographic follow up is required. If the fracture displaces or secondary congruence is lost, surgical intervention should be considered. Surgical intervention should occur within 21 days of injury, since reconstruction and results are compromised with further delay (2).

INDICATIONS FOR OPERATIVE TREATMENT

Operative treatment should be considered for all displaced fractures of the acetabulum that do not meet the criteria for nonoperative therapy as previously discussed. The vast majority of acetabular fractures reported in the literature fail to meet criteria for nonoperative care and require surgical intervention, suggesting that most acetabular fractures require surgery (31). Operative management of acetabular fractures is technically demanding. A significant learning curve exists in the management of these fractures and should only be undertaken by those with significant experience or training in the discipline (2).

CONCLUSION

An acetabular fracture represents one of the most challenging management tasks for the orthopedic surgeon. The consequences of inaccurate diagnosis and inefficient or incorrect initial management of the patient may be severe. The admitting or treating surgeon must be proficient with an efficient and accurate physical examination. Initial radiographic studies must be ordered and interpreted appropriately, and indications and tools for further investigation should be familiar. Signs of associated injury must be recognized, and a multidisciplinary approach to these difficult patients should be used whenever possible. Finally, the appropriate knowledge to classify the fracture, plan treatment, and manage the patient until definitive treatment is undertaken increase the possibility of a satisfactory outcome.

REFERENCES

1. Jimenez, ML, Tile M, Schenk RS. Total hip replacement after acetabular fracture. Orthop Clin North Am 1997; 28:435–446.
2. Letournel E, Judet R. Fractures of the Acetabulum. New York: Springer-Verlag, 1993.
3. Matta JM. Fractures of the acetabulum: accuracy of reduction and clinical results in patients managed operatively within three weeks after the injury. J Bone Joint Surg Am 1996; 78:1632–1645.
4. Advanced Trauma Life Support For Doctors Student Course Manual, 7th ed. Chicago: American College of Surgeons, 2004.
5. Chen AL, Wolinsky PR, Tejwani NC. Hypogastric artery disruption associated with acetabular fracture. J Bone Joint Surg Am 2003; 85:333–338.
6. Roise O, Pillgram-Larsen J. Fracture of the acetabulum complicated by a tear of the femoral vein—a case report after 5 years. Acta Orthop Scand 2000; 71:206–209.
7. Frank JL, Reimer BL, Raves JJ. Traumatic iliofemoral artery injury: an association with high anterior acetabular fractures. J Vasc Surg 1989; 10:198–201.
8. Ben-Menachem Y, Coldwell DM, Young JW, et al. Hemorrhage associated with pelvic fractures: causes, diagnosis and emergent management. Am J Radiol 1991; 157:1005–1014.
9. Bosse MJ, Poka A, Reinert CM, et al. Preoperative angiographic assessment of the superior gluteal artery in aetabular fractures requiring extensile surgical approaches. J Orthop Trauma 1988; 2:303–307.
10. Patel NH, Hunter J, Weber TG, et al. Rotational imaging of complex acetabular fractures. J Orthop Trauma 1998; 12:59–63.
11. Stephen DJ, Kreder HJ, Day AC, et al. Early detection of arterial bleeding in acute pelvic trauma. J Trauma 1999; 47:638–642.
12. Tabor OB, Bosse MJ, Greene KG, et al. Effects of surgical approaches for acetabular fractures with associated gluteal vascular inury. J Orthop Trauma 1998; 12:78–84.
13. Helfet DL, Anand N, Malkani AL, et al. Intraoperative monitoring of motor pathways during operative fixation of acute acetabular fractures. J Orthop Trauma 1997; 11:2–6.
14. Routt ML, Swiontkowski MF. Operative treatment of complex acetabular fractures. J Bone Joint Surg Am 1990; 72:897–904.
15. Gruson KI, Moed BR. Injury of the femoral nerve associated with acetabular fracture. J Bone Joint Surg Am 2003; 85:428–431.
16. Helfet DL, Shmeling GJ. Management of complex acetabular fractures through single non-extensile exposures. Clin Orthop 1994; 305:58–68.
17. Mayo KA. Open reduction and internal fixation of fractures of the acetabulum: results in 163 fractures. Clin Orthop 1994; 305:31–37.
18. Hak DJ, Olson SA, Matta JM. Diagnosis and management of closed internal degloving injuries associated with pelvic and acetabular fractures: the Morel-Lavallee lesion. J Trauma 1997; 42:1046–1051.
19. Parra JA, Fernandez MA, Encinas B, et al. Morel–Lavallee effusions in the thigh. Skeletal Radiol 1997; 26:239–41.
20. Hudson DA, Knottenbelt JD, Krige JE. Closed degloving injuries: results following conservative surgery. Plast Reconstr Surg 1992; 89:853–855.
21. Letts RM. Degloving injuries in children. J Pediatr Orthop 1986; 6:93–97.
22. Kottmeier SA, Wilson SC, Born CT, et al. Surgical management of soft tissue lesions associated with pelvic ring injury. Clin Orthop Relat Res 1996; 329:46–53.
23. Routt ML Jr, Simonian PT, Ballmer F. A rational approach to pelvic trauma. Resuscitation and early definitive stabilization. Clin Orthop Relat Res 1995; 318:61–74.

24. Rommens PM. Pelvic ring injuries: a challenge for the trauma surgeon. Acta Chir Belg 1996; 96:78–84.
25. Tile M. Pelvic ring fractures: should they be fixed? J Bone Joint Surg Br 1988; 70:12.
26. Hessman M, Rommens PM. Bilateral ureteral obstruction and renal failure caused by massive retroperitoneal hematoma: is there a pelvic compartment syndrome analogous to abdominal compartment syndrome? J Trauma 1998; 12:553–557.
27. Rowe CR, Lowell JD. Prognosis of fractures of the acetabulum. J Bone Joint Surg Am 1961; 43:30–59.
28. Epstein HC. Posterior fracture-dislocations of the hip. J Bone Joint Surg Am 1974; 56:1103–1126.
29. Roffi RP, Matta JM. Unrecognized posterior dislocation of the hip associated with transverse and t-type fractures of the acetabulum. J Orthop Trauma 1993; 7:23–27.
30. Matta JM. Operative indications and choice of surgical approach for fractures of the acetabulum. Techniques Orthop 1986; 1:13–22.
31. Matta JM, Mehne DK, Roff R. Fractures of the acetabulum: early results of a prospective study. Clin Orthop 1986; 205:241–250.
32. Matta JM. Operative treatment of acetabular fractures through the ilioinguinal approach: a 10-year perspective. Clin Ortho 1994; 305:10–19.
33. Collins DN, Barnes CL, McCowan TC, et al. Vena caval filter use in orthopaedic trauma patients with recognized preoperative venous thromboembolic disease. J Orthop Trauma 1992; 6:135–138.
34. Fisher CG, Blachut PA, Salvain AJ, et al. Effectiveness of pneumatic leg compression devices for the prevention of thromboembolic disease in the orthopaedic trauma patients: a prospective, randomized study of compression alone versus no prophylaxis. J Orthop Trauma 1995; 9:1–7.
35. Geerts WH, Code KI, Jay RM, et al. A prospective study of venous thromboembolism after major trauma. N Engl J Med 1994; 331:1601–1606.
36. Matta JM. Indications for anterior fixation of pelvic fractures. Clin Orthop 1996; 329: 88–96.
37. National Institute of Health Consensus Development. Prevention of venous thrombosis and pulmonary embolism. JAMA 1986; 256:744–749.
38. White RH, Goulet JA, Bray TJ, et al. Deep-vein thrombosis after fracture of the pelvis: assessment with serial duplex-ultrasound screening. J Bone Joint Surg Am 1990; 72: 495–500.
39. Fishmann AJ, Greeno RA, Brooks LR, et al. Prevention of deep vein thrombosis and pulmonary embolism in acetabular and pelvic fracture surgery. Clin Orthop 1994; 305: 133–137.
40. Salzman EW, Harris WH. Prevention of venous thromboembolism in orthopaedic patients. J Bone Joint Surg 1976; 58A(7):903–913.
41. Evarts CM, Alfidi RJ. Thromboembolism after total hip reconstruction. Failure of low doses of heparin in prevention. JAMA 1973; 225:515–516.
42. Evarts CM, Feil EJ. Prevention of thromboembolic disease after elective surgery of the hip. J Bone Joint Surg Am 1971; 53:1271–1280.
43. Webb LX, Rush PT, Fuller SB, et al. Greenfield filter prophylaxis of pulmonary embolism in patients undergoing surgery for acetabular fracture. J Orthop Trauma 1992; 6:139–145.
44. Burns GA, Cohn SM, Frumento RJ, et al. Prospective ultrasound evaluation of venous thrombosis in high-risk trauma patients. J Trauma 1993; 35:405–408.
45. Davidson BL, Elliot CG, Lensing AW. Low accuracy of color Doppler ultrasound in the detection of proximal leg vein thrombosis in asymptomatic high-risk patient. The RD Heparin Arthroplasty Group. Ann Intern Med 1992; 117:735–738.

46. Wells PS, Lensing AW, Hirsh J. Graduated compression stockings in the prevention of postoperative venous thromboembolism. A meta-analysis. Arch Intern Med 1994; 154:67–72.
47. Montgomery KD, Potter HG, Helftet DL. Magnetic resonance venography to evaluate the deep venous system of the pelvis in patients who have an acetabular fracture. J Bone Joint Surg Am 1995; 77:1639–1649.
48. Stover MD, Morgan SJ, Bosse MJ, et al. Prospective comparison of contrast-enhanced computed tomography versus magnetic resonance venography in the detection of occult deep pelvic vein thrombosis in patients with pelvic and acetabular fractures. J Orthop Trauma 2002; 16:613–621.
49. Montgomery KD, Potter HG, Helfet DL. The detection and management of proximal deep venous thrombosis in patients with acute acetabular fractures: a follow-up report. J Orthop Trauma 1997; 11:330–336.
50. Olson SA, Bay BK, Pollak AN, et al. The effect of variable size posterior wall acetabular fractures on contact characteristics of the hip joint. J Orthop Trauma 1996; 10:395–402.
51. Keith JE Jr, Brashear HR Jr, Guilford WB. Stability of posterior fracture-dislocations of the hip: quantitative assessment using computed tomography. J Bone Joint Surg Am 1988; 70:711–714.
52. Vailas JC, Hurwitz S, Wiesel SW. Posterior acetabular fracture-dislocations: fragment size, joint capsule, and stability. J Trauma 1989; 29:1494–1496.
53. Tornetta P III. Nonoperative management of acetabular fractures: the use of dynamic stress views. J Bone Joint Surg Br 1999; 81:67–70.
54. Calkins MS, Zych G, Latta L, et al. Computed tomography evaluation of stability in posterior fracture dislocation of the hip. Clin Orthop 1988; 227:152–163.
55. Moed BR, WillsonCarr SE, Watson JT. Results of operative treatment of fractures of the posterior wall of the acetabulum. J Bone Joint Surg Am 2002; 84:752–758.
56. Kreder HJ, Rozen N, Borkhoff CM, et al. J Bone Joint Surg Br 2006; 88:776–782.
57. Wolinsky PR, Davison BL, Shyr Y, et al. Predictors of total hip arthroplasty in patients following open reduction and internal fixation of acetabular fractures. Procs 12th annual Orthopaedic Trauma Association Meeting 1996; 9:29.
58. Helfet DL, Borrelli J Jr, DiPasquale T, et al. Stabilization of acetabular fractures in elderly patients. J Bone Joint Surg Am 1992; 74:753.

10

Acetabular Reconstruction: Surgical Approaches

Daniel S. Horwitz and Thomas F. Higgins
University of Utah, Department of Orthopaedics, Salt Lake City, Utah, U.S.A.

INTRODUCTION

The operative techniques used to reduce and stabilize acetabular fractures rely on adequate exposure with an attempt to minimize additional trauma to the surrounding soft tissues. With the exception of open fractures, vascular compromise, and irreducible posterior dislocation of the femoral head, most acetabular injuries permit sufficient time for a complete radiographic evaluation and a well-planned surgical approach. All the approaches we will discuss have certain advantages and limitations, but the most important factor in the decision making process is often the surgeon's experience and comfort with what may be complex and distorted anatomy. Our goal is not to discuss every potential exposure in detail but rather to focus on three fundamental approaches to the acetabulum as well as their common modifications: posterior, extensile lateral, and anterior.

The choice of approach is usually dictated by the fracture pattern, but, with the exception of posterior wall fractures, which often demand a Kocher–Langenbeck, many acetabular injuries can be reduced and stabilized from anterior or posterior, depending on surgeon's experience and associated injuries. Tranverse fracture patterns can often be reduced with a posterior or modified posterior approach utilizing back to front anterior column screws if it is necessary to stabilize the anterior column, and, likewise, posterior column injuries can be reduced from the anterior (ileoinguinal) approach with placement of front to back posterior column screws if necessary. Generalizations regarding the utility of different approaches or combinations of approaches are therefore acceptable, but absolutes in this discussion should be avoided.

POSTERIOR APPROACH

The posterior, or Kocher–Langenbeck, approach is familiar to most orthopedic surgeons from arthroplasty experience, but this can often lead to a false sense of confidence in that the technique is different when attempting to reduce and stabilize a fracture. The general indications for this approach are posterior wall and posterior column fractures and T-type and both-column fractures, which require direct posterior exposure. Visualization from the greater sciatic notch to the ischial tuberosity including the lateral aspect of the posterior column and posterior wall is usually achieved, and while palpation of the superior lateral dome is possible, visualization past the 12 o'clock position necessitates some type of trochanteric osteotomy. Fundamental to current technique is an emphasis on minimizing subperiostial and external rotator dissection and gluteal muscle damage in an attempt to avoid heterotopic ossification.

Surgical Technique

The patient is positioned either prone or lateral, depending on surgeon preference, and prepped from the iliac crest down to the knee or below. The skin incision extends from the posterior inferior iliac spine down to the posterior one third proximal femur, the actual length dictated by the fracture and patient size. The gluteus maximus is divided in line with its fibers and the tensor fascia latae is split longitudinally. Bursal tissue overlying the greater trochanter is either split or resected, and careful palpation and blunt dissection are used to identify the gluteus medius and minimus insertions onto the greater trochanter, as well as the piriformis and short external rotator insertions onto the posterior proximal femur. In most cases, these posterior tendonous structures are intact, even in the face of posterior dislocation and associated capsular tearing. The gluteus minimus often has a deep reflection, which inserts on the superior lateral capsule, and failure to recognize this can lead one to dissect between the medius and minimus rather than between the minimus and periosteum of the iliac wing. The piriforis and short external rotators are divided at their insertion on the femur and carefully tagged for retraction and later repair. It is essential that the short external rotators be identified as they serve as the primary anatomic protector of the sciatic nerve. The inferior border of the dissection is the ischial tuberosity; once it is palpated no addition inferior muscle should be divided or femoral head blood supply will be compromised as it comes through the quadratus femorus. In addition, while the sciatic nerve should not be

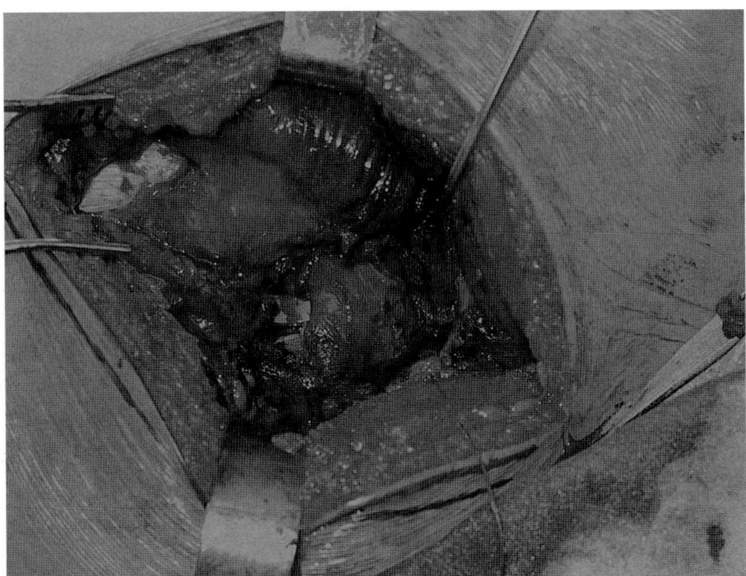

Figure 1 The posterior approach to the acetabulum can be greatly assisted by the placement of smooth Steinman pins under the abductors and above the level of the fracture.

stripped or aggressively manipulated, it should be visualized or palpated throughout the course of the exposure and carefully protected throughout the case. The placement of retractors in the lesser sciatic notch is not recommended except for brief periods of time, and the hip should be kept extended and the knee should be maintained at 90° of flexion at all times. When there is uncertainty regarding its exact location, careful deep digital palpation of the posterior structures while bringing the knee from flexion to extension will usually identify a tightening band that is the sciatic nerve. Extraperiosteal dissection of the lateral aspect of the iliac wing can usually be performed digitally, and the placement of smooth Steinman pins far superior and anterior under the gluteus minimus aids in visualization (Fig. 1). If there is a posterior wall fracture, the bony fragments are usually displaced superiorly with attached capsule, allowing a direct view into the hip joint. By applying longitudinal traction through a femoral pin or a partially threaded pin up the femoral neck, the acetabulum can be exposed and irrigated prior to fracture reduction. Alternatively, the hip can be gently redislocated for initial debridement of cartilage and bony fragments often present in the joint. Care should be taken to avoid dissecting capsular insertion from posterior wall fragments except as needed for mobilization. When a posterior wall fragment extends high onto the lateral aspect of the dome, release of the superior capsule is often necessary in order to bring the fragment inferior.

Comments

The primary structure at risk during the posterior approach is the sciatic nerve, and one cannot over stress the importance of close and careful monitoring. Peroneal palsy is often related to initial as well as iatrogenic/surgical trauma to the nerve and can result in significant morbidity. The exposure itself should rely on minimal subperiosteal stripping as already noted and minimal use of electrocautery. Reduction of posterior wall fragments often requires removal of soft tissue for several millimeters adjacent to fracture lines, but all attempts should be made to avoid complete stripping of bony fragments. Preservation of the blood supply to the femoral head contained in the quadratus femorus is essential and this muscle belly should rarely if ever be transected. The reported incidence of heterotopic ossification varies according to fracture pattern and prophylaxis following surgery, but intraoperative techniques used to minimize risk include hemostasis, debridement of nonviable muscle, aggressive irrigation, and deep drainage to avoid hematoma in the gluteal region.

MODIFICATION—GREATER TROCHANTERIC OSTEOTOMY

If a Kocher–Lagenbach posterior approach is undertaken and exposure appears inadequate, there are several tricks for adding exposure. The proximal 1–2 cm of the gluteus maximus sling may be tagged and detached, leaving a tendinous cuff to repair. This permits further posterior retraction of the gluteus maximus, may allow greater visualization and a wider field, particularly in patients who are somewhat obese.

If further extension into the superior and lateral aspects of the ilium and the lateral aspect of the dome must be obtained, greater trochanteric osteotomy may be performed. Through retraction of the skin and tensor fascia anteriorly, the anterior and posterior aspects of the greater trochanter may be visualized. The deep aspect of the gluteus medius is then identified and dissected away from the gluteus minimus right at the level of the femoral head and neck. With a combination of direct visualization laterally and use of a clamp on the deep surface of the medius, the anterior margin of the medius is better defined, particularly distally at the insertion on the greater trochanter. Once this border has been cleanly defined and the deep surface of the gluteus medius is likewise elucidated, osteotomy may be performed in a variety of ways.

At conclusion of the operation, the osteotomy may be secured with tension band, with two screws, or with any combination of these fixation methods. The method of fixation to be used at closure must be considered at the time of osteotomy. If two screws are to be used, predrilling may be employed. The intended path of the screws is from the tip of the greater trochanter to the lesser trochanter for bicortical purchase. Three-five screws, four-five screws, and six-five screws have all been employed. Ideally, screws should be evenly spaced from anterior to posterior, with full bicortical purchase to resist the pull of the abductors when the patient is awakened.

Small longitudinal incisions may be made inline with the fibers of the gluteus medius tendon down to the level of the bone prior to predrilling. Electrocautery or skin markers may be used to identify these soft tissue dissections at the conclusion of the case. Osteotomy of the greater trochanter has been described by various methods. Osteotomes, power oscillating saws, and Gigli saws have all been employed. Similarly, a wide variety of osteotomy patterns have been used. The Gigli method will be described here.

After adequate separation between the gluteus medius and gluteus minimus, a Gigli saw is passed deep to the gluteus medius tendon. It is placed down along the angle between the base of the greater trochanter and the top of the femoral shaft. Careful retraction is used to preserve soft tissues. Saw is advanced on a largely distal vector. As the visible ends of the Gigli saw appear closer to one another, signifying that the cut is nearing lateral completion, the vector is taken due laterally and the cut is completed. Before completion of the cut, an instrument should be placed over the greater trochanter by an assistant to prevent the recoil of the Gigli saw blade toward the head of the operator.

The medius is then reflected in cephalad direction. This provides extensive exposure to the lateral ilium and the lateral acetabular dome. Capsulotomy may be performed or extended if traumatic capsulotomy exists. Extending the capsulotomy in a cephalad direction will often permit dislocation at this time.

Closure of the trochanteric extension entails repair of the minimus (if taken down), closure of the capsule, and repair of the osteotomy. As mentioned previously, the osteotomy may be repaired with two screws, or this may be supplemented with a tension band wire around the heads of these two screws and introduced through drill holes in the lateral cortex of the distal greater trochanter.

Potential complications of the trochanteric osteotomy focus mostly on the osteotomy itself. Nonunion rates in the literature range from 0% to 39%. In the immediate postoperative period, patients are typically restricted from active abduction for a period of four to six weeks. Trochanteric osteotomy may be further complicated by splitting of the bony fragment or cutting too small of a bony fragment with the osteotomy. This may be addressed with supplementation of the repair with sutures through drill holes in the proximal femur and passed through the gluteus medius tendon.

The advantages of trochanteric osteotomy include greater superior and lateral exposure, more ease of dislocation and intra-articular examination, and extension of capsulotomy.

MODIFIED EXTENSILE LATERAL APPROACH

The modified extensile approach, also known as the extensile, the Maryland approach, or the Texas T, is a modification of the extended iliofemoral approach described by Letournel and Judet. This approach is first described by Reinert et al. in 1988 and provides extensive visualization of the entire lateral ilium, the inner table of the ilium, the posterior column, and intra-articular visualization of the joint.

The approach mobilizes the abductor muscles via osteotomies of their origins and insertions to yield an abductor mass pedicled on the superior gluteal neurovascular bundle at the sciatic notch. Essentially, this approach combines a Smith–Peterson and a Kocher–Lagenbach with a connection through the distal portion of the tensor fascia muscle belly. This is most useful for comminuted both-column fractures, transverse plus posterior wall with extensive anterior displacement, widely displaced transverse patterns, T-type, and anterior column posterior hemitransverse.

The patient is placed in a lateral position. An axillary roll is used and care is taken to well pad all decubitus areas. A radiolucent table is used to facilitate fluoroscopy. The operative hemipelvis and hind quarter are prepped and draped free. Cutaneous flaps are planned out with a marker prior to incision. Lying 1 cm distal to, and parallel to, the crest of the ilium, the transverse portion extends from just anterior to the posterior superior iliac spine forward to the anterior superior iliac spine. With the hip in neutral flexion, a T-perpendicular is extended in the direction of the greater trochanter, and then from the greater trochanter, extending distally down along the shaft of the femur. The transverse portion of the incision is 8 to 10 cm and the vertical limb extends to a point approximately 15 cm distal to the greater trochanter.

Dissection is taken directly down to the layer of the fascia. Full thickness skin flaps are then raised anteriorly and posteriorly. These may be then retracted with nonabsorbable monofilament suture by tacking the cutaneous flaps to the skin anteriorly and posteriorly. Damp sponges are placed over the cutaneous flaps to avoid desiccation of the exposed fatty tissues. After elevation of the anterior flap, the belly of the tensor fascia lata muscles will be evident. The Smith–Peterson interval between the sartorius and tensor fascia lata is then developed.

The hip is then flexed and a bolster is placed between the knees. The fascia lata is then opened longitudinally on the posterior margin of the femur in what would normally be the fascial incision of the Kocher–Lagenbach approach. Proximally the dissection divides between the fibers of the gluteus maximus. The most distal tendon insertion in the gluteus maximus may be partially released after being tagged to allow better mobilization of the posterior mass of the gluteus maximus.

The hip is then extended and the anterior dissection between the tensor fascia lata and the sartorius is further developed. Likewise, the division between rectus femoris and the deep aspect of the tensor fascia lata is better defined.

The ascending branch of the lateral femoral circumflex artery is identified at this time. It is divided and ligated with surgical clips. The careful marking and division of this vascular bundle has been emphasized by authors in this approach as a potential revascularization site. When the entire flap is elevated, it will be dependent upon the superior gluteal artery. If this were to fail, the only revascularization potential for the abductor mass would be through reanastamosis of the ascending branch of the lateral femoral circumflex artery.

The anterior (Smith–Peterson interval) and posterior (K–L interval) approaches are then connected. A transverse cut joins the two dissections approximately 2 cm proximal to the distal extent of the tensor fascia muscle belly. The original description of this approach describes dividing distal to the muscle belly, but the intramuscular division of this most distal aspect of the muscle is intended to help the healing of the fascia lata dissection.

Attention is then turned to mobilization of the abductor mass. The incision along the bare area of the superior aspect of the iliac crest is then elevated with electrocautery and a Cobb elevator. Abdominal and iliac muscles are elevated from the crest and inner table. From the inner table, the origin of the sartorius on the anterior–superior iliac spine is elevated. A 1 cm cut is made 1 cm posterior to the anterior–superior iliac spine. A second cut is then made at 90° to this and extended in the anterior direction. This mobilizes the origin of the sartorius on the osteotomized anterior superior iliac spine (ASIS) fragment. The sartorius is then elevated in an anterior direction.

One centimeter distal to the top of the crest on the inner table, a 90° power cutting tool such as a Midas Rex or Black Max is introduced. Mirroring the crest of the ilium, a transverse osteotomy of both tables is performed from the inside of the ilium. This extends back for 10 to 15 cm. This osteotomized piece of superior iliac crest is then elevated and Cobb is used to perform subperiosteal elevation of the abductor muscles off the lateral aspect of the ilium. This is the first of two osteotomies designed to mobilize abductor mass.

Trochanteric osteotomy is then performed. Abductor mass, specifically the gluteus medius, is elevated from the lateral capsule. Osteotomy may be performed with a Gigli saw, osteotome, or power cutting instrument. Osteotomy may be predrilled to plan for later fixation with two screws.

The entire abductor mass is then mobilized and peeled back off the ilium. The greater sciatic notch is visualized. The superior gluteal neurovascular bundle is then visualized on the underside of the abductor mass. The pulse should be easily appreciable. The abductor mass, along with the two bony osteotomized fragments, is then wrapped in a damp sponge to help prevent desiccation of this pedicled muscle flap.

The short external rotators may be released as they are in the Kocher–Lagenbach approach. Capsulotomy may be performed for visualization of the joint. This is best accomplished with a Schanz pin from the proximal lateral femur into the lesser trochanter. The hind limb may then be elevated out of the acetabulum with the use of traction table or surgical assistant.

Forward elevation of the iliopsoas off the inner table will provide visualization all the way down to the true pelvic brim and all the way back to the anterior sacroiliac joint. For further visualization of the anterior column, direct and indirect heads of rectus femoris may be released anteriorly. It has been noted that if there is a free fragment of acetabular dome and both heads of rectus are released, this may devascularize the acetabular dome fragment.

Flexion and extension of the hip will aid in extending exposure. Lateral elevation of the femur and femoral head will allow visualization of the joint space. Placement of a bolster between the thighs quite proximally will also help in lateral elevation of the femoral head.

Reduction and fixation are achieved in the usual manner. At closure, a drain is placed in the iliac fossa and a drain is placed deep to the abductor mass; both of these exit superiorly and anteriorly. All the osteotomies are repaired with 3.5 mm cortical screws. The trochanteric osteotomy or the sartorius osteotomy may be supplemented with tension band. If the rectus femoris is released, this is repaired with suture.

Interrupted figure of eight sutures are then used to repair the posterior approach as well as the tensor fascia. The corners of the distal aspect of the tensor fascia division are repaired first. Suture may be used on the deep aspect of the cutaneous flaps to close down some of the dead space. Two-layer closure of subcutaneous tissues is usually performed. Skin is closed by whatever means deemed appropriate by the surgeon.

This approach offers utilitarian access to the entire hemipelvis and may be intra-articular if deemed necessary. The most common complication reported in literature was heterotopic ossification (HO), and the Brooker grade of HO was reduced in those patients that were irradiated. There were no nonunions of the osteotomies reported.

Though not reported in Starr's paper on complications of the T extensile approach, anecdotally, several surgeons have found that this approach has a high risk of wound complications in obese patients. Perhaps this has been associated with raising thick cutaneous flaps in patients with potentially suboptimal blood supply to the skin.

Additional cautionary note on this approach concerns the blood supply to the abductor muscle mass. If the fracture being treated extends in the greater sciatic notch with significant displacement, or embolization of the superior gluteal artery has been attempted, then this approach must certainly be undertaken with great caution. The original description of this approach recommended angiography prior to undertaking this approach to confirm patency of the superior gluteal artery. This is no longer practiced very widely. In those cases where there is a high degree of suspicion of superior gluteal artery injury, however, one must certainly consider this preoperative and diagnostic option. This approach may be undertaken by two attending surgeons with one working the front and one working the back. If working alone, this will lead to a prolonged operative time, as much time and energy may be dedicated to the approach alone. In the right patient population with a fracture demanding extensive exposure, the modified extensile must certainly be considered.

ANTERIOR APPROACH

The anterior, or ilioinguinal approach, was developed by Letournel to facilitate an extensile exposure of the anterior pelvis from the SI joint to the syphysis while minimizing associated morbidity. By avoiding injury to the abductor musculature, early functional recovery is accelerated and the incidence of heterotopic bone is small in comparison to extensile lateral approaches. Its major disadvantages are potentially unfamiliar anatomy with several major structures at risk, as well as limited direct visualization of the fracture making reduction difficult. While some posterior column and transverse fractures can be reduced and stabilized through this approach, it is not possible to address posterior wall and posterior marginal impaction fractures. If significant both-column injuries exist or in combined anterior/posterior fracture patterns the ilioinguinal approach can be combined with a simultaneous or staged posterior approach. The morbidity of this combined technique is generally less than an extensile approach.

Pertinent Anatomy

Unlike the posterior approach, much of the anterior anatomy is unfamiliar to many orthopedic surgeons. Three abdominal wall flat muscles, the external oblique, the internal oblique, and the transversus abdominus are integral to the superficial approach. The three combine for a single fascial insertion on the anterior iliac crest, but, below the ASIS, the three divide to form the roof and floor of the inguinal canal. The external oblique forms the roof of the canal down to the superficial inguinal ring, and the internal oblique and transversus abdominus fuse inferiorly to form the conjoint tendon, which creates the floor of the inguinal canal. All three then rejoin to form the inguinal ligament. The inguinal canal itself permits passage of the spermatic cord (males) or round ligament (females), measures approximately 4 to 5 cm in adults, and extends from the deep inguinal ring (a defect in the fascia of the transverses abdominus) to the superficial inguinal ring.

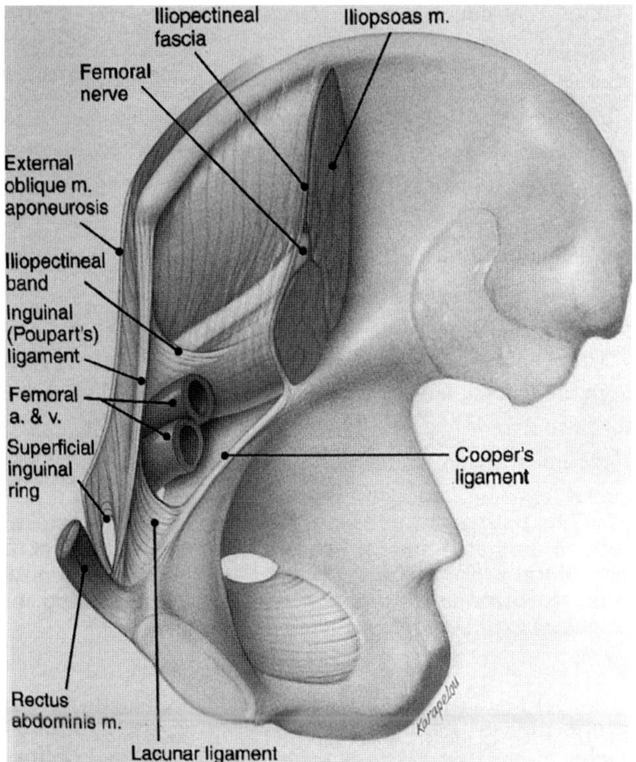

Figure 2 The anterior approach requires full comfort with the compartmentalized anatomy.

Two distinct compartments exist beneath the inguinal ligament that are fundamental to this approach (Fig. 2). The lateral compartment contains the iliopsoas and the femoral and lateral femoral cutaneous nerves, while the medial compartment contains the femoral artery, vein, and lymphatics. Dividing the two is a distinct band—the iliopectineal fascia, a vertical expansion of the fascia iliaca—extending along the pelvic brim from the anterior SI joint to the pectineal eminence. Careful identification of all these structures is essential to the ilioinguinal approach.

Surgical Approach

The patient is usually positioned either supine or floppy lateral, depending on the potential for a combined posterior approach. If a lateral position is chosen, a beanbag is most often used for stability and can be deflated, allowing the patient to fall back to a more supine position once the patient has been prepped and draped. Alternatively, the patient can be left lateral and a true simultaneous anterior and posterior dissection can take place utilizing two experienced surgeons, although the anterior anatomy is more difficult to appreciate in this position.

The skin incision extends from the lateral iliac crest inferiorly to the ASIS and then follows the inguinal ligament inferiomedially to a point one to two fingerbreadths above the syphysis. The proximal aspect of the incision should be either medial or lateral to the actual bony iliac crest, not directly over it. Deep fatty tissues are divided until the abdominal muscular fascial insertion on the crest is well visualized, and this exposure is extended to the roof of the inguinal canal and the superficial inguinal ring. The fascial insertion on the iliac crest is divided and the abdominal musculature and iliacus are mobilized from the inner table of the iliac wing. Digital dissection or dissection with a Cobb elevator is used to extend the exposure of the inner ilium back to the SI joint.

By extending the superficial dissection to the midline, the spermatic cord and superficial inguinal ring are identified along with the rectus sheath. The aponeurosis or fascia of the external oblique is incised parallel to the skin incision from the ASIS to the superficial inguinal ring. This can be done with a knife or with curved scissors inserted at the ring. It is essential that at least 1 cm of inferior fascia remains for closure, and care should be taken to avoid injury to the contents of the inguinal canal. Once the canal is unroofed, the cord or round ligament is identified and protected, and the floor of the canal and inguinal ligament are exposed from the pubic tubercle to the ASIS. By retracting the inguinal canal contents medially using a penrose drain and the inferior fascia of the external oblique caudally using nondestructive clamps (i.e., Alice), the conjoint tendon can be well visualized at its insertion onto the inguinal ligament (Fig. 3). A knife is used to carefully incise the conjoint tendon in line with its fibers, beginning laterally at the ASIS. The lateral femoral cutaneous nerve usually runs deep to this layer approximately 1 cm below the ASIS, and care should be taken to avoid cutting it accidentally. The use of a 15 blade in a "controlled plunging" technique, as opposed to a standard cutting technique, often allows one to divide the conjoint tendon while avoiding transection of the nerve running just beneath it. It is crucial that several millimeters of tendon remain inferior to this division or repair and closure will be difficult. Once the iliopsoas muscle belly is visualized, deep palpation below the remaining conjoint tendon will usually reveal the location of a deep, vertically oriented, fascial band: the iliopectineal fascia (Fig. 4). Identification at this point can aid significantly in orienting the surgeon to the location of the medial deep compartment containing the femoral vessels, thus avoiding iatrogenic injury and significant bleeding. With the hip flexed, a one-inch penrose can be passed around the iliopsoas and femoral nerve.

The conjoint tendon often thins out considerably as it extends medial to the iliopectineal fascia, and it is therefore often difficult to define and preserve a true floor to the inguinal canal at this point. What is more important is defining the iliopectineal fascia, both medially and laterally, ensuring that the pulse of the femoral artery is medial to the defined fascia. Division of the fascia is best performed using scissors, direct visualization, and minimal blind extension deep into the pelvis. Occasionally, the obturator vessels take anomalous origin from the external iliac or inferior epigastric vessels and can be in near proximity to the iliopectineal fascia, the so-called "corona mortis." For this reason, it is a safe practice to palpate the fascia closely in an attempt to identify any significant vessels and cauterize or ligate them prior to division. Another simple technique to avoid uncontrolled bleeding is to clamp the thicker anterior portion of the fascia proximally and distally, divide the fascia using electrocautery, and carefully release the hemostats under direct visualization. Once the fascia has been divided, digital dissection deep to the vessels up to the syphysis is performed, and a one-inch penrose is placed around the vessels. Depending on the degree of medial exposure

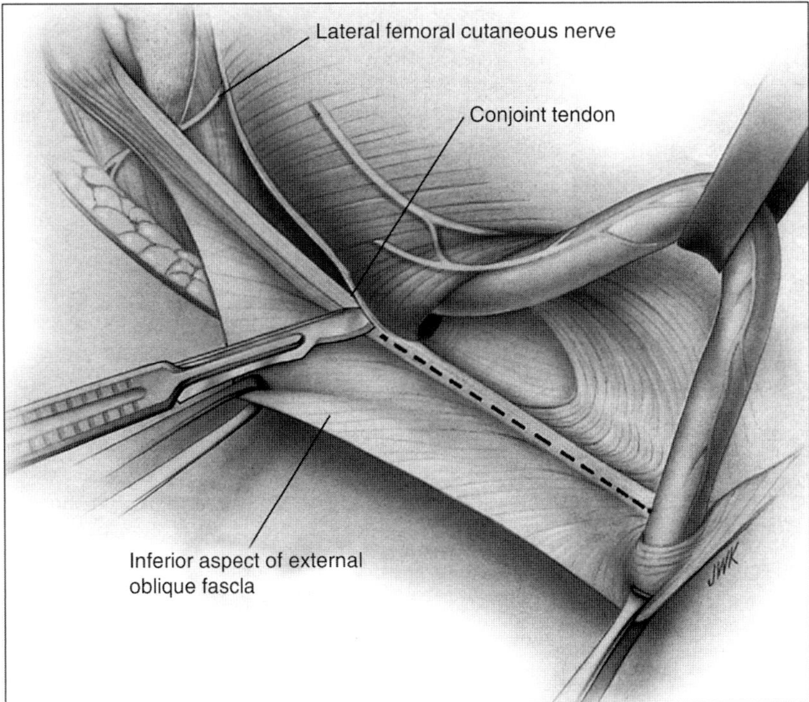

Figure 3 With the external oblique fascia retracted inferiorly, the floor of the inguinal canal is opened sharply. Retaining fascia on the superior limb greatly assists with closure.

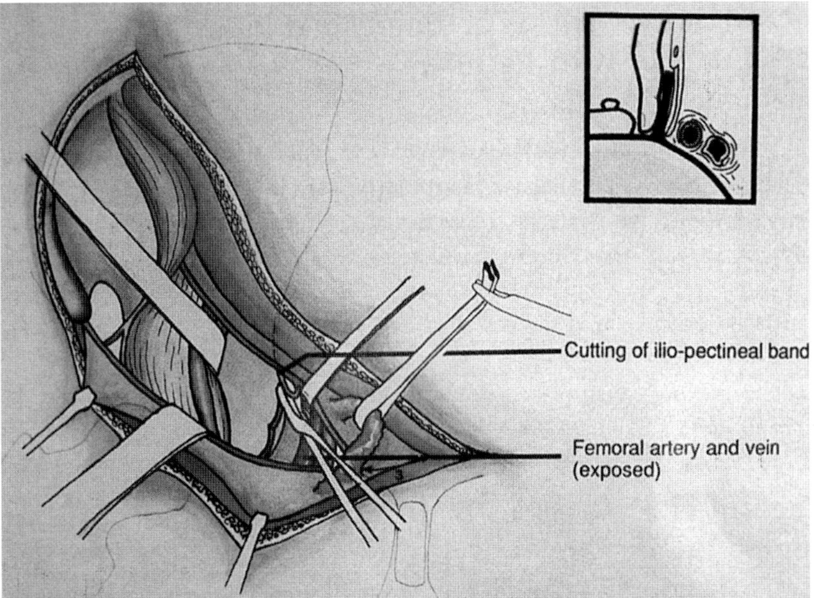

Figure 4 After dissecting medially and laterally, the ileopectineal fascias is incised under direct visualization.

necessary, the rectus fascia can be divided at its insertion onto the syphysis, making sure again tissue remains distally for closure purposes.

At this point three distinct intervals exist for visualization and reduction. By retracting the iliopsoas and femoral nerve medially, the inner table of the iliac wing and pelvic brim are exposed; the so-called first window or interval. With lateral retraction of these structures and medial retraction of the femoral vessels, the second window or interval is established. Lateral retraction of the vessels and medial retraction of intact rectus creates the third interval or window, exposing the superior pubic ramus and syphysis. Deep periosteal elevation and exposure of anterior fracture elements can be performed using a combination of direct visualization and digital palpation.

STOPPA MODIFICATION OF THE ILIOINGUINAL APPROACH

This approach was first described by Cole and Bolhofner as a limited approach through a transverse midline Pfannenstiel incision and was previously described in the hernia literature as an anterior intrapelvic approach.

This has been used both as a modified, limited intrapelvic approach or as an extension on the traditional ilioinguinal. The Stoppa approach offers good visualization of the true pelvic rim and quadrilateral plate in patterns that include significant protrusion and low pelvic comminution, which must be approached anteriorly.

The standard ilioinguinal approach, which is 2 cm proximal to the pubic symphysis at the midline, is extended across the midline in slight cephalad curve as it proceeds toward the contralateral hip. Typically, the incision is taken 3 cm across the midline.

The third window of the ilioinguinal approach is defined medially by the lateral margin of the rectus abdominus and rectus insertion on the pubic tubercle. The rectus abdominus is then split vertically along the linea alba up to 5 cm above the pubic symphysis. Care is taken to stay extraperitoneal at the proximal extension. The rectus insertion is carefully defined from the medial border of the third window to the base of the vertical midline incision. Nonabsorbable, large diameter sutures are then used to tag the medial and lateral edges of this hemirectus insertion. These will be used as tagging sutures after retraction of the rectus in the cephalad direction. Rectus insertion is then divided, with a small cuff tissue left to facilitate repair. A working knowledge of the anatomy of rectus insertion is helpful at this time. The rectus inserts at the top of the pubis and insertion envelopes the cephalad and ventral aspects of the entire pubic tubercle.

Malleable retractor is then placed to protect the bladder. For examination of the fracture within the true pelvis and for reduction, the operating surgeon then stands on the opposite side of the table from the affected hip. This allows the surgeon to "look back" inside the true pelvis from the contralateral side. The retractors will be held by an assistant physician on the side of the table ipsilateral to the fracture.

Along the lateral border of the rectus, inferior epigastric or external iliac vessels will have been identified and must be ligated. An anastamotic connection ("corona mortis") between inferior epigastric or external iliac and obturator vessels, if present, must also be ligated.

As with the ilioinguinal approach, the Stoppa modification requires the hemipelvis and hind limb on the affected side to be draped free. Flexion of the hip on this side reduces tension on the iliopsoas, femoral nerve, and external iliac vessels to allow better access to the upper pelvis and iliac wing.

Of the acetabular approaches, the Stoppa approach shares with the ilioinguinal that it is the only approach that is intrapelvic, but likewise it is exclusively extra-articular. No direct visualization of the joint can be accomplished. Further exposure of the iliopectoneal and obturator fascias and the quadrilateral plate are afforded by this modification, but further dissection of the external vessels also must be undertaken with care and the obturator nerve must be visualized and respected. Furthermore, care must be taken not to extend too proximal or to become intraperitoneal with the approach. Posterior retraction must also be careful to avoid the lumbosacral trunk.

Closure is performed over drains. A drain is placed in the space of Retzius as with a standard ilioinguinal approach. Large diameter nonabsorbable sutures are used to repair the medial and lateral aspects of the rectus origin from the affected side. Interrupted figure of eight nonabsorbable sutures are then used in an interrupted fashion between these two corners. Interrupted figure of eight nonabsorbable sutures are used to repair the midline split of the linea alba. The remainder of the closure proceeds as per standard ilioinguinal approach.

The main advantage of the Stoppa modification or extension of the ilioinguinal approach is for further visualization of the true pelvic brim and quadrilateral plate. This may be helpful in especially low fractures that are being repaired from the front, and in the obese patient where adequate visualization is difficult.

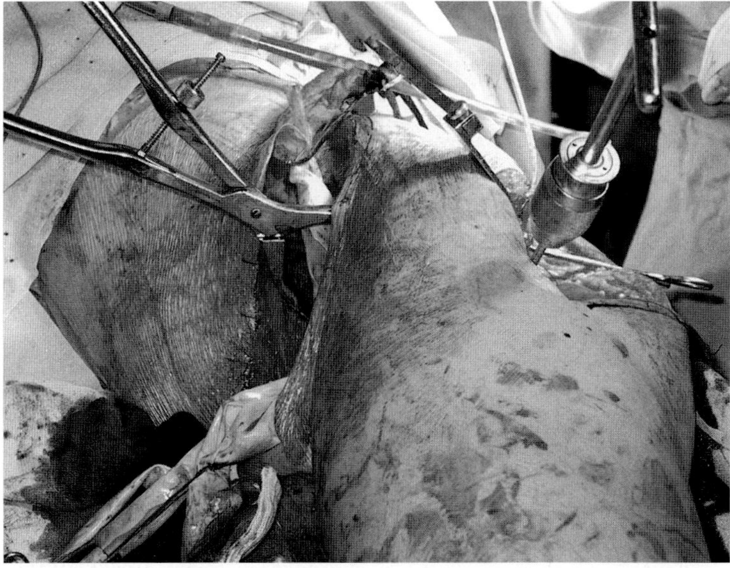

Figure 5 The patient positioned in a sloppy lateral allows simultaneous anterior and posterior approaches. The morbidity of this technique is significantly less than an extensile lateral approach.

Modified Anterior Approach

Occasionally it is necessary to obtain more direct exposure to the anterior wall or femoral head and this can be accomplished by combining the ilioinguinal approach with the Smith–Peterson iliofemoral approach. A vertical extension to the skin incision is made just distal to the ASIS, and the interval between the sartorius and the tensor fascia latae is developed. If visualization of the anterior femoral head is required, the rectus femoris origin may be divided. In addition, if exposure of the lateral ilium is desired, the sartorius origin may be osteotomized and the anterior lateral musculature can be stripped. Unfortunately, these maneuvers significantly increases the incidence of heterotopic ossification.

COMMENTS

Modifications of the ilioinguinal approach and combined anterior/posterior techniques continue to gain in popularity as extensile lateral approaches have a significantly higher morbidity (Fig. 5). Unfortunately the dissection and visualization using the anterior approach can be extremely difficult and has a fairly steep learning curve. One problem associated with a simultaneous anterior/posterior approach in the sloppy lateral position is the tendency of gravity to displace the femoral head medially. This can be overcome by utilizing a modified lateral traction apparatus to unload the acetabulum.

BIBLIOGRAPHY

Cole JD, Bolhofner BR. Acetabular fracture fixation via modified Stoppa limited intrapelvic approach. Clin Orthop 1994; 305:112–123.

de Ridder VA, de Lange S, v. Popta J. Anatomical variations of the lateral femoral cutaneous nerve and consequences for surgery. J Orthop Trauma 1999; 13(3):207–211.

Gautier E, Ganz K, Krugel N, et al. Anatomy of the medial femoral circumflex artery and its surgical implications. J Bone Joint Surg 2000; 82B(5):679–683.

Gorczyca JT, Powell JN, Tile M. Lateral extension of the ilioinguinal incision in the operative treatment of acetabulum fractures. Injury 1995; 26(3):207–212.

Hospodar PP, Ashman ES, Traub JA. Anatomic study of the lateral femoral cutaneous nerve with respect to the ilioinguinal surgical dissection. J Orthop Trauma 1999; 13(1):17–19.

Kloen P, Siebenrock KA, Ganz R. Modification of the ilioinguinal approach. J Orthop Trauma 2002; 16(8):586–593.

Letournel E. The treatment of acetabular fractures through the ilioinguinal approach. Clin Orthop 1993; 292:62–76.

Matta JM. Operative treatment of acetabular fractures through the ilioinguinal approach. Clin Orthop 1994; 305:10–19.

Reinert CM, Bosse MJ, Poka A, et al. A modified extensile exposure for the treatment of complex or malunited acetabular fractures. J Bone Joint Surg 1988; 76A(3):329–337.

Routt MLC, Swiontkowski MF. Operative treatment of complex acetabular fractures. J Bone Joint Surg 1990; 72A(6):897–903.

Starr AJ, Watson JT, Reinert CM, et al. Complications following the "T extensile" approach: a modified extensile approach for acetabular fracture surgery—report of forth-three patients. J Orthop Trauma 2002; 16(8):535–542.

11

Acetabular Reconstruction: Fixation Methods in Simple Fracture Patterns

Bruce H. Ziran
Department of Orthopaedic Trauma, St. Elizabeth Health Center and Department of Orthopaedic Surgery, Northeastern Ohio Universities College of Medicine, Youngstown, Ohio, U.S.A.

Daniel R. Schlatterer and Robert M. Harris
Atlanta Medical Center, Department of Orthopaedic Trauma, Atlanta, Georgia, U.S.A.

INTRODUCTION TO SIMPLE FRACTURE PATTERNS OF THE ACETABULUM

Acetabular surgery is one of the more intensive and complex surgeries performed in orthopaedics. This includes the complexity of the surgical dissection, the significant risk of neurovascular and or visceral injury, and the three-dimensional challenge of reducing and fixing the fracture itself. An important aspect of acetabular fracture surgery should be the establishment of expectations for both the surgeon and the patient. Surgeons should be expected to have dedication to improving their skills and be diligent about analyzing and monitoring their own results, in an effort to learn, and improve, their outcomes. So, prior to embarking on such an endeavor, and during their careers managing acetabular fractures, surgeons should make efforts to learn from their own experiences, as well as those of others. The patient's expectations should also be established. They should be informed that even in the hands of subject-matter experts, the outcomes are not uniformly excellent. Preoperative counseling with the patient and family members should include a discussion of expected outcomes. In this section, we review techniques used for obtaining reduction, as well as propose a method of fixation.

PLANNING AND OPERATIVE TACTIC

The simple acetabular fractures, while basic in their pattern, are not always the simplest fractures for treatment. After careful preoperative evaluation and planning, the fixation methods usually employ some type of screw or plate fixation. The amount of fixation required is variable, and there will be many opinions. There is no set rule, except to make sure there is stable fixation of the essential elements of the reduced fracture. Whether this is achieved percutaneously, or with extensile approaches, the goals are an acceptable reduction and a stable fixation until healing. With regard to approaches, we have found that the vast majority of fractures with simple patterns can be fixed through one approach. Recently, adjunctive techniques and new "windows" have been developed that help preclude the necessity for more extensile approaches. Occasionally, a second simultaneous or sequential approach is needed, but rarely are extensile approaches required for simple fracture patterns.

An important aspect of acetabular fracture surgery should be the establishment of expectations for both the surgeon and the patient. Surgeons should be expected to have dedication to improving their skills and be diligent about analyzing and monitoring their own results, in an effort to learn, and improve, their outcomes. Acetabular surgery is one of the more intensive and complex surgeries performed in orthopedics. This includes but is not limited to the complexity of the surgical dissection, the significant risk of neurovascular and or visceral injury, and the three-dimensional challenge of reducing and fixing the fracture itself. So, prior to embarking on such an endeavor, and during their careers managing acetabular fractures, surgeons should make efforts to learn from their own experiences as well as those of others. The patient's expectations should also be established. They should be informed that even in the hands of subject-matter experts, the outcomes are not uniformly excellent. Preoperative counseling with the patient and family members should include a discussion of expected outcomes. The avascular structure of cartilage limits its reparative potential. Thus, the combination of articular damage, slightly imperfect reductions, extensive surgical exposures, and load requirements of the hip joint will frequently result in some dysfunction. This may lead to early and rapid post-traumatic arthritis requiring secondary intervention. Thus, the goals of the surgeon and patient should be set at reasonable levels for each patient and fracture. For example, in the elderly, a lengthy operation and exposure to achieve perfection may be at too great a cost because of the associated and increased morbidity in this population. Some acetabular surgeons argue that restoration of the bony architecture and a "good enough" reduction may be all that is necessary, in anticipation of arthroplasty. Even so, many of the elderly are very resilient and may not require arthroplasty even in the face of significant post-traumatic arthritis.

The implants used for fixation will most frequently be some type of bendable reconstruction plate. The authors typically have a pelvic reconstruction set and a small fragment set open and available during the surgery. Recently, newer versions of reconstruction plates were introduced that allow the use of locked screws. While rarely needed, there are certain situations where locked screws may be beneficial, such as with osteoporotic bone and, for example, with long posterior column screws. The one instance where the authors have found locking plates to be very helpful has been for combined approaches (for example, a posterior approach followed by an ilioinguinal approach). This is because shorter screws can be used in the locking mode. Shorter locked screws in the posterior column have less of a chance of interfering with hardware placement in the ensuing anterior approach. Keep in mind that bending locking plates can alter the locking mechanism, and it is easier to redirect a nonlocking screw into good bone. Also, acetabular exposures are often confined spaces and the locking guides can be challenging to thread into the locking plate. Finally, despite the theoretical advantages of locking plates, clinical outcome studies are lacking. There are specialized pelvis/acetabular systems available that provide appropriate instrumentation including long screws, long drill bits, and plates. The workhorse plates are the 3.5 mm reconstruction plates, both straight and curved. The curvature has been determined from previous cadaveric work and approximates that of most pelvic brims. Other instruments include an assembly of appropriate reduction clamps, from standard bone forceps to the specialized pelvis and acetabular versions. The ball spike pusher is an invaluable tool, and we recommend two: one with a standard point, and the other with a spiked washer, which will help prevent iatrogenic fractures by distributing the reduction force. The authors recommend putting a saw bone pelvic model into a clear plastic sterile bag for intraoperative referencing. The model can be used for plate contouring and as a reference for safe screw placement.

Regarding the operative table and positioning, it is important to ensure adequate visualization of the entire fracture and the ability to have visual or digital palpation of the fracture reduction. Some of the specialized fracture tables are impractical and costly to obtain, but a radiolucent table is an essential element of this type of surgery. We have found that the radiolucent Jackson flat top table (OSI, Union City, California, U.S.A) is an excellent choice and can also be utilized for most other orthopedic fracture cases, which makes it cost-effective as well. It can be supplemented with various traction setups in order to achieve both longitudinal and lateral traction. We have been able to obtain longitudinal and lateral traction in supine, lateral, and prone positions with this system.

Surgical tactic has many variables, not the least of which is the number and experience of the assistants. A surgeon at a training program may have two to three extra pairs of hands and essentially an endless supply of "traction." Others practicing in a community setting must be more mindful of ergonomic factors. In either case, the surgeon must understand that traction for long periods of time has well-described complications. With regard to positioning of the patient, the ilioinguinal approach will necessitate a supine position. If exposure of the outer aspect of the ilium or placement of an ipsilateral iliosacral screw is required, the patient should be positioned closer to the edge of the table. Bean bag use is minimized as it can interfere with fluoroscopy. An appropriate "mini" bowel prep with a lower abdominal radiograph (KUB) before surgery is also recommended to ensure adequate visualization of the sacrum if percutaneous fixation is a possibility. If traction is used and the pelvis and limbs become somewhat "statically" positioned (as compared to free), then we recommend distal femoral traction and some pads under the thigh to allow hip flexion. Flexing the hip will help relax the iliopsoas muscles and greatly facilitates exposure (Fig. 1). Use of manual traction is performed by pulling on the leg or with use of a temporary 5-mm Schantz pin at the level of the lesser trochanter. Use of a radiolucent triangle is used for hip flexion

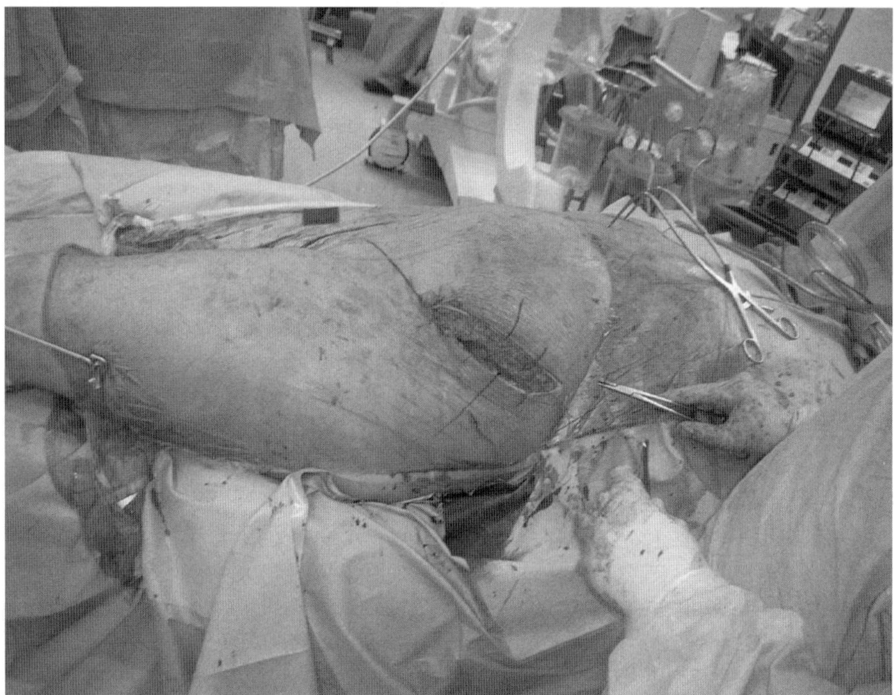

Figure 1 Supine positioning for ilioinguinal approach. Distal femoral traction can be employed. Alternatively, flexion of the hip (supported by a radiolucent triangle) will relax the iliopsoas muscle to facilitate exposure during reduction and fixation.

(thus relaxing the iliopsoas muscles). If an extensile approach such as the triradiate or the extended iliofemoral is used, the lateral position is most suitable. This will provide access to all aspects of the ilium and joint, but this approach is rarely done.

For the posterior approach, there are two alternatives for patient positioning, both with strong proponents. The traditional position for the Kocher–Langenbach approach has been prone with flexed knee traction. Proponents of this tactic cite a better access to the sciatic notch and a better ability to work through the notch for the "felt but not seen" portion of the pelvis. Also, the fact that the weight of the leg is not a force vector into the acetabulum medially or posteriorly (e.g., the femoral head is not opposing the reduction) is cited as an advantage. Placement of an anterior column screw or a sacroiliac screw is also permissible with prone positioning. However, access to more anterior structures is significantly limited as is the ability to perform an extended trochanteric osteotomy. Proponents of the lateral position cite ease of set up and access to the anterior structures. Those who are comfortable with a floppy lateral may also propose that it allows for simultaneous posterior and anterior approaches. A detriment to this tactic is the need for an extra assistant to neutralize the weight of the femoral head into the acetabulum. One of us (B.Z.) feels that the lateral position, when used with fixed (but adjustable) traction, provides the best of both methods. The perineal post and longitudinal femoral traction both neutralize the weight of the femur, and allow for subluxation of the joint. Note that the Jackson apparatus has an attachable arc that allows for traction and extension of the hip and a leg holder to allow flexion of the knee. These tactics allow for relaxation of the sciatic nerve (Fig. 2). Alternatively, others (D.S.) utilize a five to six-inch stack of folded towels placed deep into the groin between the legs. Gentle downward pressure at the flexed knee reduces the weight of the femoral head on the acetabulum. The stack of towels combined with longitudinal and lateral traction via the trochanteric Schantz pin results in very good joint exposure for many posterior fractures (Fig. 3). The lateral position also allows "neutralization" of the weight of the gluteal musculature and does not require an assistant for retraction. While proponents of the prone approach state that access to the notch and inner pelvis is difficult with the lateral approach, we have not found this to be the case. Also, if the need for an extended trochanteric flip osteotomy is needed, it can be done easily, and the spectrum of treatable fractures with this tactic is extended. Finally, if needed, the traction can easily be relaxed to allow minor positional changes.

We are not proponents of simultaneous front and back approaches because there is a distinct loss of visualization and access when the patient cannot be fully supine and fixed traction cannot be used (thus losing a major advantage of each approach). So, if front and back access is needed, we recommend sequential (do one, close, and flip over), and not simultaneous approaches. While these issues have been covered elsewhere, we believe it is salient to the discussions in this chapter and the next chapter,

(*Text continues on page 192.*)

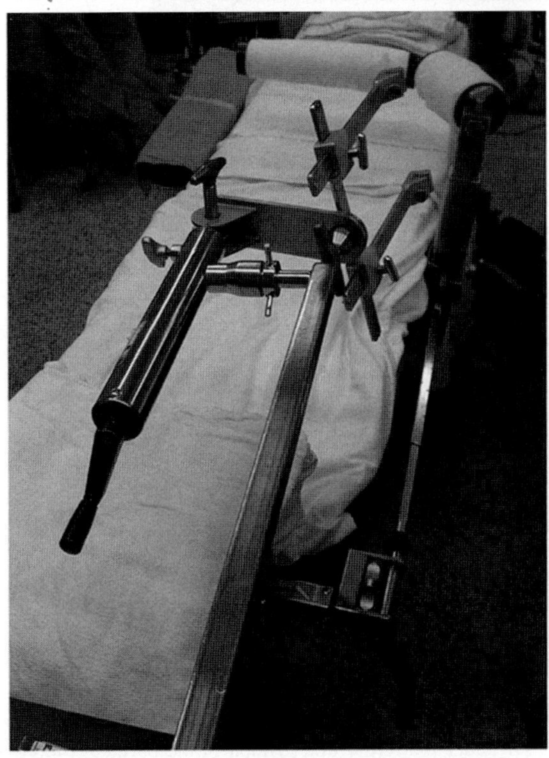

(A)

Figure 2 (**A**) The flat top Jackson table with longitudinal traction and perineal post. The perineal post can move vertically and thus provide a "lateral" vector to overcome the weight of the leg. Setup shown without patient. (*Continued*)

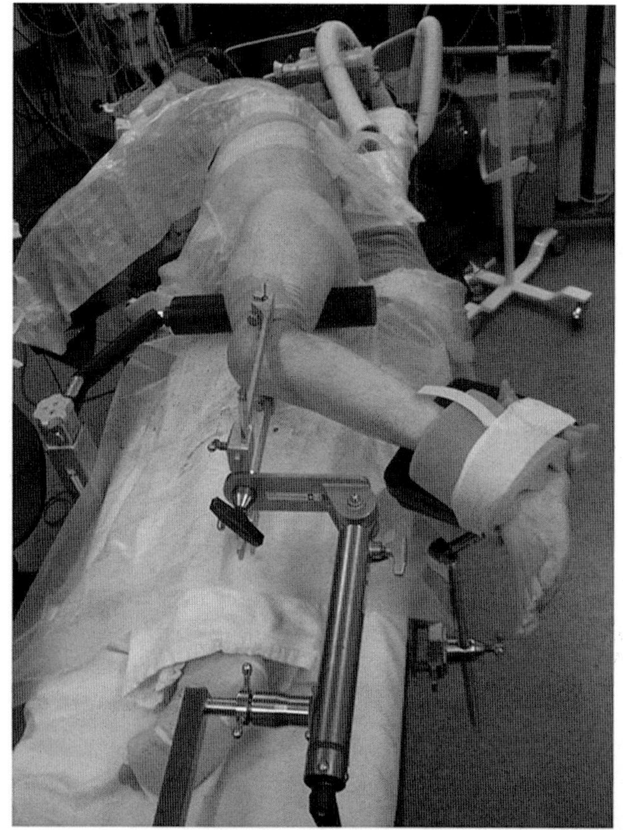

(B)

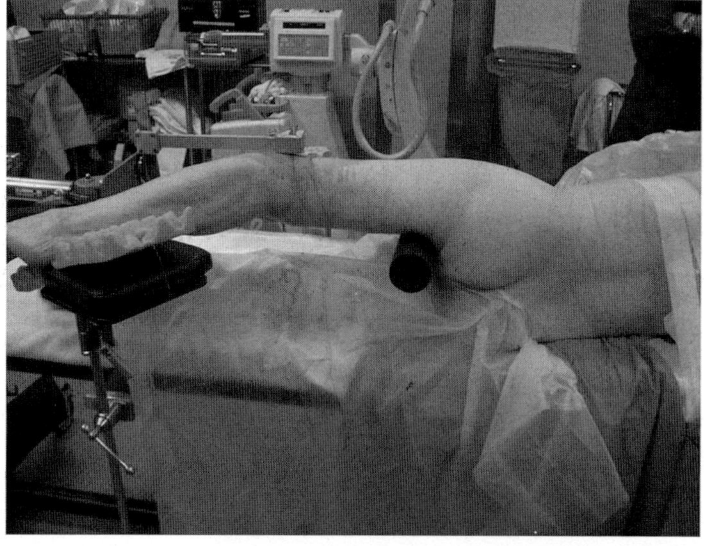

(C)

Figure 2 (*Continued*) (**B** and **C**) The patient in lateral position with longitudinal traction via femoral traction. The perineal post is set under the femur and padded in the perineum to counter the longitudinal force of the femoral traction, as well as provide a vertical lift. It can actually distract the joint laterally and lift the patient. For this reason, the patient has to be bound down to the table via taping and strapping.

(A)

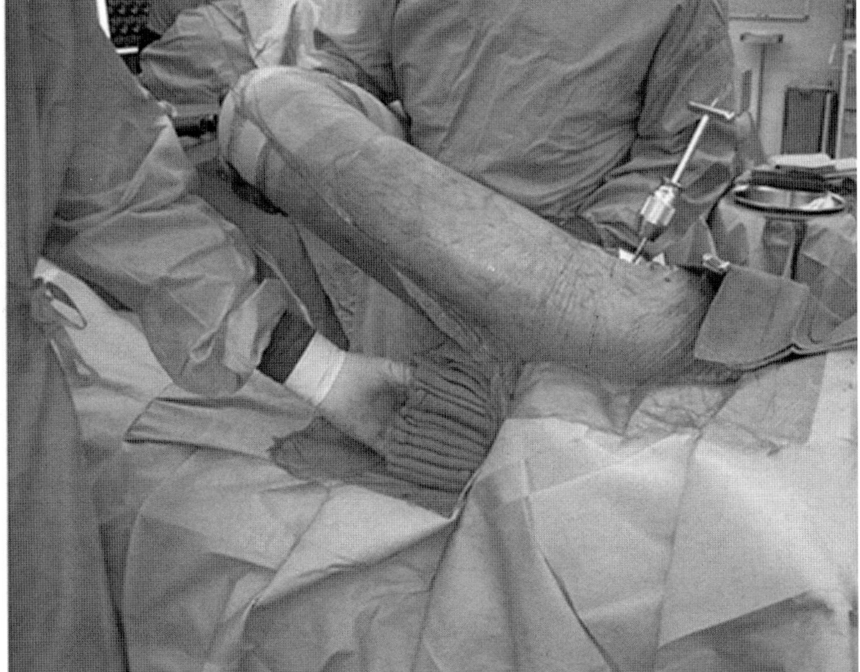

(B)

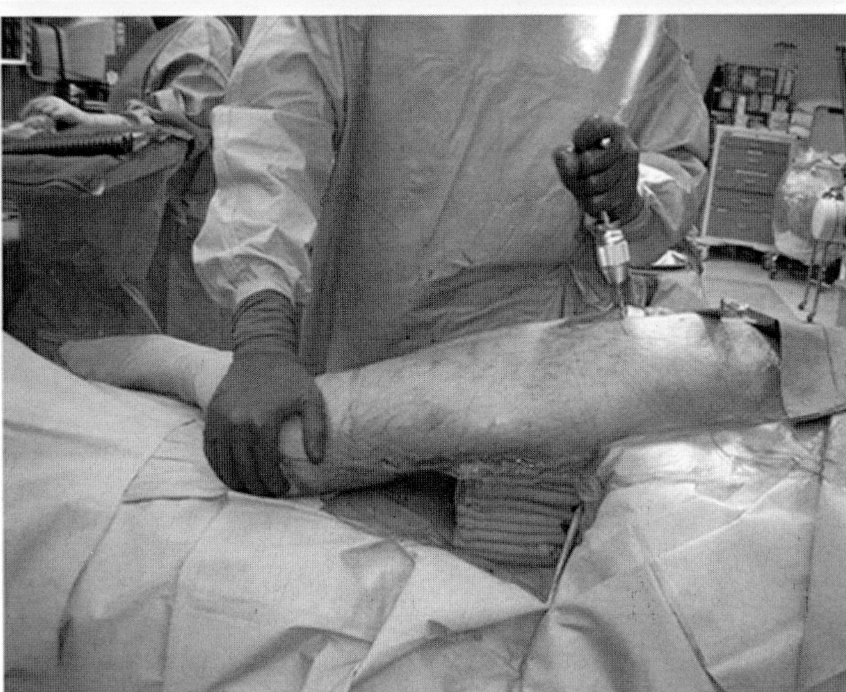

Figure 3 The patient in the lateral position with no fixed traction. A stack of towels tucked under the thigh acts as a fulcrum to assist with hip subluxation. Longitudinal traction is provided manually via the Schanz pin placed into the femur at the level of the trochanters. The extremity and hip are free for repositioning as needed.

and have included our personal views to facilitate discussion. As in many fractures, there are very strong opinions on indications, approach, and tactic, and the reader is referred to the literature for a more comprehensive view for each school of thought.

ANTERIOR WALL ACETABULAR FRACTURES

Isolated anterior wall fractures are relatively rare, and these fractures are usually a part of a more complex pattern. Normally, the ilioinguinal approach will be used to operate on anterior wall fractures with the patient in supine position on a radiolucent table. Unlike the posterior wall, access and fixation of the anterior wall may be a bit more difficult. In 2002, Kloen et al. reported their favorable experience in treating 15 patients with a modified ilioinguinal approach, which was combined with a Smith–Petersen anterior approach. An anterior superior iliac spine (ASIS) osteotomy is a component of this modified approach, and it greatly enhances access to the anterior wall (Fig. 4). In some cases of femoral head lesions with anterior or superior wall lesions, this approach can be very useful (Fig. 5).

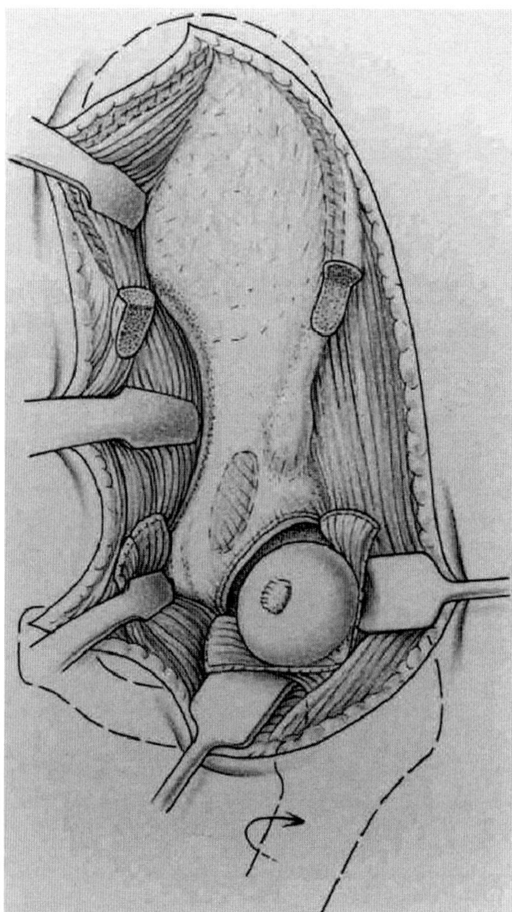

Figure 4 Schematic illustration of modified anterior approach for treatment of anterior wall fractures. Note anterior superior iliac spine osteotomy and release of rectus femoris insertion.

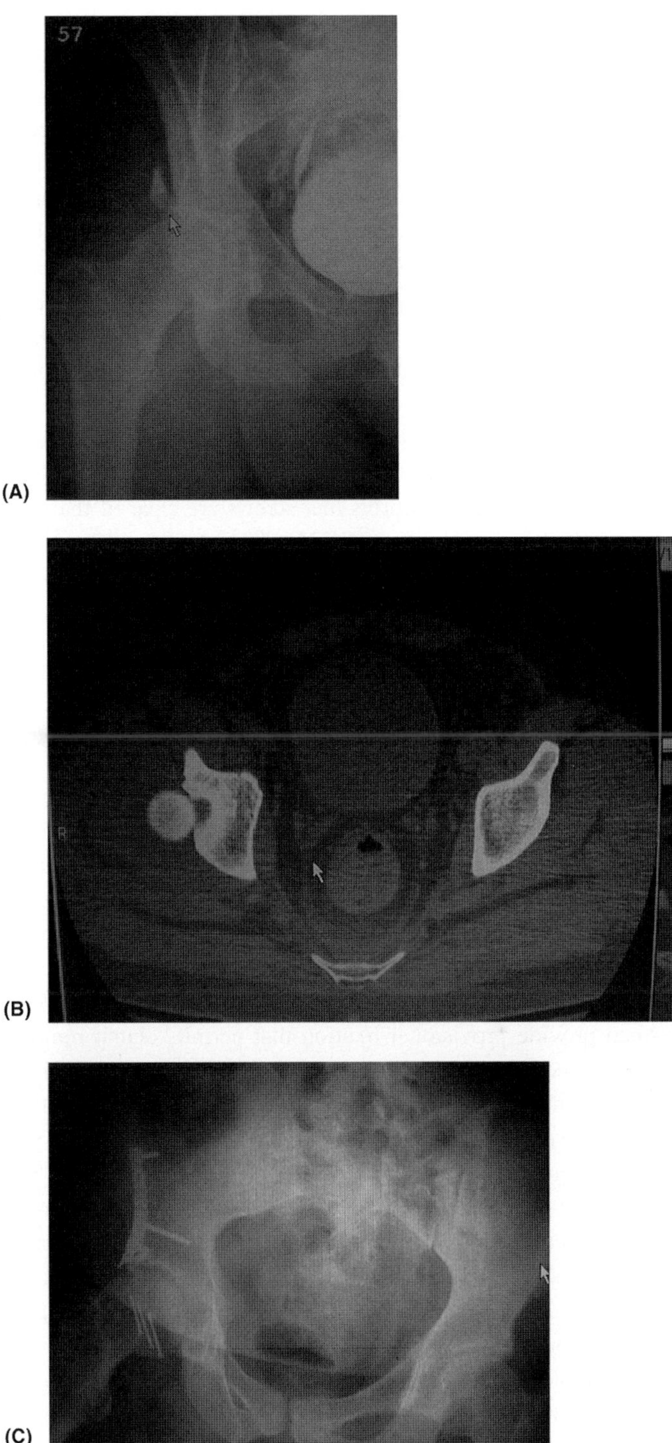

Figure 5 Use of an anterior approach for a superior wall fracture with femoral head fracture. Exposure of the external aspect of the iliac wing provides additional access to the superior anterior wall. (**A**, **B**) Radiograph and axial CT scan of the lesion. (**C**) Demonstrates repair of head and use of buttress plate using distal radial T plate to distribute force on small wall fragment.

If the wall is comminuted or with impaction, smaller implants (hand and foot) may be necessary for stabilization. In cases where the wall involves a portion of the quadrilateral surface there is more bone to consider, and adjunct screws along the corner of the brim or plates can be used. Use of a ball-spike pusher and clamps will generally be enough to reduce and hold the fragment. Kirschner wires can then be placed for provisional fixation, which permits removal of the clamps and facilitates plate positioning. A standard curved plate placed along the pelvic brim will frequently be enough to hold the wall in place. Similar to the posterior wall, the plate provides a buttressing effect. Screws are placed at the ends of the plate, and the mid-portion of the plate is the buttress with unused screw holes. Unlike the posterior wall, fixation directly into the wall fragment is problematic. Usually, screws have to be angled into the pelvis and catch the corner of the pelvic brim. These screws actually course behind the articular surface of the acetabulum. In the area of the pectineal eminence, usually only a short screw (approximately 12–18 mm long) can be placed to avoid entering the joint (Fig. 6). After fixation, the reduction can be checked using an image intensifier, which additionally confirms that screws are clear of the joint. The provisional Kirschner wires (K-wires) can give invaluable clues as to the safe position and direction of screws. When checking the reduction on fluoroscopy and prior to definitive fixation, use the K-wires as references to identify safe zones for hardware placement.

ANTERIOR COLUMN ACETABULAR FRACTURES

The anterior column is more common than the anterior wall and will frequently be accompanied by an incomplete hemitransverse component. Some anterior column fractures can be rather extensive and comminuted and can be as challenging as more complex associated patterns. In general, the approach will be some anterior exposure, followed by systematic reduction and fixation. With more extensive patterns, the fixation usually progresses from posterior (intact component) to anterior (fracture component). For the crest, both large and small tenaculums can be used to effect a reduction of the crest. Kirchner wires can then provide provisional fixation that permits clamp removal and plate or screw placement. If needed, the exposure can be extended over the ASIS to allow placement and use of the Farabeuf clamp, which can help control rotation of the wing. The ball spike pusher is a very effective reduction tool but care is necessary to prevent iatrogenic fracture propagation in thin areas (Fig. 7). Once reduced, 3.5 mm reconstruction plates or judiciously placed screws will suffice to provide stabilization.

The low anterior column fractures will frequently have a portion of the quadrilateral surface attached. In these cases, it is important to recognize if there is any instability from the central component of this fracture, especially in osteoporotic bone. If so, fixation of the anterior column alone may leave the central portions unstable, and can potentially allow a protrusion of the femoral head. In these cases, a standard plate can be placed along the pelvic brim, but attention to the quadrilateral surface is needed. While standard spring plates can be used, they can be difficult to contour and, due to the thin plate profile, may be overcome by the high forces in the hip. We have used an alternate method of fixation that has the plate along the quadrilateral surface in the inner portion of the brim. The plates and screws are oriented about 90° to normal. In

(A)

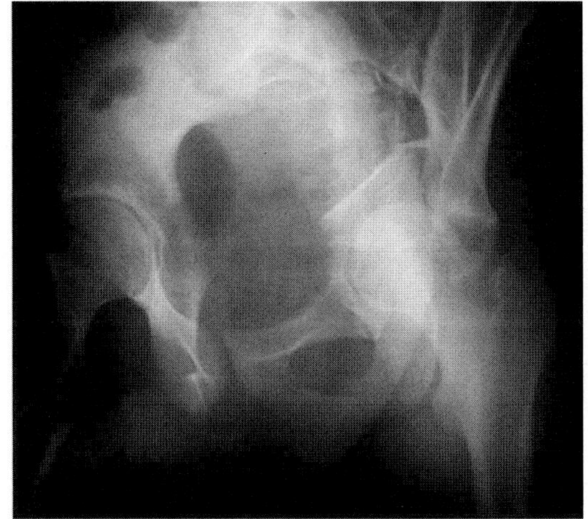

(B)

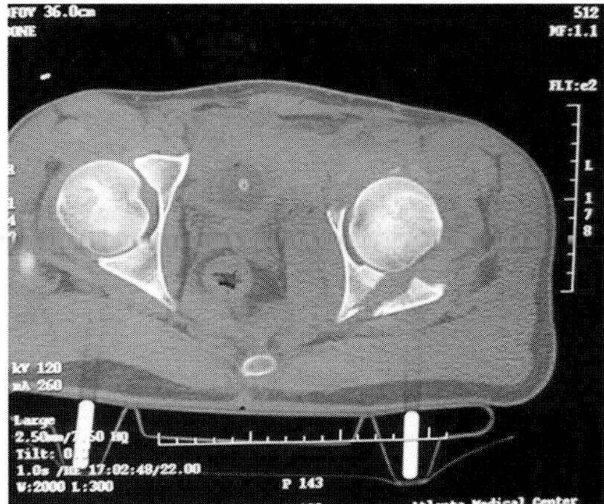

(C)

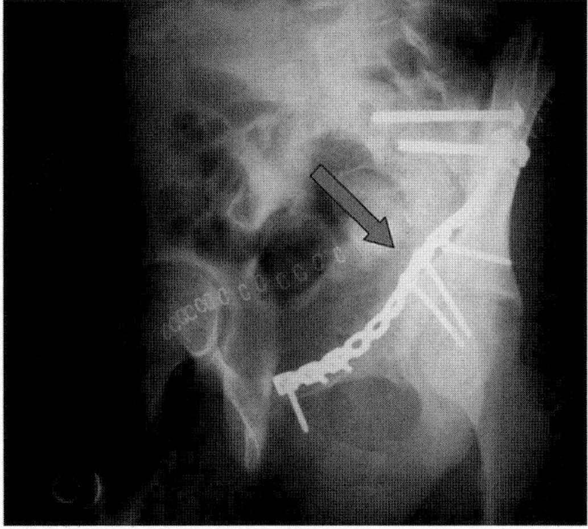

Figure 6 (**A**, **B**) Anterior wall fracture radiograph and axial CT scan. (**C**) The buttress plate spans the fracture, but also uses screws directed behind the joint (*gray arrow*) into the quadrilateral surface bone outside of the joint.

(A)
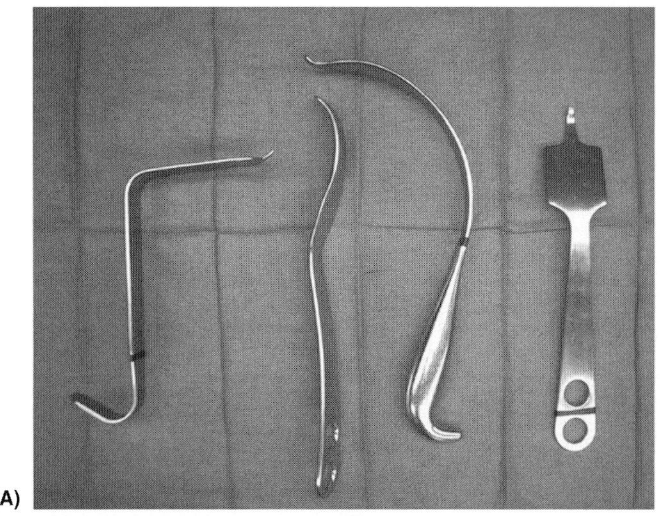

(B)
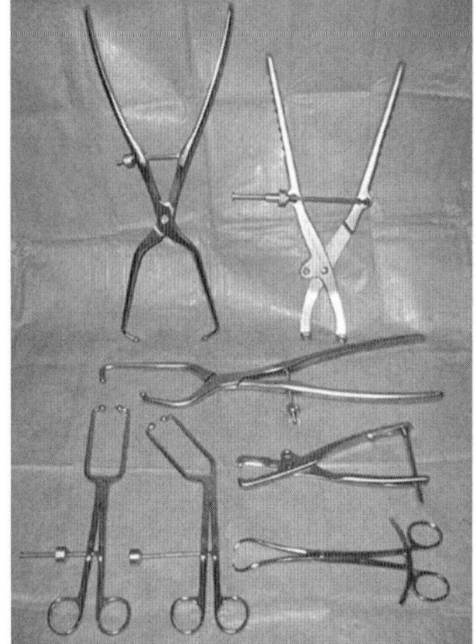

(C)
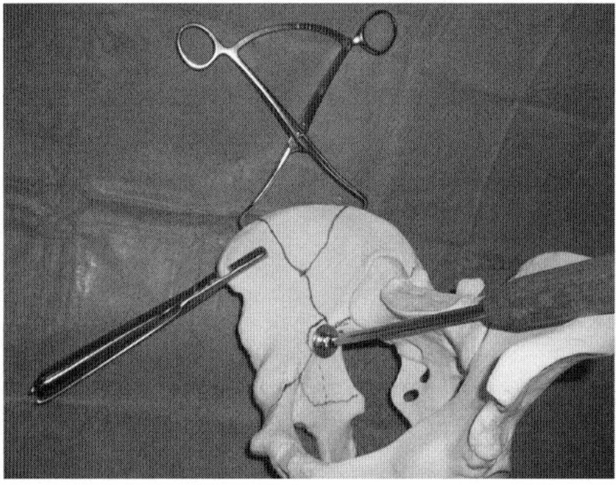

Figure 7 (**A**, **B**) Various retractors and equipment useful during surgery of the acetabulum. (**C**) Illustration on a sawbone model showing the various clamps and assistive devices that can be used to help effect a reduction.

order to accomplish this, we have used the subinguinal window for visualization and access. We began using this modification in the late 1990s and it was described formally by others. The approach involves the surgeon moving to the opposite side of the table and working through the medial window of the ilioinguinal approach but under the vessel and muscle sheath. Once the bladder is moved, there is direct access to the quadrilateral surface, posterior column, and anterior ramus (Figs. 8 and 9).

For middle and high anterior column fractures, the options are more plentiful. In these fracture patterns, where the required access is high on the ilium, the iliofemoral approach may be considered. We typically prep and drape for a full ilioinguinal approach, though the lateral window is often all that is needed. Working in the lateral window can be very tight quarters, and determining the best direction for screws that are safely out of the joint and in an ideal orientation for secure fixation can be challenging. One can place a finger along the inner iliac table to get proprioceptive feedback during drilling and screw placement. Slowly advance the drill, and leave your fingers of one hand on the inside of the anterior column for feedback on the exit point of the drill. Redirect the drill as necessary to get a screw through the best bone. The use of the obturator-outlet view can also provide an end-on view of the screw pathway between the iliac tables, which will identify the axis for screw placement. Once reduced, a long screw across the anterior column fracture heading towards the sacroiliac joint and above the sciatic notch is usually sufficient for fixation (the so called LCII screw) (Fig. 10). Plating along the superior ramus can be achieved by developing the medial window of the ilioinguinal approach. An alternate method would be to use percutaneous methods, described elsewhere in this book. Keep in mind that the fracture hematoma becomes more mature daily and delayed operative treatment results in a more challenging closed reduction and percutaneous fixation. For the purposes of this chapter, we discuss open fixation techniques.

With all such fractures, the reduction should be verified in two locations: the crest (if the fracture exits the crest in high fractures) and the articular surface (which is the essential element). Methods to effect a reduction include use of tenaculums, pelvic clamps, and direct pressure from a ball spike pusher. With the hip flexed and the iliopsoas muscles relaxed, placement of the longer limb of an offset clamp low on the anterior column or on the medial wall is achievable. The shorter limb of the offset clamp can be placed on the outer table after lateral release of the fascia on the iliac crest (Fig. 11). Occasionally there will be marginally impacted segments or small articular osteocartilagenous fragments. In these cases, the fracture can be "booked" open to gain access to the joint. In cases where there is an extended plate of quadrilateral surface involved, a more invasive approach with an ilioinguinal is needed. Care should be taken when reduction is difficult, so that forceful maneuvers with a pelvic clamp on the quadrilateral surface do not create a fracture, thus destabilizing the area even further. The spiked washer can be used to distribute forces and minimize the risk of fracture comminution. This is where a Schantz pin in the lesser trochanter, with a laterally directed pull, helps to reduce the "protrusio" significantly. Finally, high anterior column fractures that exit the iliac wing require stabilization. Plates along the inner table or individual screws along the iliac crest are advisable. A plate along the iliac crest may utilize longer screws through a plate and achieve

(*Text continues on page 203.*)

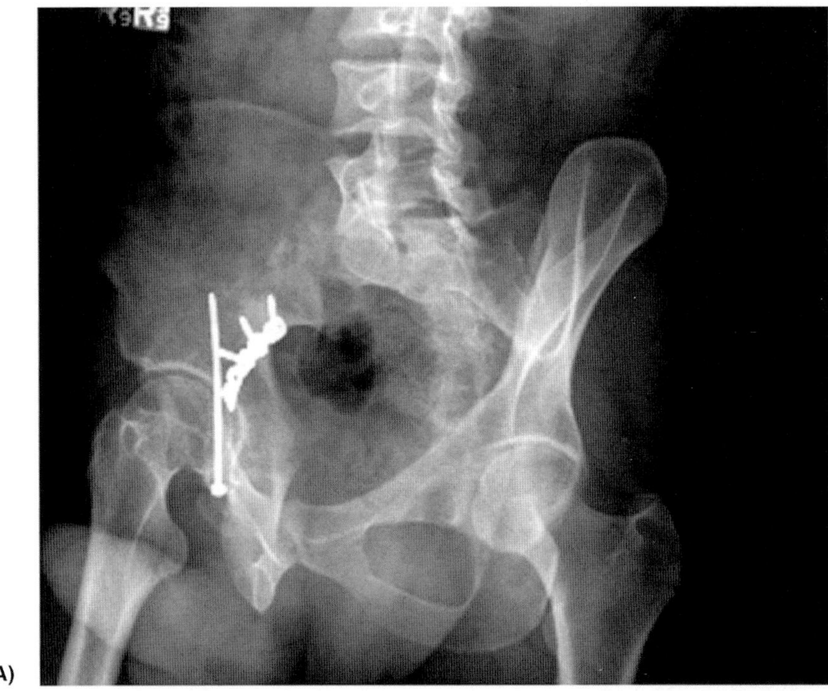

(A)

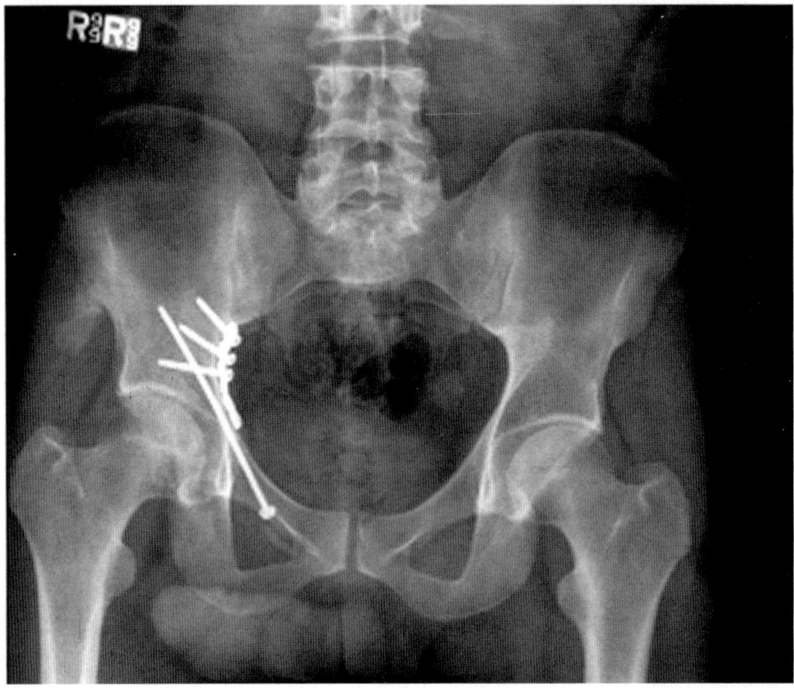

(B)

Figure 8 (**A**) Iliac oblique and (**B**) AP view of anterior wall and column involvement of a transverse fracture. The anterior wall component was the predominant characteristic with a protrused quadrilateral surface. It was treated with a retrograde ramus screw and a quadrilateral plate. The plate buttresses the quadrilateral surface directly with excellent inside out screw placement.

(A)

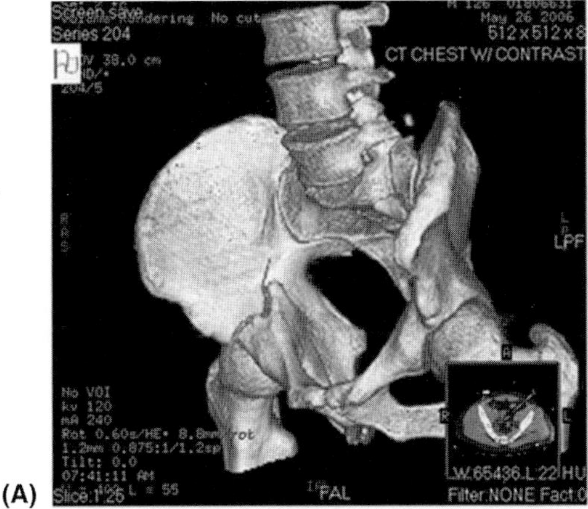

(B)

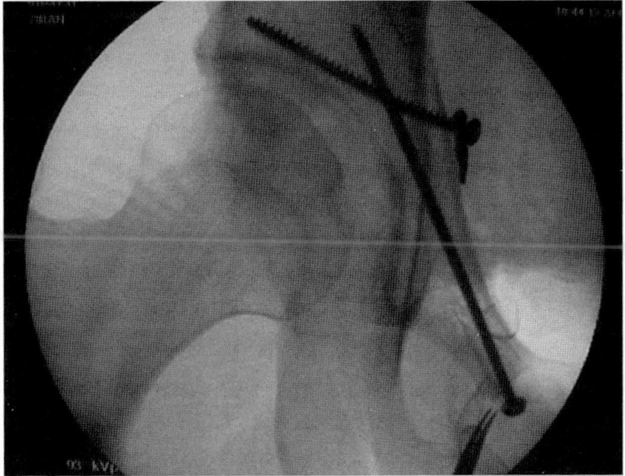

(C)

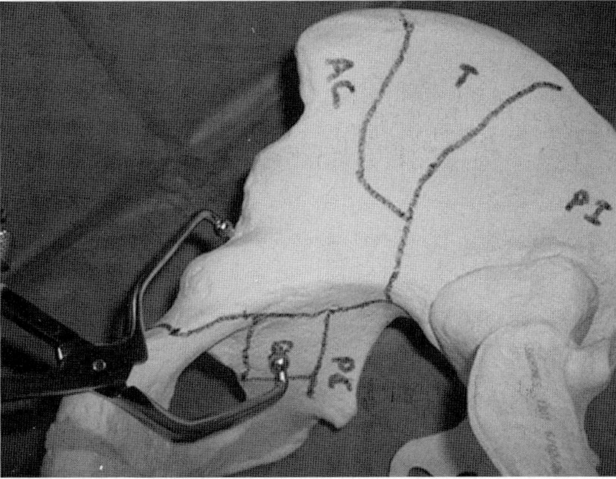

Figure 9 (**A**) Low anterior column fracture with quadrilateral surface involvement. (**B**) The "inside-out" screw with a small plate is used to prevent protrusion. (**C**) Demonstrates clamp placement if necessary.

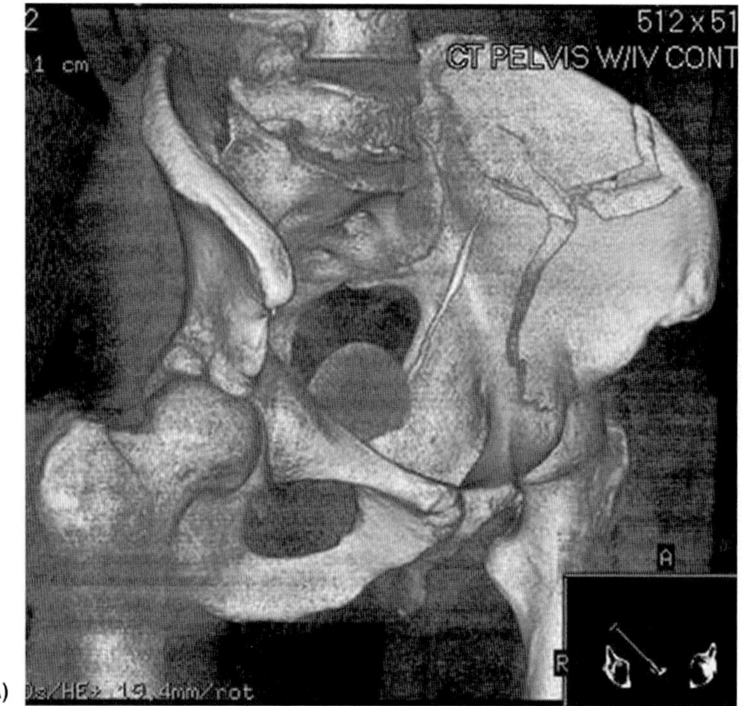

(A)

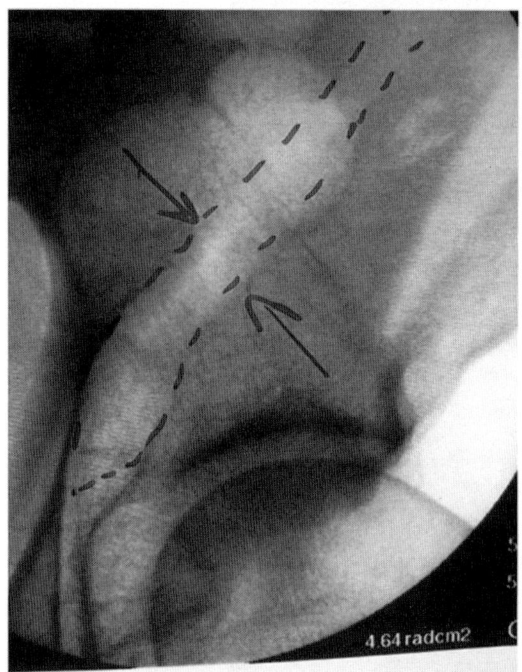

(B)

Figure 10 (**A**) High anterior column fracture with rotation. (**B**) highlights the pathway of the screw seen in (**E**) placed between the inner and outer iliac tables (*arrows*). (*Continued*)

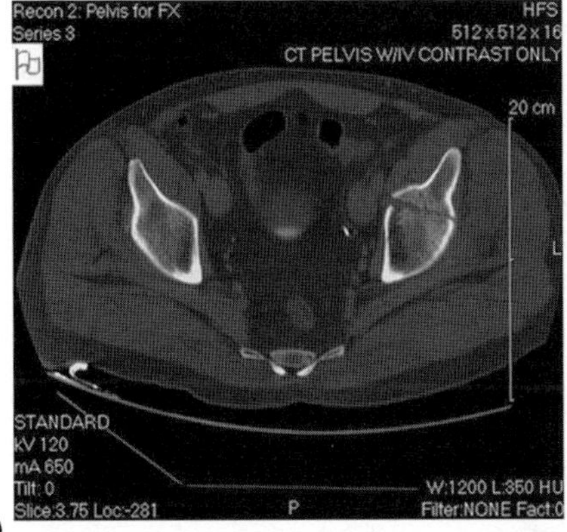

(C)

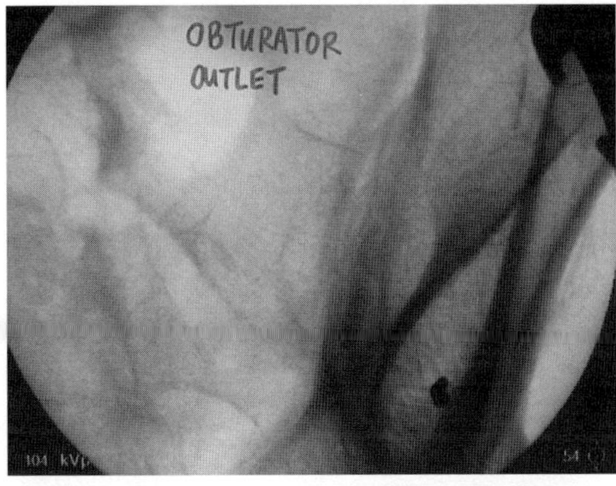

(D)

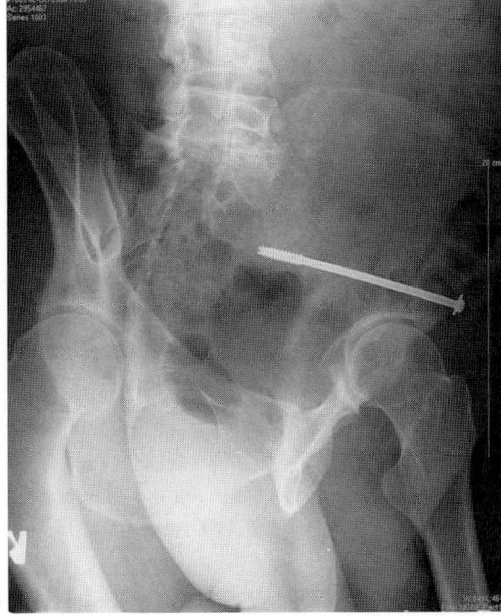
(E)

Figure 10 *(Continued)* (**C**) Axial CT scan at level of anterior inferior iliac spine. Note how a screw placed at this level will be nearly perpendicular to the transverse fracture line. (**D**) Obturator outlet fluoroscopy image demonstrating guide wire position within iliac inner and outer tables and just cephalad to the hip joint. The Farabeuf clamp is used to effect a reduction (not shown), and the iliac oblique view (**E**) can provide an end-on view of the anterior column to facilitate screw placement. Note the start point of this screw at the level of the anterior inferior iliac spine.

(A)

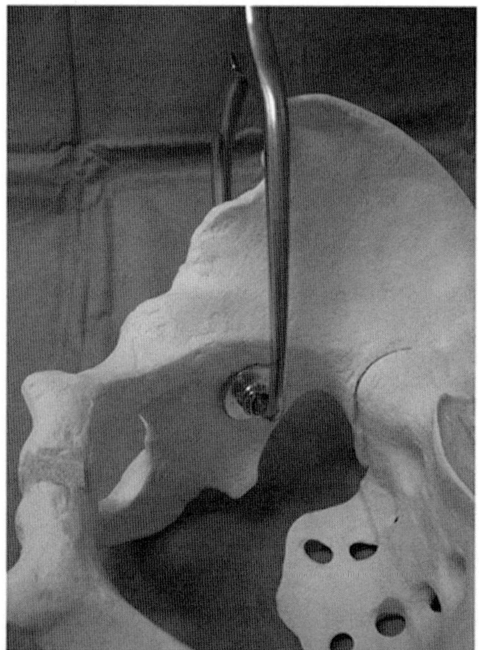

(B)

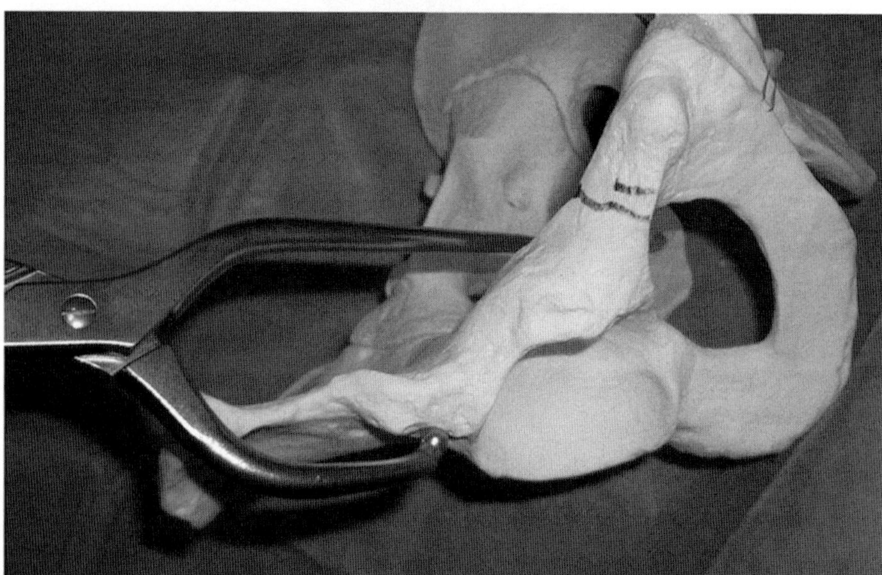

Figure 11 (**A** and **B**) Even with the iliac portion of the fracture reduced, the quadrilateral surface may still have some displacement due to rotation. The offset pelvic clamp can be placed to reduce the quadrilateral surface component of the fracture. Because of the thin bone, it is possible to create an iatrogenic fracture. For this reason, the use of a disk and lateral traction of the femur is recommended.

better fixation, but the hardware can be prominent and may require removal soon after the fracture heals.

POSTERIOR WALL ACETABULAR FRACTURES

Posterior wall fractures are the most common acetabular fractures but unfortunately are associated with higher rates of poor outcomes. The hip usually dislocates with isolated posterior wall lesions and may spontaneously relocate or will require manual relocation. There is a small but definite incidence of sciatic nerve injury, which should be well documented prior to reduction and surgical reconstruction. The peroneal division of the sciatic nerve is more frequently injured than the tibial division. This may be due to the more lateral position of the peroneal nerve and being more in line with the dislocation vector. This is similarly true for all posterior acetabular fracture patterns, as an injured but incomplete nerve lesion may progress to a complete nerve lesion from surgical intervention. This documentation is needed to help surgical tactic as well as establish a baseline of function and help guide patient expectations. Keep in mind that knee flexion during surgery lessens the tension on the sciatic nerve, and retractor position should be monitored closely. Special sciatic nerve retractors are available and intermittent periods of retractor removal can help minimize iatrogenic injury.

Surgical tactic will require a few decisions regarding position and traction. The posterior surgical approach is the commonly accepted approach, but there is much heated debate on the best patient position for such fractures. One school of thought utilizes the prone position, which removes the effect of gravity. In the lateral decubitus position the effect of gravity tends to pull the femoral head posteriorly and medially into the acetabulum. The weight of the femoral head with the patient in the lateral decubitus position tends to displace the fracture. In the prone position, reduction maneuvers are less hampered by the weight of the femoral head. Also, the proponents of the prone position state that this approach provides better access to work around the sciatic notch into the pelvis

The other school of thought utilizes a lateral position with or without some type of traction. If the lateral position without traction is used, any visualization of the hip will require some type of manual traction. If fixed continuous traction is used, then some form of counter traction is required (e.g., a perineal post or taping), otherwise the patient can gradually migrate, and thus make sustained traction maneuvers difficult (Figs. 2 and 3). If lateral positioning is combined with a traction apparatus, however, such as one that provides both longitudinal and laterally based traction, then all features of the prone position can be achieved while still providing more access to the anterior structures. This is beneficial when such access to more superior or anterior structures via an extended trochanteric osteotomy (the trochanteric flip or slide) is needed. We have utilized both prone and lateral positioning with traction and have found that the lateral position provides the most access and is more versatile. For this setup, we use a Jackson radiolucent table with distal femoral skeletal traction, as well as a padded perineal post. The perineal post is adjustable in the vertical direction and provides the lateral force while the longitudinal traction distracts the joint (Fig. 2). Furthermore, with the traction setup, rotation, flexion, and abduction of the femur are possible. With this setup, we have been able to visualize all aspects of the hip joint from behind, and have found that access via the sciatic notch to palpate and place clamps over the pelvic brim to be easier because the posterior soft tissues do not require active retraction and are gravity assisted. In the absence of fixed traction, one can place a five- to six-inch stack of folded towels deep into the groin between the legs. Gentle downward pressure at the flexed knee reduces the weight of the femoral head on the acetabulum. The stack of towels combined with longitudinal and lateral traction via the trochanteric Schantz pin results in very good joint exposure for posterior fractures (Fig. 3). Whatever the position, it is highly recommended that if any traction be applied, the hip should be neutral or extended and the knee should be flexed. Even Letournel himself recognized that, during the times he used straight leg traction, there was a postoperative palsy rate of about 18%, while after flexing the knee the incidence fell to under 4%.

Prior to embarking on surgical fixation, it is important to recognize the nature of the posterior wall fracture. There are differences between the inferior, middle, and superior wall patterns, and the potential need for special devices and a trochanteric slide osteotomy will require appropriate surgical planning. Recognition of the articular comminution and presence of marginal impaction are necessary for proper equipment selection and restoration of a stable joint. During surgical exposure, we recommend partial detachment of the gluteal insertion along the back of the femur. There is always a perforating vessel in this area, but release of the gluteus maximus insertion greatly facilitates the posterior soft tissue envelope retraction. Release the gluteal sling 1.5 cm from the bone and this will facilitate identification and coagulation of the perforating vessels. Repair at the time of closure with #1 Vicryl or other heavy suture. Another important anatomic recognition is the variants of the piriformis and sciatic nerve (split nerve, split muscle, or both). While in the majority of cases the nerve courses anterior to the muscle, there are cases of variants that require appropriate maneuvers to protect the nerve (Fig. 12).

Once the posterior acetabular area is reached, it is important to maintain the capsular attachments of the posterior bone fragment so that vascularity may be maintained. There is always the need to trim the edges and even the labral tear, but the hinge of capsule should be maintained. It can usually be flipped up and held during reduction maneuvers. To facilitate retraction of this fragment, consider placing a suture through the soft tissue of this fragment. Then secure the suture line with a clamp to the Charnley retractor. Prior to definitive reduction, we recommend inspection of the joint for loose bodies and fracture lines. Some small fragments are inevitably discarded, but an effort should be made to save and reduce all fragments, because discarding fragments can lead to defects in the posterior wall. In cases of associated fracture or transverse fractures, the inspection of the joint with traction will show the quality of articular reduction (Fig. 13). Once reduction has been verified and the joint has been cleaned, the femoral head is gently placed back into the acetabulum and used as a template, around which small detached osteocartilagenous fractures can be placed. At that point, the femoral head can be drilled on the edge of the articular surface to assess for bleeding. It has been postulated that lack of bleeding is a poor prognosticator for avascular necrosis (AVN). This technique of femoral head drilling has been reported as a negative predictor for AVN (Gill et al.) for femoral neck fractures but is yet to be demonstrated for acetabular fractures.

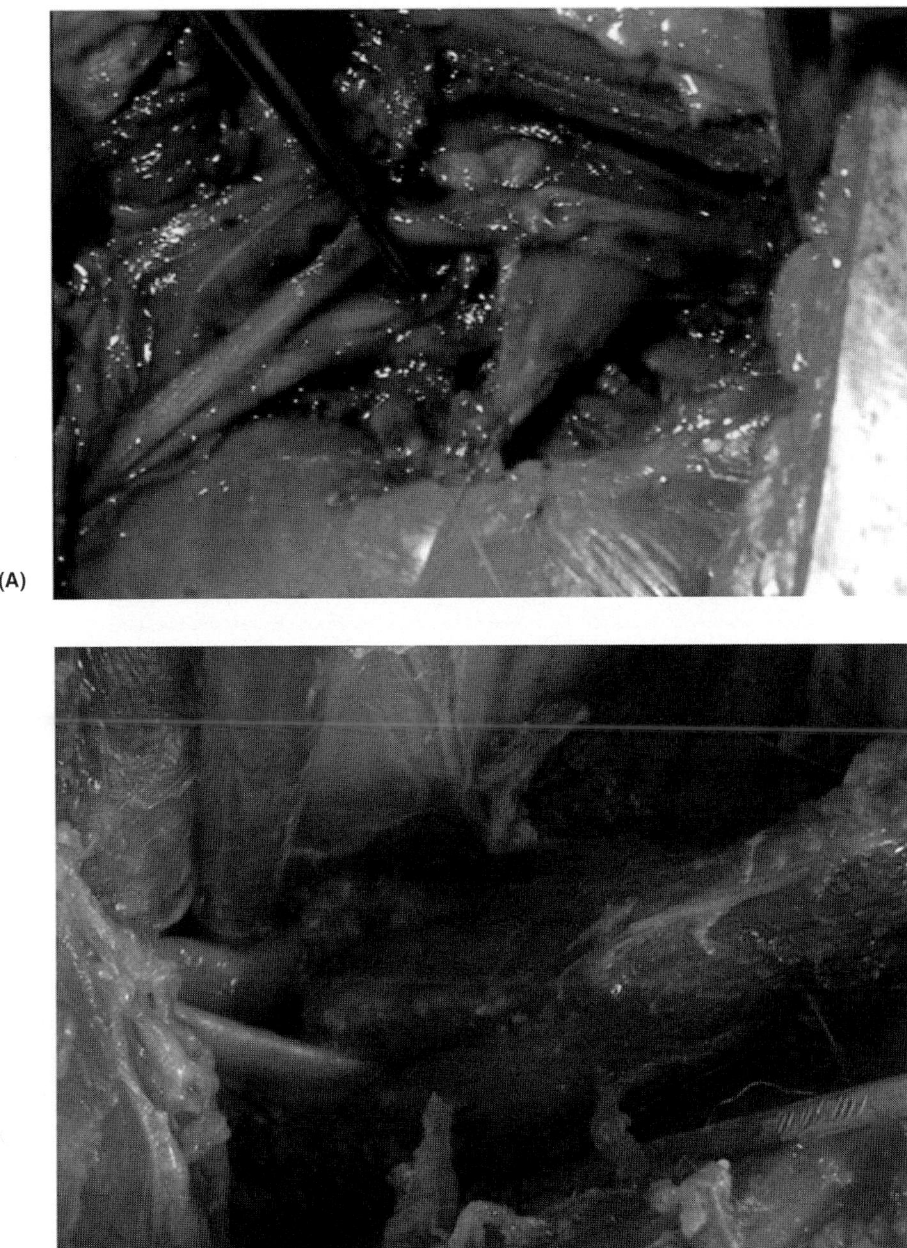

Figure 12 Two sciatic nerve variants to recognize. In (**A**) the nerve splits around the piriformis muscle and in (**B**) the nerve splits into the muscle. Recognizing the presence of each variant will help avoid inadvertent nerve injury.

Marginal impaction destabilizes the joint and will need to be recognized and addressed. It is considered another poor prognosticator but should nonetheless be elevated and stabilized as anatomically as possible. The disimpaction technique uses an appropriately sized osteotome to lift the cartilaginous fragment, if possible, as one main

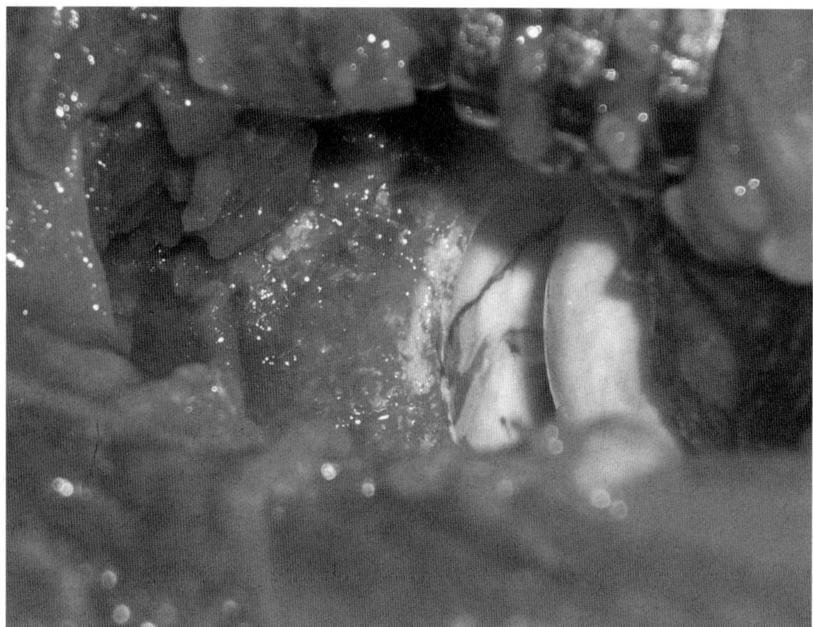

Figure 13 A posterior wall fracture viewed from behind and with the joint distracted. The subtle crack in the articular surface was identified intraoperatively. The posterior wall fragment is being held up with the retractor in the foreground and maintained on its capsular hinge. Visualization of the joint is excellent and can be increased as needed.

unfragmented piece. The osteotome is placed behind a portion of the subchondral cancellous bone bed in an added attempt to reduce a sizable and more stable piece. The reduced femoral head serves as a template around which the fragment is placed. Then, any defects are back-filled with some type of graft material, which can be synthetic, autogenous, or allogenic. Our preference is the use of a demineralized bone matrix with fine (1–3 mm bone chips). For younger patients and patients requesting autograft, cancellous graft can easily be harvested from the lateral aspect of the exposed greater trochanter. Following grafting, the posterior wall is replaced. We prefer to slightly overpack the defect, and then use the natural wall to impact the graft in its tissue bed. Use of a ball spike pusher with a disk attachment will minimize the risk of iatrogenic fragmentation of the exiting wall fragment. Thereafter, temporary stabilization using small wires allows contouring and placement of appropriate plates for fixation (Fig. 14).

Fixation is generally accomplished by buttressing the posterior wall with the use of 3.5 mm reconstruction plates (6–8 holes are usually sufficient). The plate is placed along the posterior column from the ischial prominence over the posterior wall and up onto the superior acetabular surface. Exposure can be facilitated by placing a cobra retractor anterior to the ischial tuberosity, a cobra retractor anterior to the obturator internis tendon and in the lesser sciatic notch, and a Taylor retractor up under the gluteal musculature and gently hammered into the outer iliac table. Contouring of a curved plate will frequently require a few distinct bends (Fig. 24). The superior aspect of the plate will be twisted to sit along the superior wall, the inferior portion will often be acutely bent at the second or third screw hole to fit in the infracotyloid groove, and

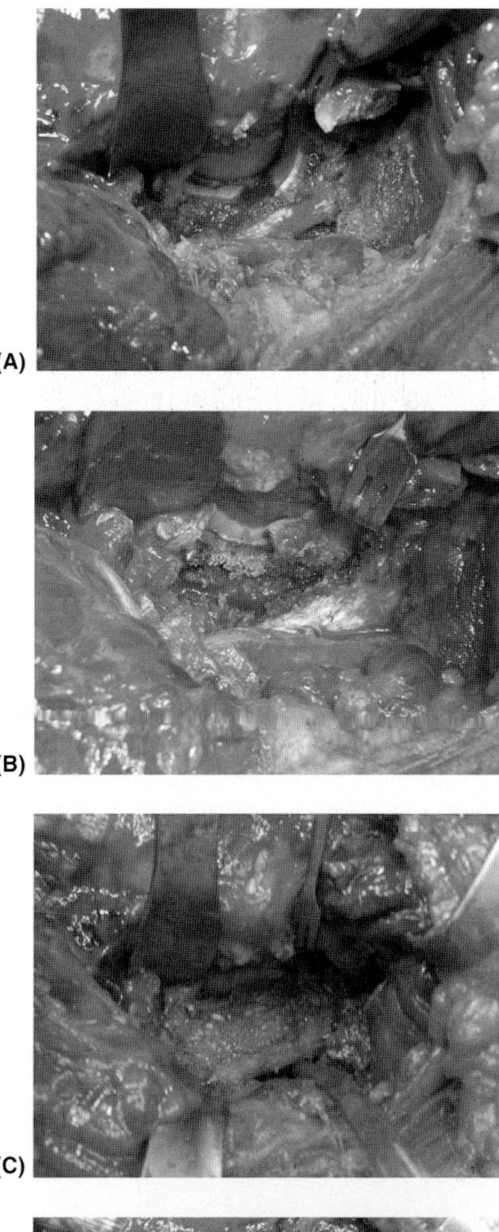

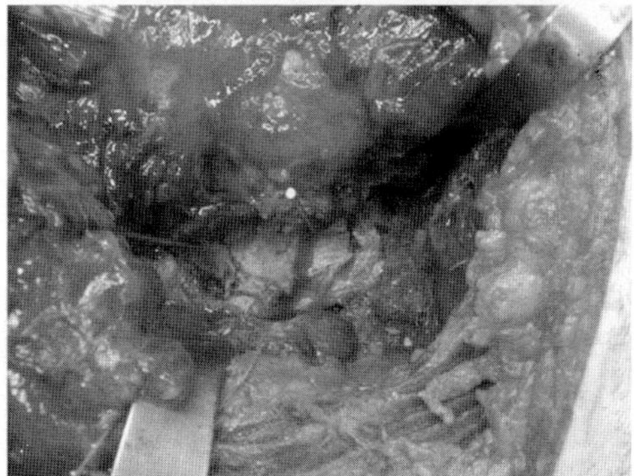

Figure 14 Example of marginal impaction with posterior wall fracture. (**A**) After joint inspection, the femoral head is placed into the hip socket and used as a template. (**B**, **C**) The impacted fragments are elevated to the head and the space behind them is packed with graft, after which the posterior wall is reduced. (**D**) Once reduced and impacted, the wall is temporarily held with K-wires strategically placed to allow plate placement.

the mid-portion of the plate will be bent along its major axis to match the curvature of the posterior wall. Release of the hamstrings at their ischial tuberosity origin may be necessary to provide increased area for plate and screw placement. It is recommended that the plate be slightly under bent in this aspect, so that it provides a compressive effect to the posterior wall fragment when finally fixed. Once the plate contour is established, the first screw placed is inferior (usually the second hole) to secure the plate into the infracotyloid groove. This area usually has better quality bone and can provide excellent fixation. The screw is not fully tightened to allow adjustments in plate position. The under contouring of the plate will be evident superiorly, wherein a ball spike pusher in the last screw hole can be used to push the plate into position and allow provisional fixation of the plate (Fig. 15). Once acceptable, these two screws are tightened. In the past, numerous screws were placed along the plate, but currently we find that two good screws on each side are generally sufficient. In some cases we place a single screw in the posterior wall fragment through the plate to augment fixation. If the posterior wall is rather large, then separate 3.5 mm cortical screws can be placed prior to placement of the buttress plate. These screws invariably are adjacent to or come to rest under the buttress plate but can also be placed through the plate. These screws must be angled posteriorly and away from the hip joint. The provisional K-wires can give invaluable clues as to the safe position and direction of these screws, but with experience, the surgeon should become aware of the "windows" of appropriate screw placement (Fig. 16).

If the posterior wall is rather comminuted, smaller plates placed under the reconstruction plate to hold the small comminuted pieces are used. These "spring" plates are made from the 1/3 tubular plates and placed before application of the 3.5

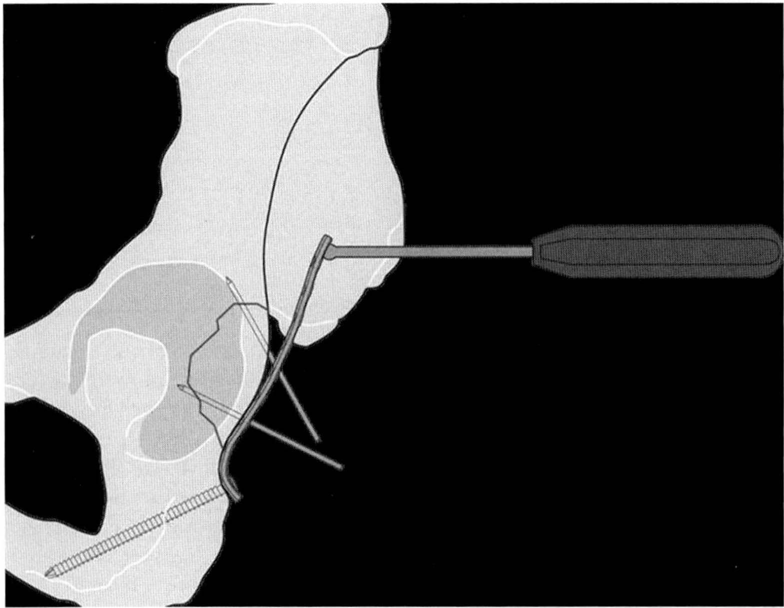

Figure 15 The plate should be slightly under-contoured to provide a compressive effect when fixed on both sides.

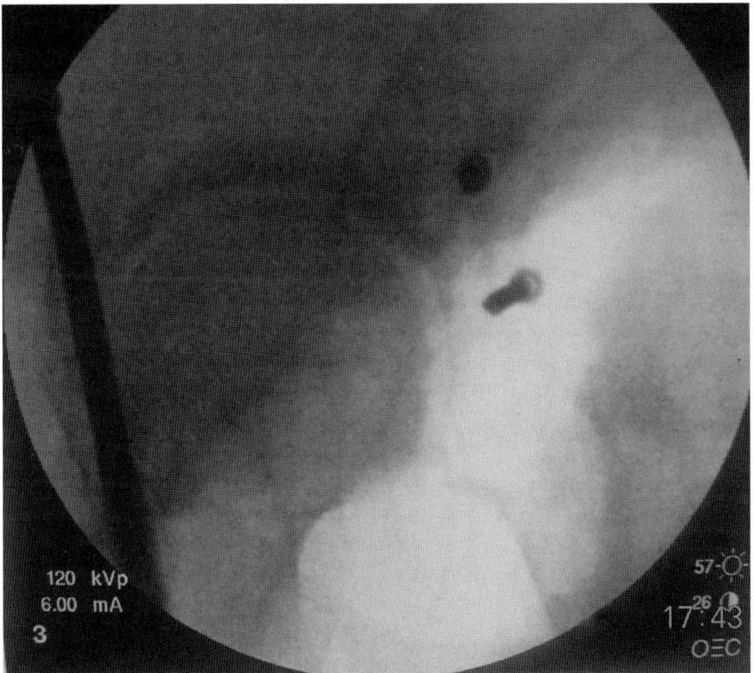

Figure 16 Operative acetabulum is to the left. Note extra-articular position of the screws in the posterior wall. This is important to confirm prior to placement of a buttress plate, which may overlap these screws. K-wires (not seen in this image) provide provisional fixation, but they can also serve as a reference for subsequent screw placement after checking the reduction on fluoroscopy.

reconstruction plate. This plate should be placed with independent fixation along the posterior column, and then the recon plate is placed on top. The independent fixation of these small plates prevents any chance of plate migration. Some authors advocate cutting the end of the 1/3 tubular plate through the end hole. Then the tips of the plate are bent for theoretical added fixation. Sometimes more than one spring plate is required. In such cases, the authors have modified the technique by substituting a distal radius T plate, which can be used in the same context (a spring plate), but, because of the T shape, it can spread its effect over a greater distance and can be use instead of two 1/3 tubular plates (Fig. 17).

There are two distinct fracture patterns worthy of mention. The superior posterior wall fracture tends to be highly unstable and very difficult to access. The difficulty arises with exposure because of the limiting gluteal musculature. While tempting to increase retractile efforts, we believe that excessive traction may potentially cause damage to the musculature as well as the superior gluteal neural trunk as it exits the greater sciatic notch. Additionally, the increased surgical trauma may cause muscle damage, leading to heterotopic ossification. Therefore, we advocate the use of the extended trochanteric osteotomy, also called the trochanteric flip osteotomy. This has been described by Seibenrock and later by our group for such fractures and provides

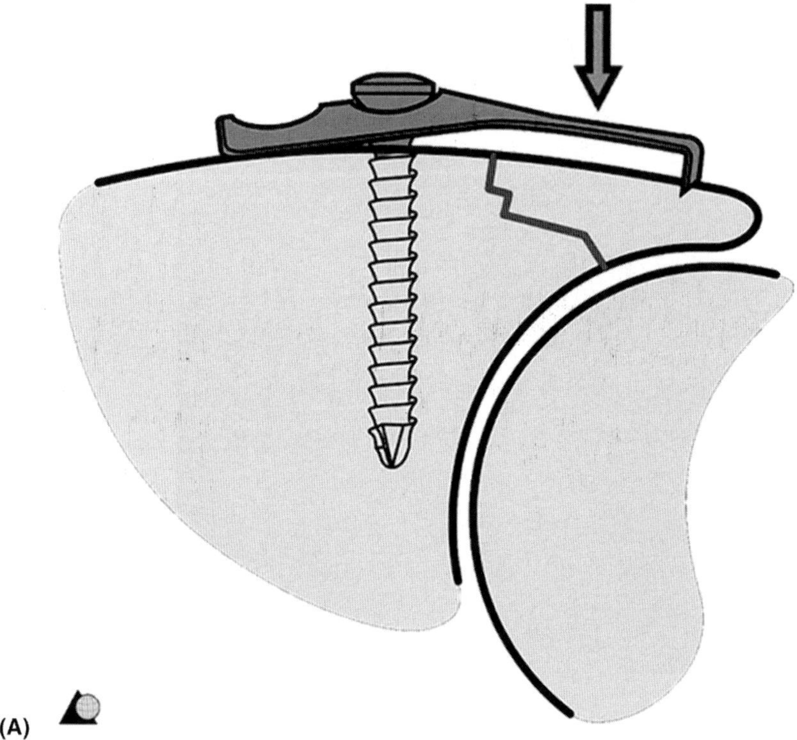

(A)

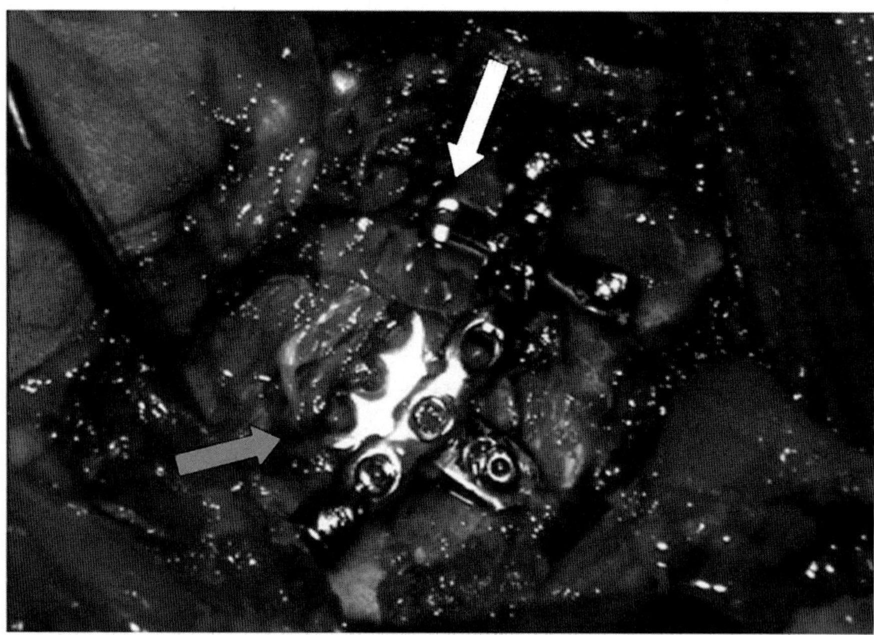

(B)

Figure 17 (**A**) The concept of a spring plate that pushes and holds small fragments. (**B**) Posterior wall of Fig. 14 fixed with use of spring plates. The superior plate (*white arrow*) is a standard 1/3 tubular plate, but the inferior one (*gray arrow*) is a modified distal radial T plate. The T plate is now our preferred plate because of the wider surface area of contact.

excellent view of the superior acetabular surface with a controlled and less damaging surgical exposure. Once exposure is obtained, the superior wall can be addressed with standard plating as described previously. Because of the large biomechanical forces in this area, we have occasionally utilized an antiglide plate for the superior wall that is straddled by a recon plate. The osteotomy is fixed with two 3.5 mm screws and, because it maintains the vastus attachment distally, there is little risk of proximal migration and has had little to no complications associated with its use (Fig. 18). It has recently been described for use when there is an associated posterior wall and femoral head fracture. In this case, the osteotomy permits dislocation of the femoral head and provides sufficient exposure to the anterior aspect of the hip joint and femoral head where pathology is typically located.

The second fracture pattern is the posterior wall that extends all the way across the posterior column. This extended posterior wall fracture displaces the entire retroacetabular surface and involves the greater or lesser sciatic notch. It is probably a transitional fracture pattern that represents something between a posterior wall and posterior column fracture. Nonetheless, it is a very challenging fracture because of the logistics of fixation and especially difficult when accompanying an associated fracture pattern (PC/PW, T/PW). Many authors report that the prone position is the most suitable position for this fracture so that the gravitational effect on femoral head can be neutralized. We have not found this to be problematic in the lateral position when the methods described previously were used to offset the weight of the leg (and femoral head) and when traction is used to distract the joint for inspection. The fracture may not be amenable to hinging open to inspect the joint without risk to the sciatic nerve. Efforts should be made to correct any marginal impaction and intra-articular fragmentation. Fixation is accomplished with the usual recon plates, but in these cases we believe that there should also be direct fixation of the fragment through the plate. This is in direct contrast to our previous recommendation for two screws in the superior and inferior aspects of a buttress plate for a posterior wall fracture. In all cases, after final reduction and fixation, fluoroscopic verification and debridement of the gluteal and the short external rotator musculature (to prevent heterotopic ossification) should be performed.

POSTERIOR COLUMN ACETABULAR FRACTURES

The posterior column fractures are operated on using a Kocher–Langenbeck approach. Again, there remains controversy about patient positioning, but both lateral and prone positions are acceptable. What is most important is not the patient position but the surgeon's ability to achieve the desired result of an anatomic reduction with stable fixation and minimal biologic cost. After the same exposure as noted above, the fracture can be distracted using either the pelvic clamps with a Cobb elevator or with careful use of a lamina spreader. Hematoma and any small fragments that may impede reduction are removed. Thereafter, reduction can be obtained with several methods. If a pelvic clamp was used to distract the fracture, it is now used to reduce and hold the fracture. Tenaculums, Matta clamps, and Farabeuf clamps can all be utilized for the same purpose. The authors have also found great utility in strategic

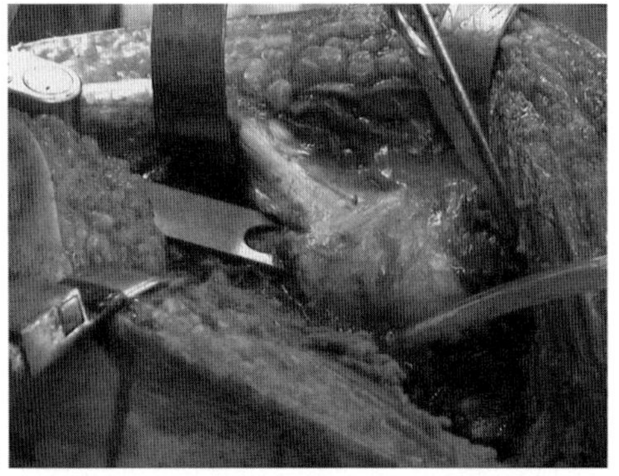
(A)

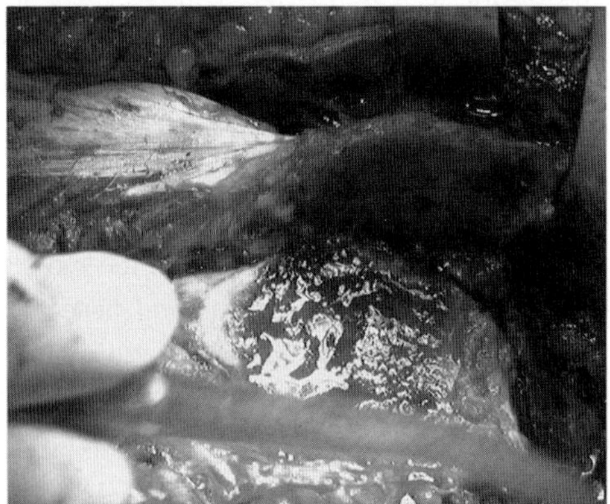
(B)

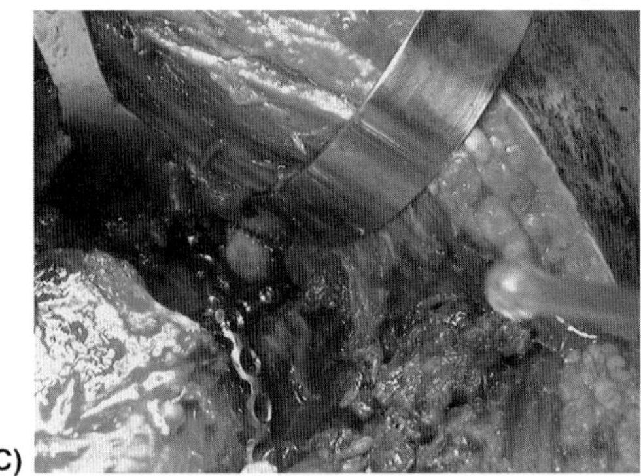
(C)

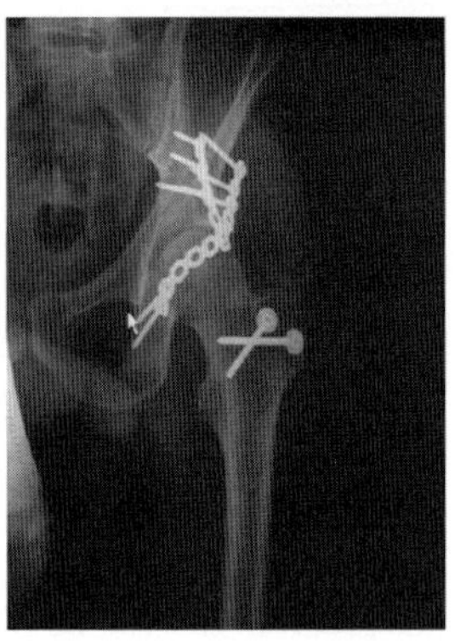
(D)

Figure 18 Use of trochanteric slide osteotomy as described by Seibenrock et al. and later by us. It provides excellent and controlled access to the superior aspects of the acetabulum and as far anterior as the anterior inferior spine. (**A**) The vastus is elevated to identify the "plane" of the lateral femur. A saw is passed along this plane toward the greater trochanter. (**B**) A desired thickness for the trochanteric fragment is about 1.5 cm. It is "flipped" anterior and the dissection is completed. Gluteus medius and capsule can be detached as needed. (**C**) A view of the superior acetabular area and outer iliac wing. The top left retractor is in the notch of the inferior iliac spine. Excellent exposure is possible without the need of a second approach. Luxation of the hip allows for joint inspection. In such cases, we recommend a single dose of therapeutic radiation to prevent heterotopic ossification. (**D**) Post operative radiograph. The osteotomy can usually be fixed with two 3.5 mm or 4.5 mm lag screws. *Note*: The proximal extention of the hardware exposure of this magnitude without an osteotomy requires aggressive gluteus medius retraction and increases risk of injury to the superior gluteal neurovascular bundle.

placement of a three-hole plate. The plate is secured with a 3.5 mm screw on one side of the fracture line. The second screw, on the opposite side of the fracture, is drilled eccentrically as much as possible to achieve a compressive effect. A bit of residual gapping at the fracture is typically still noted despite the compression screw. This is where the third screw is also drilled eccentrically to further add compression. Before this third screw is tightened, the second screw is loosened slightly. This sequence achieves an excellent closure of the fracture gap. Further fixation can be added with a longer recon plate along the posterior column. It is important to note that the column frequently will have a rotational component that may be hard to identify from the posterior fracture line. It may appear perfectly reduced along the posterior column, but the part of the fracture that extends to the quadrilateral surface may remain unreduced. Digital palpation through the sciatic notch is needed to determine the accuracy of this part of the reduction. Rotation may be hard to control with simple clamps, so if such a maneuver is needed, use of a Schanz pin into the ischial tuberosity or angled clamps (Matta) may be placed through the notch to effect a reduction of the anterior aspects of the fracture. Once reduced, one or two strategically placed screws can be placed to provisionally secure the fracture, after which a neutralization plate is applied across the fracture. We find that if the first two screws have excellent purchase and provide good interfragmentary compression, then a short spanning plate is all that is required (Figs. 19 and 20).

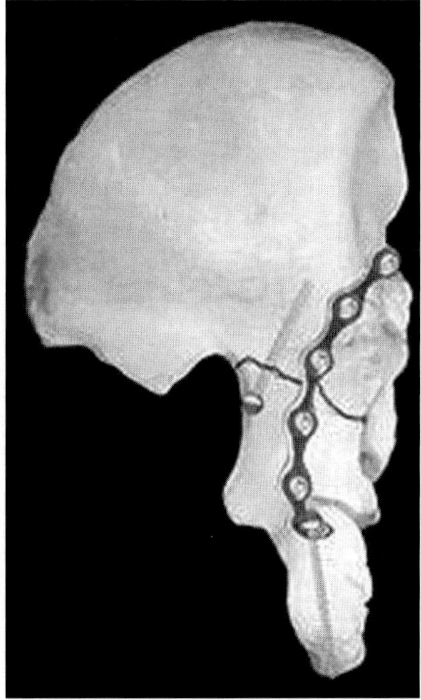

Figure 19 Reduction of a displaced posterior column acetabular fracture can be facilitated in several ways, including a Schanz pin into the ischial tuberosity to control the inferior segment (Fig. 20A and B). Alternatively, a Farabeuf clamp placed around temporary screws in each bone segment can achieve provisional reduction (Chapter 12, Fig. 2). The sciatic notches are digitally palpated to assure acceptable reduction. This figure illustrates a compression screw near the sciatic notch, which then permitted removal of the provisional fixation clamps and compression plating.

Also, in these fractures, as in T fractures or some transverse fractures, a carefully placed screw along the medial wall of the acetabulum may provide added fixation. This screw begins along the most posterior aspect of the column, very close to the notch or spine, courses behind the acetabulum, and may just cross the fracture towards the pelvic brim. Whatever the case, fixation should be sufficient to prevent redisplacement. The posterior column usually rotates along its longitudinal axis as it displaces. It is imperative to correct this displacement. A femoral head corkscrew or a Schantz screw placed into the ischial tuberosity will likely correct this displacement (Fig. 20).

TRANSVERSE ACETABULAR FRACTURES

The transverse fracture is another very common fracture pattern but requires careful assessment to identify the most appropriate surgical tactic. Most of these fractures remain hinged at the symphysis pubis, a feature that can be capitalized upon during surgical reduction. In cases of anterior ramus or symphyseal disruption, the technical difficulty of the fracture reduction is much greater. As noted in other chapters, Letournel described this fracture in three varieties: the high or transtectal fracture, the middle, and the low transverse fracture. The description and radiographic features have been described elsewhere. In general, most of these fractures can be addressed via a posterior approach, except in the occasional circumstance where the majority of the fracture displacement is anterior. In these cases, the ilioinguinal approach is most suitable. The transtectal fracture deserves special mention because of its involvement in the weight-bearing region of the hip joint. Letournel and others recommended that an extensile approach be considered so that direct visualization of the joint be performed to ensure a perfect reduction. We are in agreement that a perfect reduction be achieved, but do not believe that every transtectal fracture requires an extended ilioinguinal approach. We have found that the use of an extended trochanteric osteotomy and luxation of the hip provides the needed requisite visualization of the hip, and if an appropriate reduction is obtained, then an extensile approach can be avoided. However, if there is impaction of the dome with a transtectal fracture, then a truly extensile approach is needed to allow the correction of the articular surface, and for these rare cases we perform an extended iliofemoral approach.

When a posterior approach is used, whatever the position of the patient, it is imperative that the anterior aspect of the fracture along the pelvic brim be reduced and verified with digital palpation through the notch. Techniques used to help with reduction include traction and via ligamentotaxis of the hip joint, Schanz pins in the ischium, and pelvic reduction clamps. In this particular fracture, the angled reduction clamps (Matta) can be placed through the notch to effect a reduction (Fig. 20). In fractures that are transtectal, Letournel recommended an extensile approach so that the joint could be visualized for a perfect reduction. While we agree with the need for a perfect reduction in these cases, we believe that it may be possible to do so without incurring the morbidity of an extensile approach. If a posterior approach is used and arthrotomy can be performed with traction, a suitable amount of traction will distract the joint sufficiently to allow visual inspection of the tectum

(Fig. 13). We have found this to be easiest in the lateral position. Once appropriate reduction is achieved, fixation can follow one of several tactics. The anterior column screw is an excellent option and begins directly superior to the acetabulum about 4 to 6 cm. It is directed anteriorly and distally along the pelvic brim into the superior pubic ramus. This can be a very difficult and dangerous screw because of the vascular structures

(*Text continues on page 221.*)

(A)

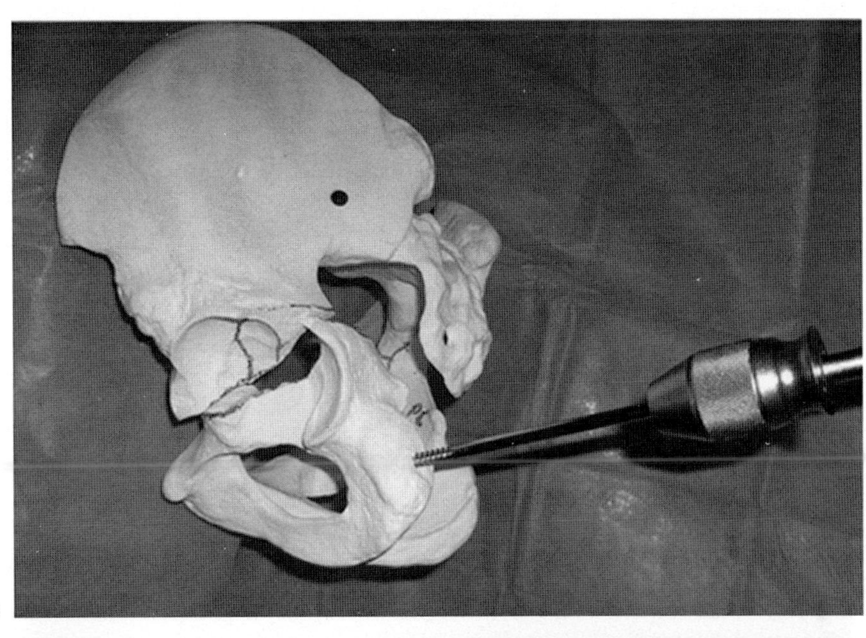

(B)

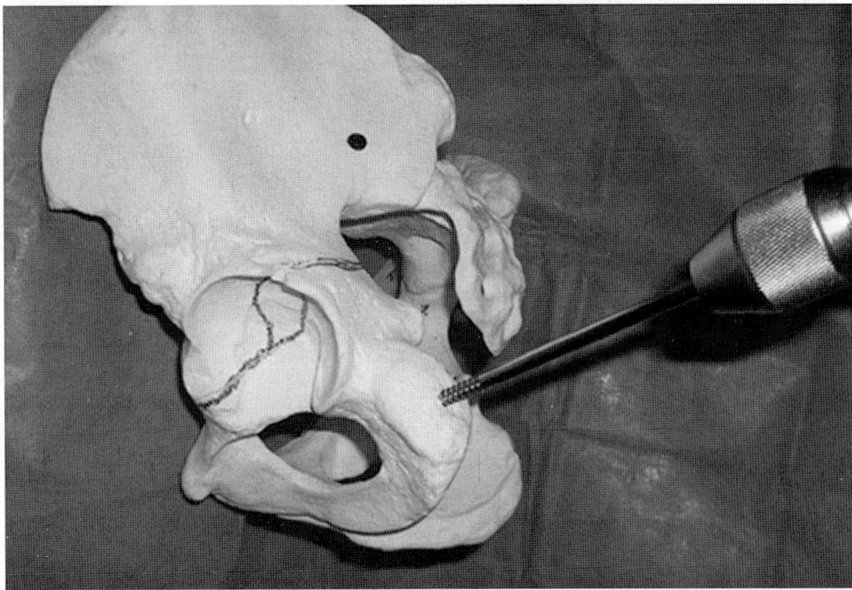

Figure 20 Reduction of the transverse fracture. (**A**,**B**) Using a Schanz pin to correct displacement and rotation. (*Continued*)

(C)

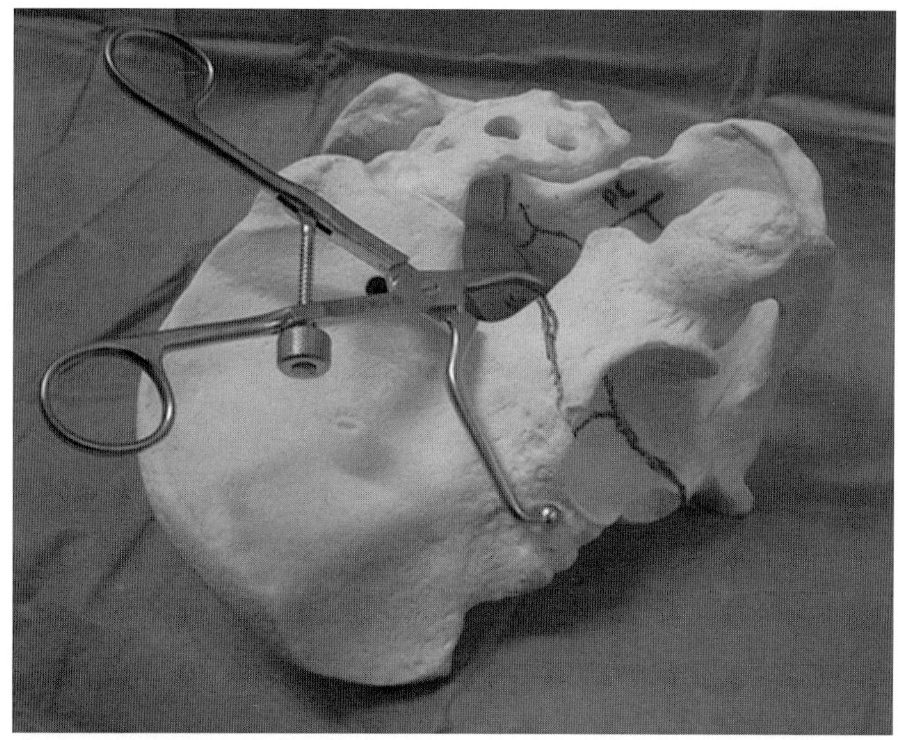

(D)

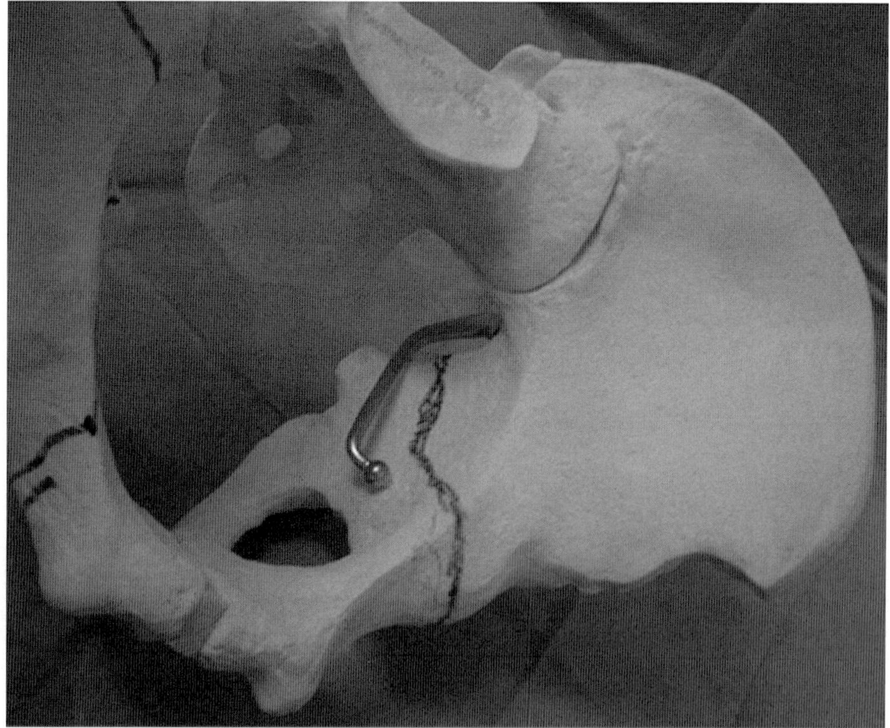

Figure 20 (*Continued*) (**C**,**D**) Use of the angled pelvic clamps (Matta) through the notch.

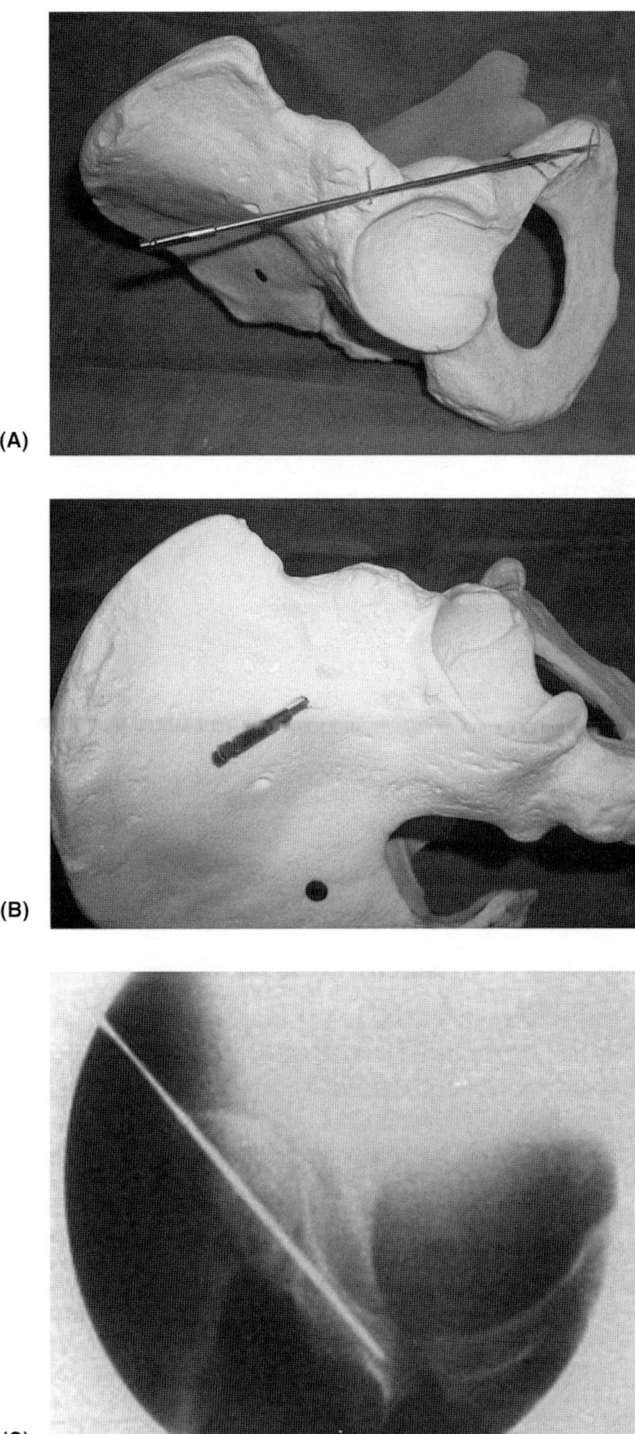

(A)

(B)

(C)

Figure 21 The anterior column screw. (**A**) A drill superimposed over its intended trajectory. (**B**) Entry point of the drill is about 3 to 4 cm directly superior to the acetabulum. (**C**,**D**) The trajectory can be viewed with a number of different image intensifier positions including an iliac-oblique inlet and obturator oblique outlet. *(Continued)*

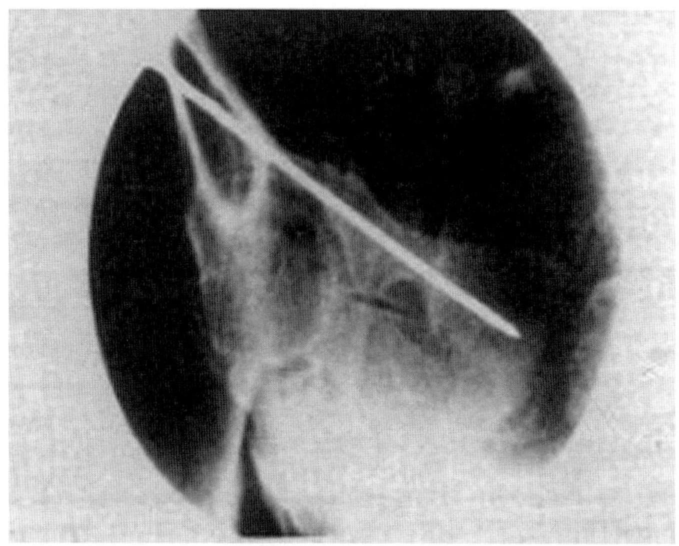

(D)

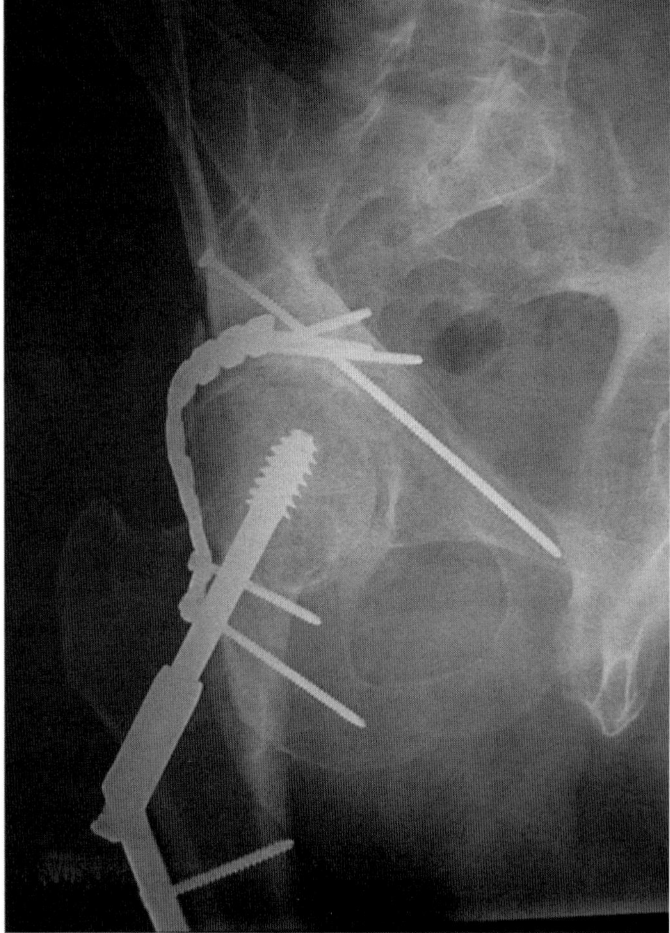

(E)

Figure 21 (*Continued*) (**E**) Radiographic appearance of the screw.

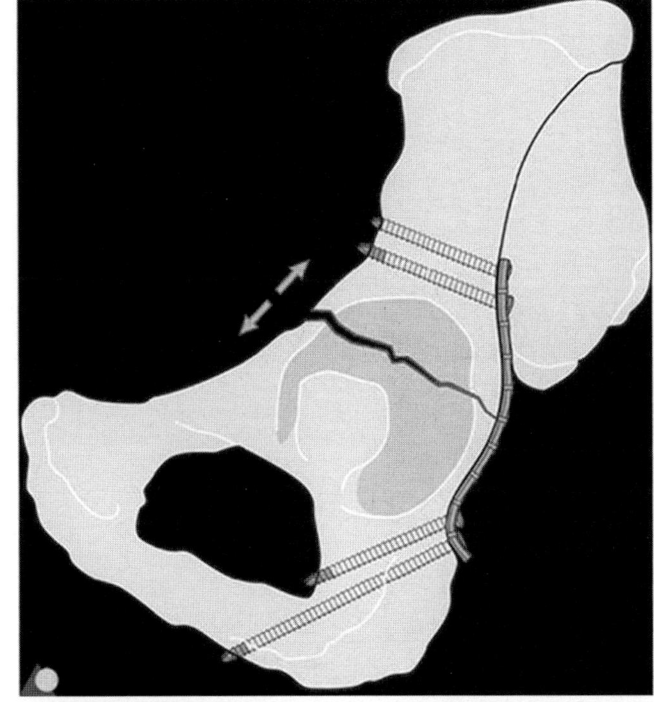

(A)

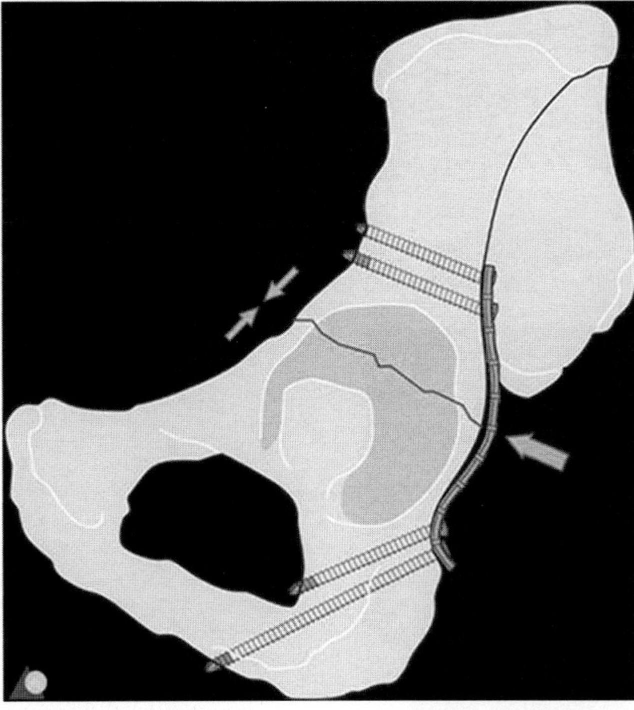

(B)

Figure 22 An underbent plate will have a tendency to gap open the fracture at the anterior column (**A**). For this reason, unlike posterior wall fractures, the plate used for the transverse fracture is slightly overbent (**B**). In cases where both a posterior wall and a transverse fracture exist, two plates may be used and contoured for their respective fracture.

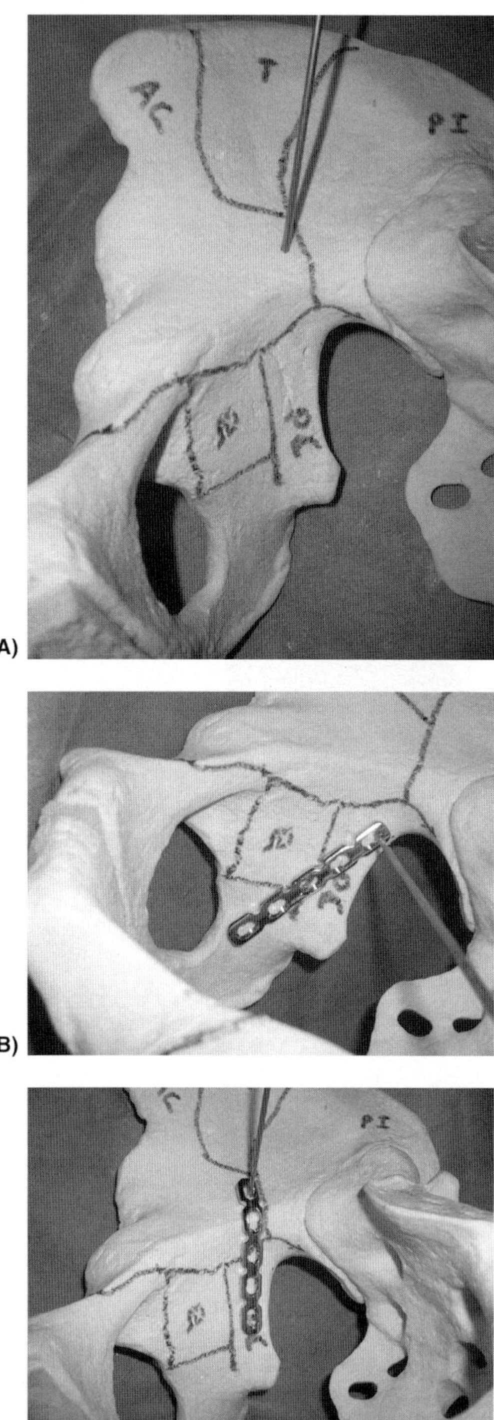

Figure 23 Placement of posterior column fixation devices. In the sawbones models, differing fracture lines have been drawn, but the use of (**A**) posterior column screws and (**B**,**C**) direct column plating from the subinguinal window is the same for any fracture pattern that requires posterior column stabilization.

anteriorly and the joint below. This was another reason stated by Letournel for use of the extensile approach (Fig. 21).

Alternatively, standard posterior plates can be utilized. However, unlike pure posterior wall fractures, the plate is overcontoured (e.g., larger hump over the posterior wall segment and you will note that this overcontoured plate does not sit flush against the posterior wall, and it does not have to be flush since it is not a buttress plate) slightly to help maintain the anterior reduction (Figs. 22 and 24). Occasionally, two plates are required, while on other occasions well-placed screws may suffice. Most importantly, the surgeon must be willing to acknowledge their inability to achieve a suitable reduction using a single approach. In cases where this occurs, it is far better to accept this fact and proceed with a sequential reduction from an alternative exposure (e.g., posterior approach followed by an ilioinguinal) than to struggle fruitlessly with a

(A)

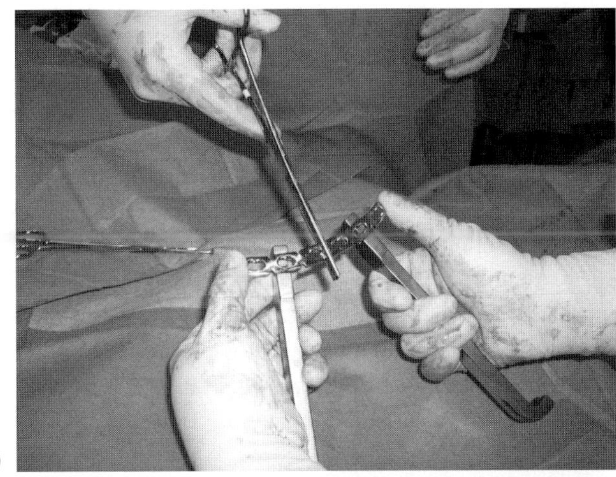

(B)

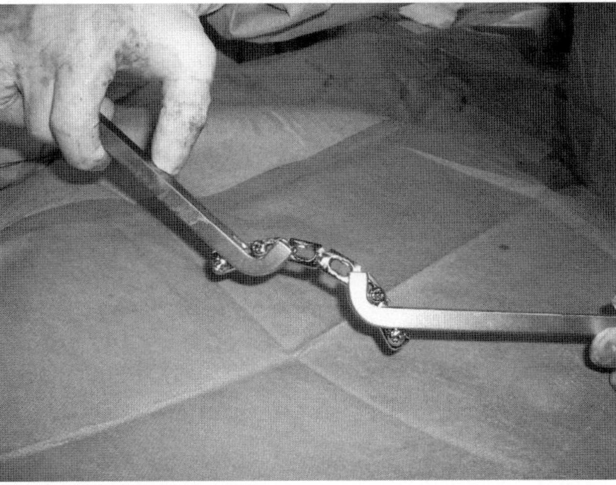

Figure 24 (**A**) Use of standard off-axis plate benders to increase or decrease "curve." The plate should be well stabilized as it has a tendency to fly out of the bending irons. (**B**) An alternate method where two screws are placed into the end holes and the bending irons are used like "crowbars" to effect a bend.

single approach. While uncommon, this can occur even in the most experienced hands. When a second approach is needed, the fixation during the initial approach should be modified so as not to impede reduction and fixation during the second approach. This is one instance where two of our authors (D.S. and R.H.) have found utility in using shorter locking screws in a locking plate during the initial posterior approach. Alternatively, fixation anteriorly can be achieved with a percutaneous anterior column screw, followed by fixation posteriorly with standard Kocher approach and plating. Prior to prepping and draping, ipsilateral lower extremity traction and reduction maneuvers under fluoroscopy will indicate if percutaneous anterior column fixation is feasible. If the anterior column screw is obtainable, then one sequence of management could be the following: patient supine for percutaneous cannulated anterior column screw placement. Close the small incision with staples and cover with Ioban. Reposition the patient in a lateral position for a posterior approach. During the posterior exposure it is sometimes noted and necessary to achieve a better reduction. If necessary, the guide wire can be passed down the cannulated screw and the screw threads can be backed up proximal to the fracture line. The posterior and anterior columns can be rereduced, fixed posteriorly, and then readvancement of the guide wire readvancement of the anterior column screw can be done. Anterior column screws are very challenging in the lateral position because fluoroscopy imaging is limited; again, this is not an issue with the prone positioning. The authors have found that the time spent in repositioning, re-prepping, and re-draping between the anterior column screw placement with the patient supine and the switch to the lateral decubitus position is marginal.

If the transverse fracture is treated with an anterior approach alone, the posterior portion of the fracture can be treated with a posterior column screw placed through the lateral window of the ilioinguinal or via the subinguinal window (described previously). The posterior portion of the fracture can be directly visualized, reduced, and stabilized. These methods can also be used for associated fracture patterns (Fig. 23) described in Chapter 12.

SUMMARY

In this chapter, we reviewed some of the fixation methods for simple patterns. While the complex fracture patterns will follow in the next chapter, many of these methods are applicable to them as well. There are many more "tricks" and methods possible and each surgeon should develop their own specific routine. We outlined some of the more common methods as well as some of our own. We hope they will be useful to anyone contemplating treatment of such complex injuries.

BIBLIOGRAPHY

Benedetti JA, Ebraheim NA, Xu R, Yeasting RA. Automatic considerations of plate-screw fixation of the anterior column of the acetabulum. J Orthop Trauma 1996; 10(4):264–272.

Gill TJ, Sledge JB, Ekkernkamp A, Ganz R. Intraoperative Assessment of Femoral Head Vascularity After Femoral Neck Fracture. J Orthop Trauma 1998; 12:474–478.

Hardy SL. Femoral nerve palsy associated with an associated posterior wall transverse acetabular fracture. J Orthop Trauma 1997; 11:40–42.

Kloen P, Siebenrock KA, Ganz R. Modification of the ilioinguinal approach. J Orthop Trauma 2002; 16(8):586–593.

Ziran et al. OTA, Archdeacon.

12

Acetabular Reconstruction: Fixation Methods in Associated Fracture Patterns

Bruce H. Ziran
Department of Orthopaedic Trauma, St. Elizabeth Health Center and Department of Orthopaedic Surgery, Northeastern Ohio Universities College of Medicine, Youngstown, Ohio, U.S.A.

Daniel R. Schlatterer and Robert M. Harris
Department of Orthopaedic Trauma, Atlanta Medical Center, Atlanta, Georgia, U.S.A.

INTRODUCTION TO ASSOCIATED FRACTURE PATTERNS OF THE ACETABULUM

The associated patterns of acetabular fractures were described by Letournel and are described elsewhere in this text. They tend to be more severe in nature and require very thorough planning to ensure appropriate access. In all but the posterior column/posterior wall fracture pattern, both anterior and posterior aspects of the acetabulum are involved and need to be considered when planning. While the definition of each fracture pattern is well described, there will be frequent situations where the fracture pattern is transitional. It is important to try to understand the essential features and behavior of each pattern, the so called "personality" of the fracture, so that an appropriate tactic can be performed. An example of fracture personality is the presence of intra-articular foreign bodies. A fracture pattern amenable to an anterior approach may not permit adequate access to the joint to remove joint debris. This "personality" of the fracture may mandate a sequential or extensile approach as opposed to a standard approach. Osteopenia and concomitant pelvic disruption are further characteristics of the fracture personality. These two issues are addressed in this chapter. Finally, many of the concepts of the previous chapter are applicable in this chapter and appropriately referenced.

POSTERIOR COLUMN AND POSTERIOR WALL ACETABULAR FRACTURES

This pattern is relatively rare. Often a posterior wall fracture will be found to have a minimally displaced or occult column fracture (or transverse fracture). These fractures behave and are better classified as posterior wall fractures, as recommended by Letournel, since the essential lesion is the posterior wall. True posterior column fractures have definite displacement. Nonetheless, the treatment paradigm is similar and will utilize a posterior approach. The options of positioning and traction for the posterior approach have been described in the preceding chapter. The preferred method of one author (B.Z.) is with a lateral position and the use of skeletal traction, both longitudinal and lateral, as previously described in the section on "Simple Fracture Patterns" (Chapter 11, Fig. 2). The other authors (D.S., R.H.) also prefer a lateral position, but uses a five- to six-inch stack of folded towels tucked deep into the groin between the legs. Gentle downward pressure at the flexed knee reduces the weight of the femoral head on the acetabulum. The stack of towels, combined with longitudinal and lateral traction via the trochanteric Schantz pin, results in very good joint exposure for posterior fractures (Chapter 11, Fig. 3). Reduction techniques for an associated posterior wall and column fracture will be similar to a simple posterior column and a simple posterior wall fracture. For this associated pattern, it is most logical to begin with column fixation first, followed by the posterior wall. This sequence (column first then wall) permits restoration of a "foundation" upon which to restore the posterior wall. With the column reduced and the wall not reduced, an opportunity exists to widely inspect the reduced column through the joint surface. The position of the column can be modified if need be, and then one can proceed with the posterior wall. Keep in mind that operative management of displaced posterior column fractures have a higher risk of injury to the sciatic nerve, especially in patterns involving the sciatic notch (Fig. 1). In all cases, a good documentation of any

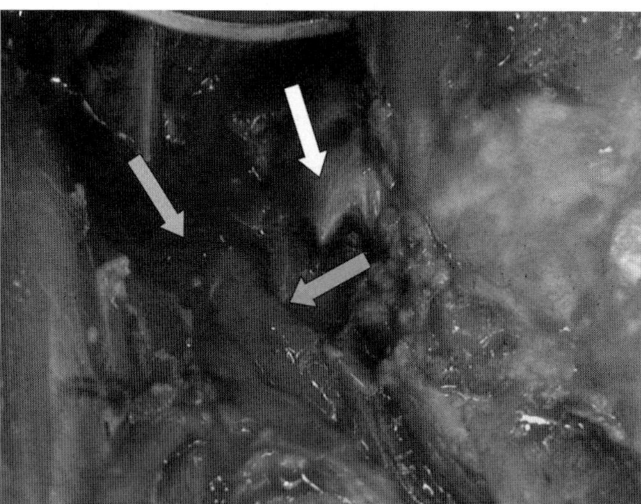

Figure 1 Intraoperative view of impingement of sciatic nerve by posterior fragment. The posterior column fracture is close to the sciatic notch and may damage the sciatic nerve, especially with an associated posterior wall fracture.

dysfunction prior to surgery is essential to avoid any misunderstandings if postoperative dysfunction is encountered. For severely displaced fractures and in cases of subtle deficits, consideration should be given to nerve monitoring, mostly to document a deficit prior to surgical intervention, but also to ensure that surgical tactic does not worsen the problem. Some centers utilize intraoperative neuro-monitoring, but this has not been routine in our practices. Equally important during operative management of fracture patterns involving the sciatic notch are the superior gluteal vessels and nerve. Overzealous retraction can injure these structures. Hemostasis can be very challenging as the vessels are prone to retract into the pelvis. Debriding intervening fracture hematoma and periosteum at the notch level is also very dangerous. Care should be taken to visualize these neurovascular structures as they exit the notch and come "around the corner." Judicious use of Cobb elevators and curettes is imperative.

Depending on the level of the posterior column fracture and the body habitus of the patient, the exposure may require more cephalad exposure, in which case, implementing the trochanteric slide, or flip osteotomy is recommended. The reduction of the posterior column needs to be ensured and can be determined by viewing and palpating the posterior cortical borders and by palpation through the greater and lesser sciatic notches into the area of the quadrilateral surface. In some cases, provisional fixation can be obtained via lag screws, especially when there is an extensive posterior wall fracture, wherein use of a plate for the column might interfere with reduction of the wall segment. In these cases, logical surgical tactic to sequence the reduction steps is critical to ensure an anatomic reduction. An example may be a situation where a single lag screw cannot be used for temporary stabilization. In this situation, use of reduction clamps that engage screws placed on each side of the fracture (Farabeuf or pelvic reduction) is needed (Fig. 2). In these cases, reduction is achieved, but the clamps can obstruct free access to the posterior wall elements, and in cases where there is marginal impaction the reduction and fixation tactic may be difficult. In such cases of potential clamp obstruction, treatment of the wall first and then addressing the posterior column second is sometimes the easier sequence to follow. Kirshner wires can then provide provisional fixation after finalizing the posterior wall reduction. The final step of stabilizing both with a spanning plate may be more elegant than struggling with exposure and access. To assist with the rotation and reduction of the column fragment, a Schantz pin can be placed into the ischial tuberosity and used as a "joystick" to effect a reduction (Chapter 11, Fig. 20). Alternatively, use of angled pelvic reduction clamps placed through the sciatic notch may achieve and maintain reduction of the more anterior parts of the column. The advantage of pelvic reduction clamp or Farabeufs that engage separately placed screws is that they can help with translational maneuvers and then compress the bone directly. The second author, D.S., frequently implements a flattened three hole 1/3 tubular plate (or 3.5 mm reconstruction plate) for the posterior column component. The advantages of this method are many and include compression across the fracture. In addition, pelvic clamps and screws are not typically necessary after fixation with the 1/3 tubular plate. Partial fixation with a thin plate permits clamp removal, which in turn improves access and options to overlay a longer 3.5 mm reconstruction plate for additional fixation. Care must be taken when using this method that the corners of the plate do not overhang either sciatic notch. This runs the risk of irritating the neurovascular structures and the short external rotator tendons. The plate

(Text continued on page 230.)

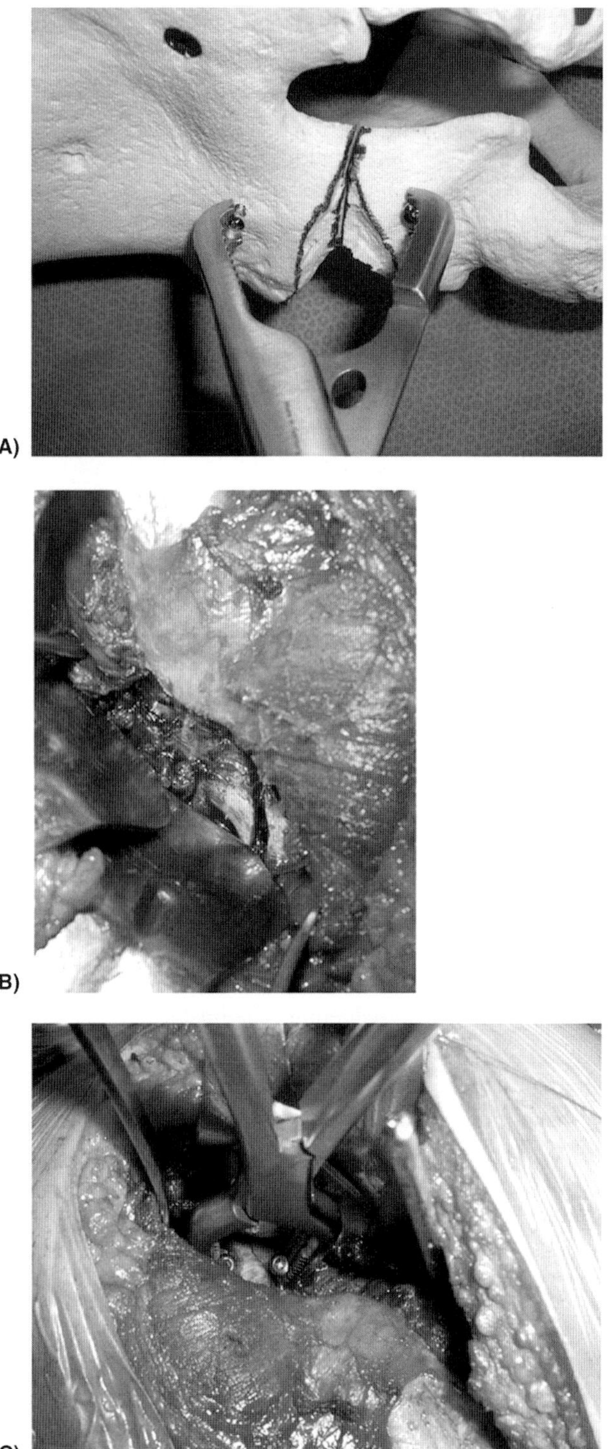

Figure 2 (**A**) Demonstration of reduction clamps around screws to help reduce column fragments. (**B**) Patient in prone position with fracture of posterior column. (**C**) Intraoperative view of Farabeuf clamps and reduction. Note that space is tight. (*Continued*)

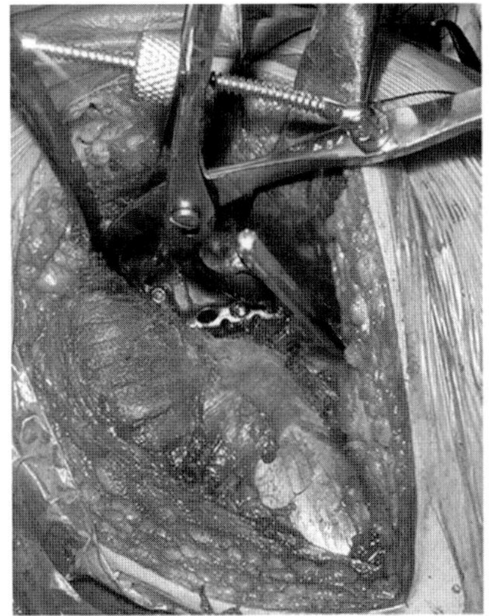
(D)

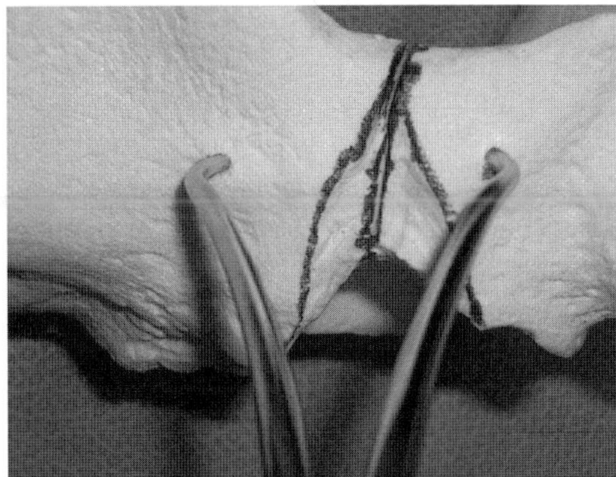
(E)

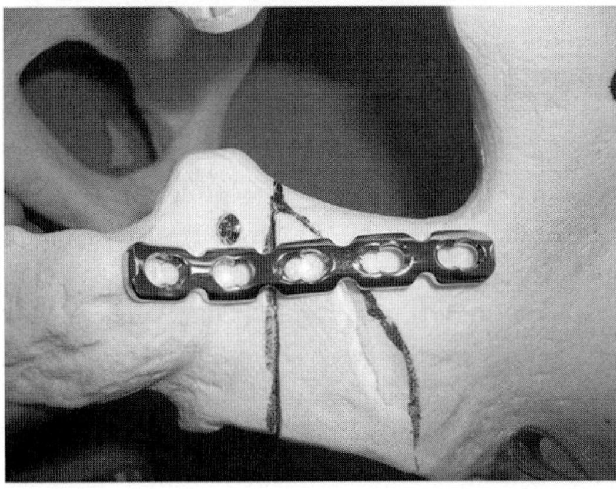
(F)

Figure 2 *(Continued)* (**D**) Alternative method of using same post screws but now placing a plate in position and using a Verbrugge clamp to effect a reduction with plate in place (images courtesy of Rodrigo Pesantez, MD). (**E**) Alternate method using tenaculums. (**F**) Bone model showing temporary screw and a posterior column plate over an extensive posterior wall fracture. *(Continued)*

(G) 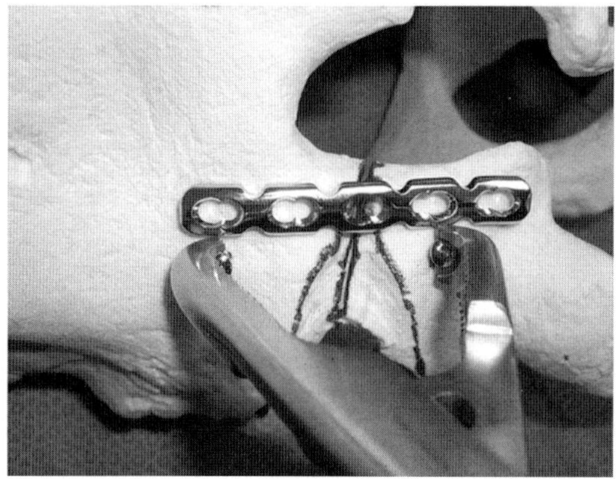

Figure 2 *(Continued)* A buttress plate would be required to adequately stabilize the posterior wall component. In some cases, the screws can be placed surrounding the posterior wall segment to allow space for the posterior column plate (**G**).

corners can be cut and then smoothed with the knurled portion of a "quick connect" or other power drill adapter with a knurled portion. Simply turn the drill on and use the knurled portion as a grinder.

As in most situations, two good screws (in the plate) on both sides of the fracture are generally enough to ensure fixation. In cases where the fracture of the posterior column extends cephalad to the hip joint or into the angle of the sciatic notch, fixation of the column to the posterior ilium may be performed with lag screws. Depending on the quality or amount of bone available for fixation, one should consider use of two screws with or without washers. The plate used for the posterior wall fracture will supplement these screws, as the screws are generally not sufficient by themselves. In cases where the vertical component of the posterior column fracture enters the obturator foramen and through the ischial ramus, reduction of the cephalad portion of the column may not be sufficient to ensure a congruent joint reduction, and the inferior portion needs to be evaluated. In these cases, pelvic reduction forceps through the sciatic notch may help pull the column into place. If there is a tendency towards rotation, slight overrotation of the plate may assist in maintaining the reduction.

Once the posterior column is satisfactorily secured, the posterior wall can be addressed as described in Chapter 11 in the section on "Posterior Wall Fractures." An advantage of addressing the column fracture first is that it allows easier visualization of the articular surface to ensure a satisfactory reduction of the articular surface. This can be done with in line traction. In such cases, however, care should be taken if the hip is subluxed with traction to make sure the posterior column fracture and fixation is not disrupted. If there is comminution of the posterior wall that requires a "spring" plate, anticipation of this technique should be considered during fixation of the column so that the column fixation does not interfere with the placement of the spring plate. Ideally, the spring plates are placed first and the reconstruction plate overlaps the spring plates.

There are cases where the posterior wall fracture extends very posteriorly. As the posterior wall fracture line approaches the sciatic notches, less posterior column is available for fixation without interfering with reduction of the posterior wall. In these extreme cases, the fracture may appear to be nearly segmental, where the posterior wall exits via part of the column. These fractures can be very difficult to reduce and fix because of the lack of access to posterior column surface. In these cases, lag screw fixation, either from column to ilium or vice versa, should be considered for fixation of the posterior column. Alternatively, if the posterior wall is one large piece, the order of fixation may be reversed, such that the wall is fixed provisionally to the column, thereby simplifying the fracture, and then reducing and fixing the column. Another upside of this fracture pattern is that the wall fragment is large and amendable to lag screws and/or buttress plating. Finally, another technique to consider in such cases is to (*i*) ensure that the wall can be reduced, (*ii*) reduce and plate the posterior column, and then (*iii*) remove a small portion of the most posterior extent of the wall fragment (which is not articular or structural) to allow the wall to seat along side the column plate. A second reconstruction plate can then be placed (adjacent to the first posterior column recon plate) over the posterior wall for buttressing purposes (Fig. 3).

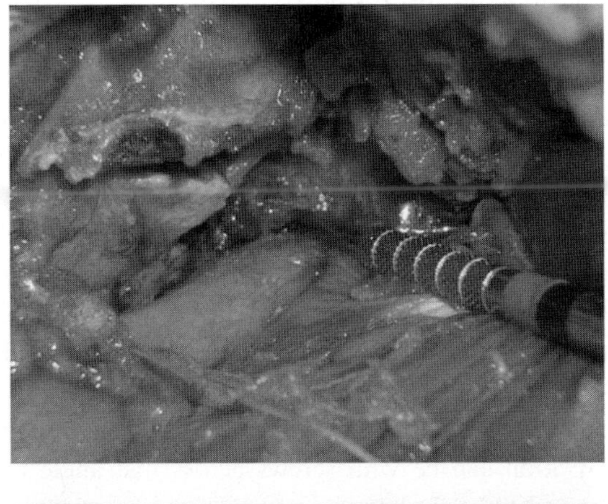

(A)

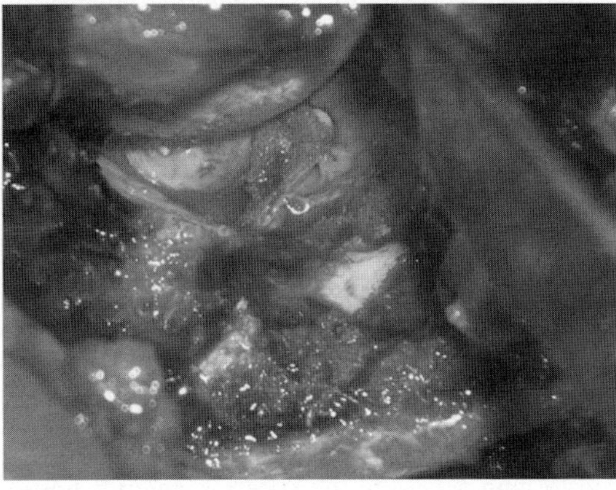

(B)

Figure 3 (**A**) A posterior column and wall fracture showing the extent of posterior wall injury and the little remaining space available in the posterior column for fixation. In this case, the column was plated first, and then the posterior cortex of the posterior wall was trimmed to allow reduction of the wall next to the plate. (**B**) A fragment of bone from the same fracture impinging on sciatic nerve and incarcerated in the greater sciatic notch.

TRANSVERSE ACETABULAR POSTERIOR WALL FRACTURES

The surgical approach for an isolated transverse fracture varies. High-fracture patterns can be approached anteriorly and a low-fracture pattern can be approached posteriorly. The preoperative planning to a transverse posterior wall fracture begins with determining if the posterior wall is unstable and operative. If so, then some form of a posterior approach is mandatory. The decision that follows is whether a simple approach, an extensile approach, or a combined posterior and anterior approach is indicated. In Letournel's original text, he occasionally described the use of an extended iliofemoral approach for transtectal transverse fractures with anterior displacement and an associated posterior wall fracture. However, as the use of this approach diminishes, some advocate a sequential approach if needed, and few advocate simultaneous approaches. Frequently, the transverse fracture is most displaced posteriorly and can be hinged back, as described for the simple transverse pattern. The reduction maneuvers and techniques used for this component of the fracture are similar to those described in the individual sections of the previous chapter dedicated to posterior column and transverse fractures. Again we use the lateral position for this fracture.

In these cases, it is important to digitally palpate the pelvic brim via the sciatic notch to ensure that the anterior portions of the fracture are sufficiently reduced. Plate contouring is a subtle but important point in posterior plate fixation of a transverse fracture. An under-contoured plate can result in anterior fracture line gapping. Over-contouring the reconstruction plate used for the transverse fracture will minimize anterior fracture line gapping. This point is nicely demonstrated on saw-bone models of transverse fractures (Chapter 11, Fig. 20). Use of the Schantz pin inserted into the ischial tubersosity and angled pelvic reduction clamps through the notch will assist in the reduction of this fracture. Since the posterior wall is fractured, visualization of the reduction via inspection of the joint is facilitated, and acceptable reduction ensured. As in posterior column/posterior wall fractures, the posterior fixation should be addressed elegantly. The column fixation can be with screws across that angle of the sciatic notch or a slightly over-bent and twisted plate to assist with the anterior portion of the reduction. If it is determined that the anterior segment of the fracture cannot be adequately reduced, or stabilized, then we recommend addressing the anterior component with a separate (sequential) surgical approach. In these cases, the fixation of the posterior elements must be performed in such a manner that they do not interfere with the anterior elements. As such, keeping screws more posterior and using a more flexible construct (longer plate, wider separation of screws) will facilitate the anterior reduction. This may be one indication for locking plates with locking screws short of the anterior column.

In transtectal transverse fracture patterns, we have not reflexively opted for an extended iliofemoral approach. Instead, we used the posterior approach and ensured that the fracture line is accurately reduced via direct visualization. In some cases, the trochanteric flip osteotomy was used to gain access to the superior/anterior portions of the acetabulum, as well as allow access as far anterior as the anterior inferior iliac spine. We feel that this approach, while a more extensile posterior approach, is preferable to an extended iliofemoral. Also, it allows easier placement of the anterior column screw, which can be fairly difficult to place. This screw, as described previously, begins in the superior aspect of the acetabulum and courses along the anterior column and provides sufficient "intramedullary" fixation of the anterior column (Chapter 11, Fig. 21). It can be placed in a retrograde fashion as well but would require a separate surgical prep and drape. It should be noted that placement of this particular screw in the lateral position without an extensile approach is fairly difficult. Most surgeons prefer to place this screw supine, prone, or with use of an extensile approach. However, good knowledge of the pelvic anatomy and appropriate visualization with an image intensifier will facilitate this screw in the lateral position.

The posterior wall fracture will be addressed as described in the previous section on "Posterior Column and Posterior Wall Acetabular Fractures." The elements of the wall fracture will be varied, and fixation will depend on the morphology and location of the fracture. In superior fracture patterns, the quality of reduction is most important since this area is the primary load-bearing section of the acetabulum. Again, a trochanteric flip of greater trochanter osteotomy can be utilized to gain access for visualization and stabilization. In the more inferior fracture patterns, this technique is obviated and more conventional methods can be used (Fig. 4).

T-SHAPED ACETABULAR FRACTURES

The T-shaped fracture can be one of the most challenging and difficult of the acetabular fractures to treat. It is also a fracture that will incur numerous varying opinions on surgical tactic, but most agree that an accurate reduction is the key to success. The radiographic features that distinguish the T-fracture from its analogs [a low anterior column, posterior hemitransverse, a transverse with pubic fracture, and posterior column-anterior hemitransverse (which Letournel lumped with T-shaped)] have been discussed elsewhere but include a fracture that involves or exits via the ischial ramus. The surgical tactic for T-fractures begins with identifying the essential pathology to be addressed. The transverse component and the stem, along with the presence or absence of an operative posterior wall and the nature of the displacements, will guide the surgeon toward the optimal surgical approach. The axial CT scan can facilitate examination of the posterior wall and overall fracture pattern. Involvement of the posterior wall can rule in or rule out the need for a posterior approach. For fractures with operative posterior wall involvement, the decision is then either sequential approaches or an extensile approach with the possibility of a trochanteric osteotomy. Unlike a transverse fracture or a both-column fracture, in T-shaped fractures the femoral head is usually completely separated from the columnar segments, either by dislocation or protrusion into the pelvis (Fig. 5). Also, there is usually loss of the ligamentous attachments that facilitate reduction of each segment using ligamentotaxis. This feature makes choosing the correct surgical approach and having tools available to facilitate reduction very important.

In general, the segment with the most displacement or location of the transverse component will dictate the preferred approach. If the posterior approach is chosen, the posterior fragment can be reduced and stabilized to the posterior iliac segment at the sciatic angle. Use of a few screws will allow the removal of the reduction clamps. It is important to verify that the posterior segment is reduced, not just along the posterior cortical border, but also along the quadrilateral surface and up to the pelvic brim. This

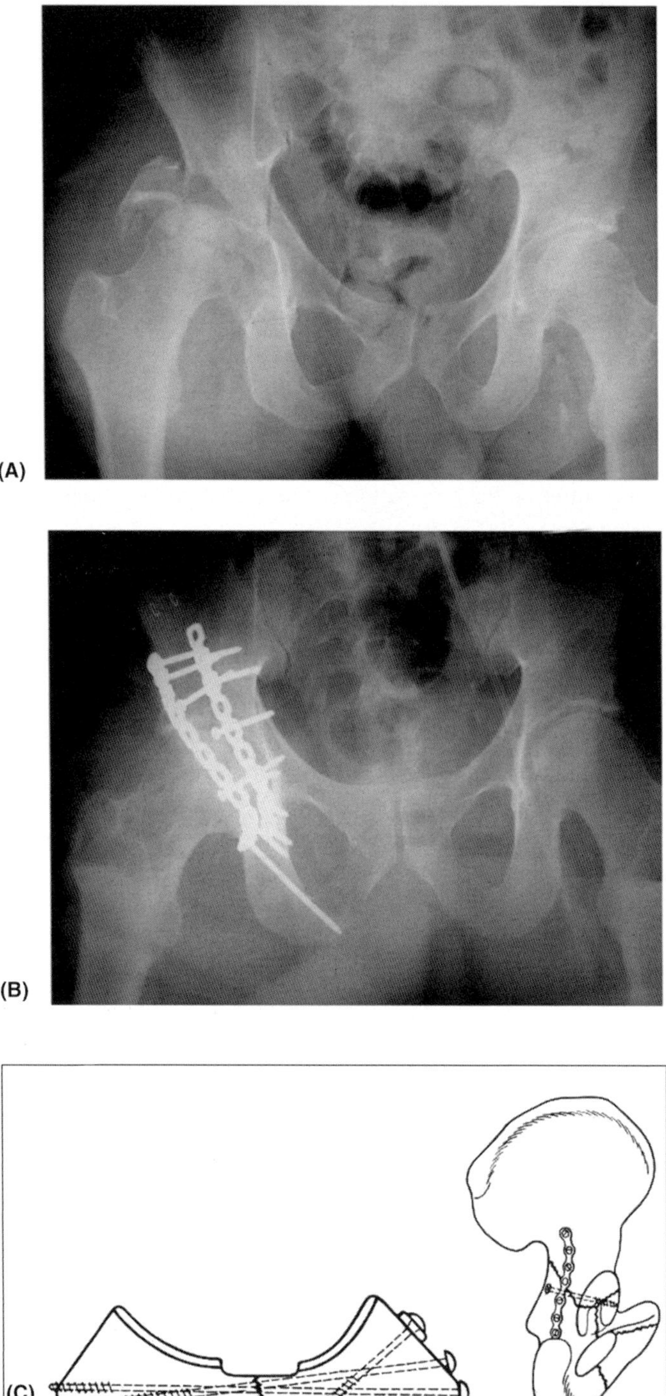

Figure 4 (**A**) Pre- and (**B**) postoperative radiographs of a transverse posterior wall fracture. Note the individual screws placed behind the acetabulum that capture some of the anterior transverse component. (**C**) Schematic of screw trajectory. *Source*: From Ref. 2.

(A) 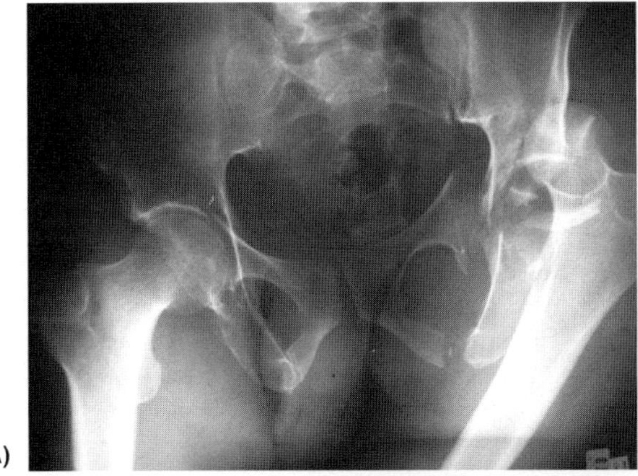

(B) 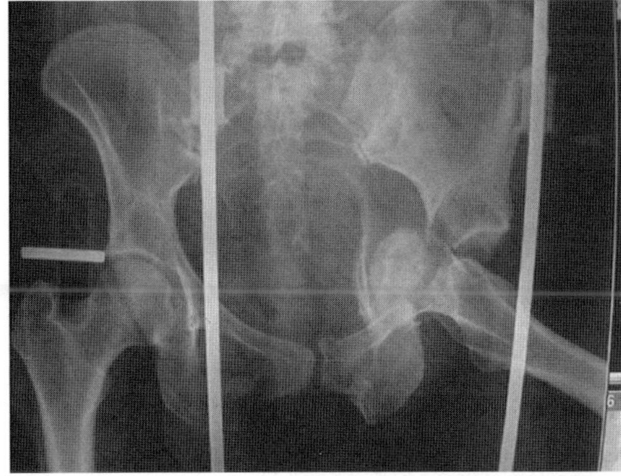

Figure 5 (**A**) T-fracture with posterior dislocation and posterior wall fracture. (**B**) T-fracture with central protrusion and impaction. The T-fracture can be one of the most difficult acetabular injuries to treat and has a relatively poor prognosis.

is best done with digital palpation. Also, it is important to ensure that the provisional fixation of this segment does not exit the posterior segment and interfere with reduction of the anterior segment. Again, as mentioned earlier in this chapter, this may be an indication for short locking screws in locking plates.

To reduce the anterior segment, angled pelvic clamps (also called the Matta clamps) are carefully placed through the notch to reduce the anterior segment. It is important to place one tine on the anterior fragment and the other on the intact iliac bone. If excessive force is placed on the provisionally fixed posterior segment, it can cause displacement or, worse, further comminution. Once reduced, there are several options for fixation. For the anterior segment, screws placed along the posterior border of the posterior segment can course behind the acetabulum and, depending on the location of the stem of the T, may secure the anterior fragment. Alternatively, these screws may be placed through a plate as well (Fig. 6). In many circumstances, the anterior column screw is desirable because of the stability afforded by its intramedullary position. This screw can be placed percutaneously or with some added dissection through the exposed but remaining transmuscular. It is usually not necessary to detach any of the abductor mechanism for this screw. The

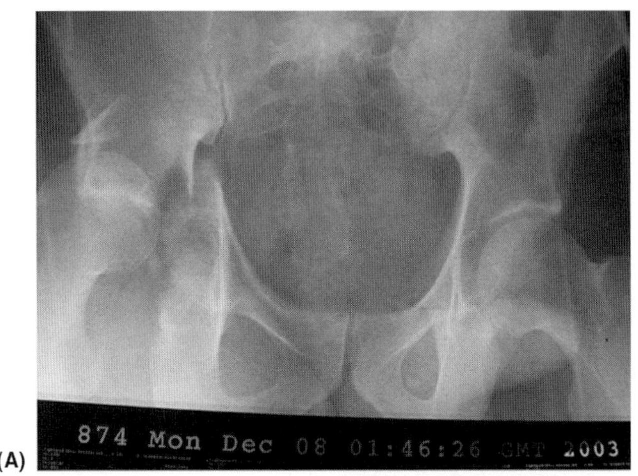

(A)

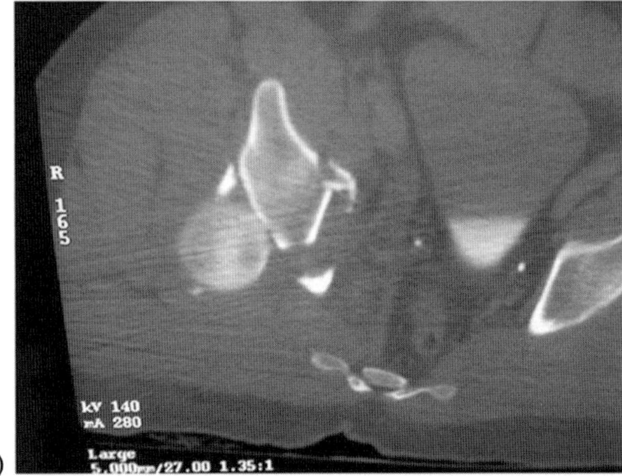

(B)

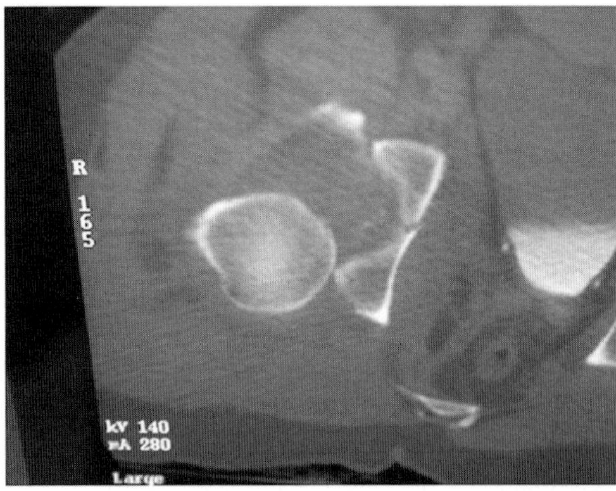

(C)

Figure 6 (**A**–**C**) Radiographs and CT scan of a transischial T-fracture dislocation with posterior wall fracture. (*Continued*)

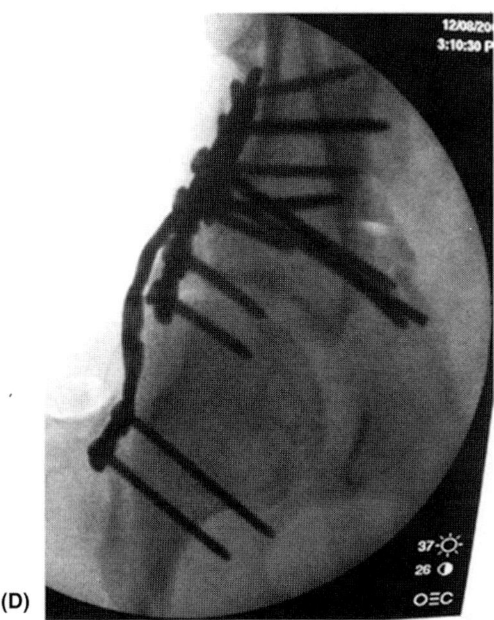

(D)

Figure 6 (*Continued*) In this case, screws through the plate provided fixation to the anterior column (**D**).

cutaneous entry point for this percutaneous screw is a position midway between the greater trochanter and iliac crest. The osseous insertion site is 4 to 6 cm superior to the acetabular roof. Fluoroscopic guidance is imperative with this screw to ensure that it does not enter the joint or injure the anterior vascular structures. Please see Chapter 6 on percutaneous fracture management for optimal fluoroscopic imaging. Regarding definitive fixation, a plate traversing the posterior segment will generally be sufficient, along with any supplemental screws that have been placed (Fig. 7).

In some cases, the posterior fragment may not be the first to be reduced and stabilized, and it can be pulled out a bit to visualize the anterior reduction directly. If there is a posterior wall fracture, it will need to be addressed as a separate entity. Because the plating of the T-fracture will often have the plate in a more posterior position (to allow placement of the screws into the anterior fragment), this plate may not sufficiently cover the posterior wall fragment. In this case, the use of a spring plate or two may provide the stability needed. If after all maneuvers the anterior fragment is either insufficiently reduced or stabilized (drifts after fixation, indicating insufficient fixation), then the patient should be considered for a sequential anterior approach that addresses the anterior problem directly. Prior to doing so, the surgeon should ensure that none of the posterior fixation interferes with reduction of the anterior fragment (Fig. 8). This may require removal of several posterior screws and further destabilization of the overall fracture. However, since the anterior fragment will be addressed definitively with an anterior approach, it is of little consequence to remove several posterior screws.

Alternatively, a transverse fracture can be approached anteriorly first followed by a posterior approach. The second author, D.S., has found utility in placement of a percutaneous anterior column screw with the patient supine. The patient is then repositioned and redraped for a more formal posterior approach. The supine position (or prone) is ideal for fluoroscopic imaging of the anterior column screw. In acute fractures (prior to organization of the fracture hematoma), closed reduction of the anterior portion of the fracture is often possible with manipulation of the ipsilateral lower extremity. The added time for repositioning, prepping, and draping is about 20 minutes and this is more than offset by the fluoroscopic imaging permitted. Furthermore, through the

(*Text continued on page 242.*)

(A)

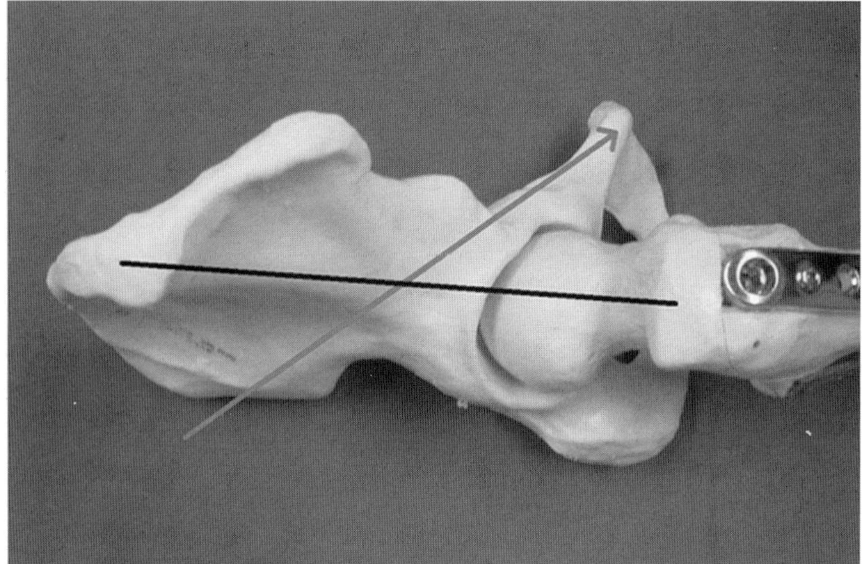

(B)

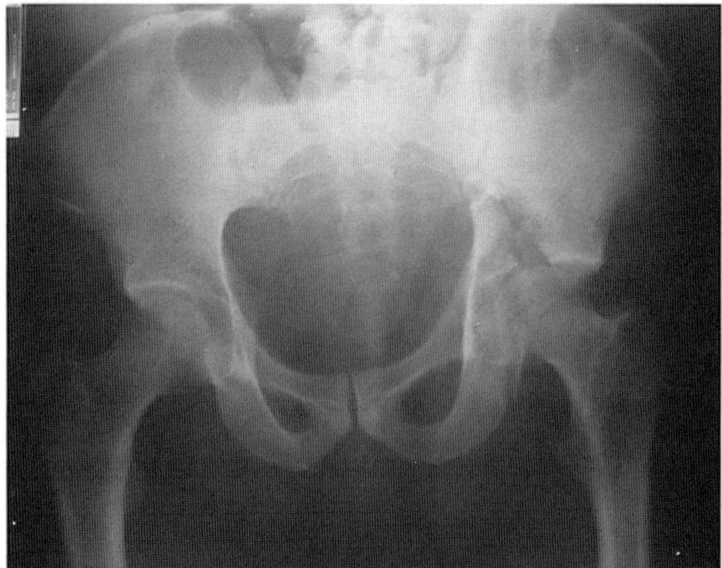

Figure 7 (**A**) The trajectory of the anterior column screw in a pelvis model. This screw should be placed with fluoroscopic guidance as described in a previous chapter. (*Continued*)

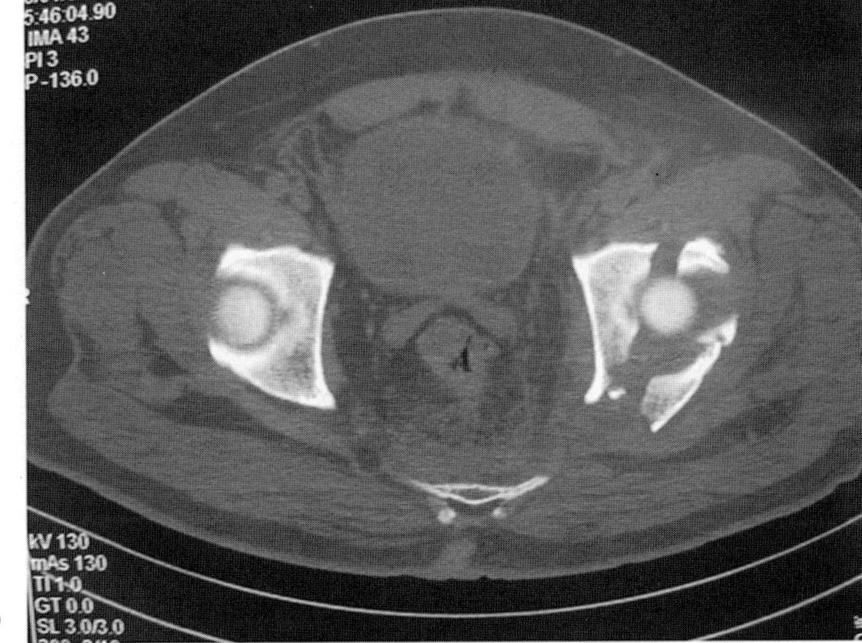

(C)

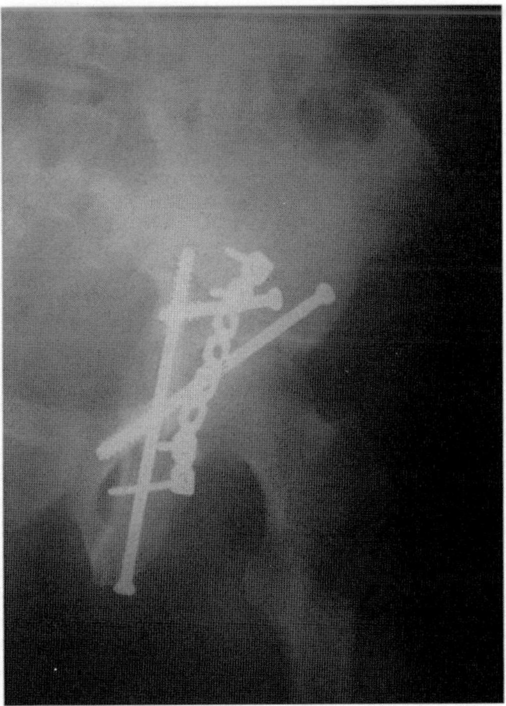

(D)

Figure 7 (*Continued*) (**B–D**) A severe transverse-posterior wall fracture with an extended transischial stem. While technically not a T, it is probably a transitional variant, and demonstrates the use of a plate for posterior fixation and the anterior column screw for the anterior segment of the transverse acetabular fracture.

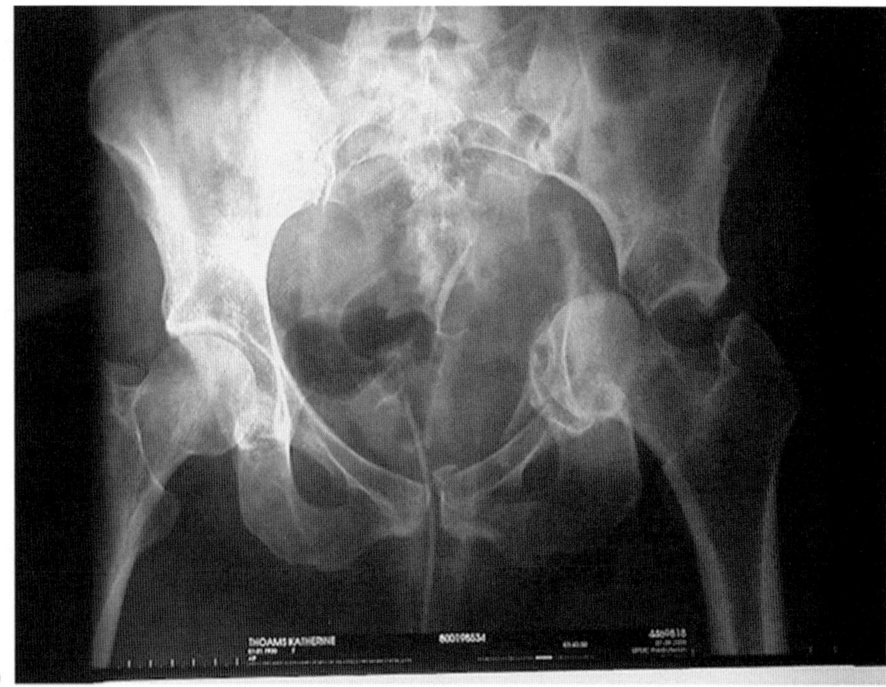

(A)

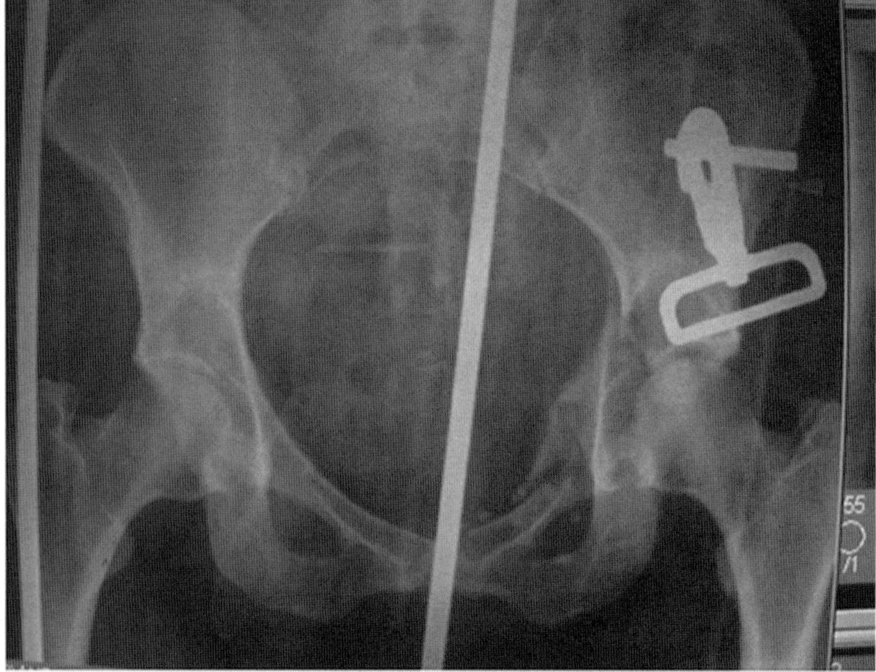

(B)

Figure 8 (**A**, **B**) A T-fracture that required a sequential anterior then posterior approach. This is the same fracture depicted in Figure 5B. The fracture had anterior impaction of the dome as well the femoral head. (*Continued*)

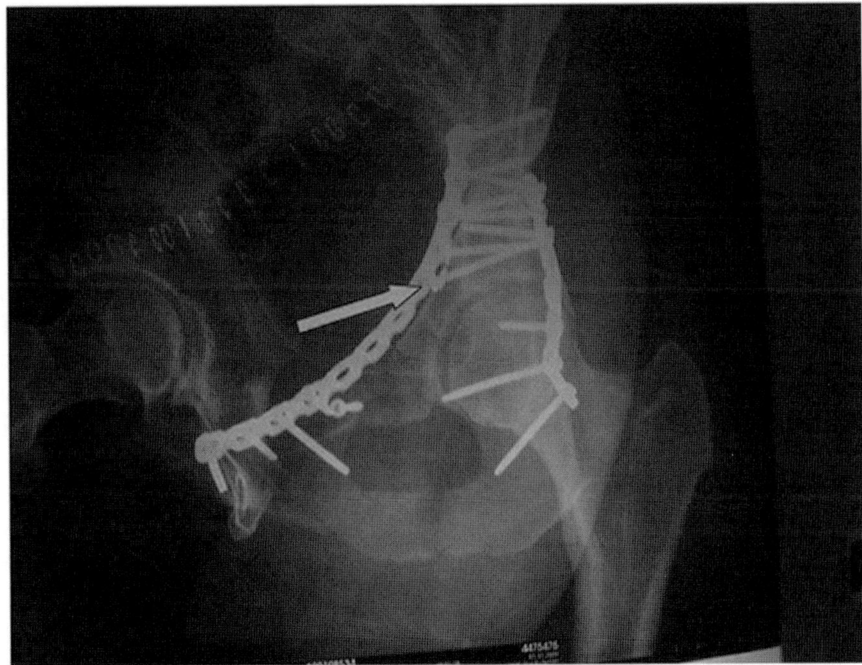

(C)

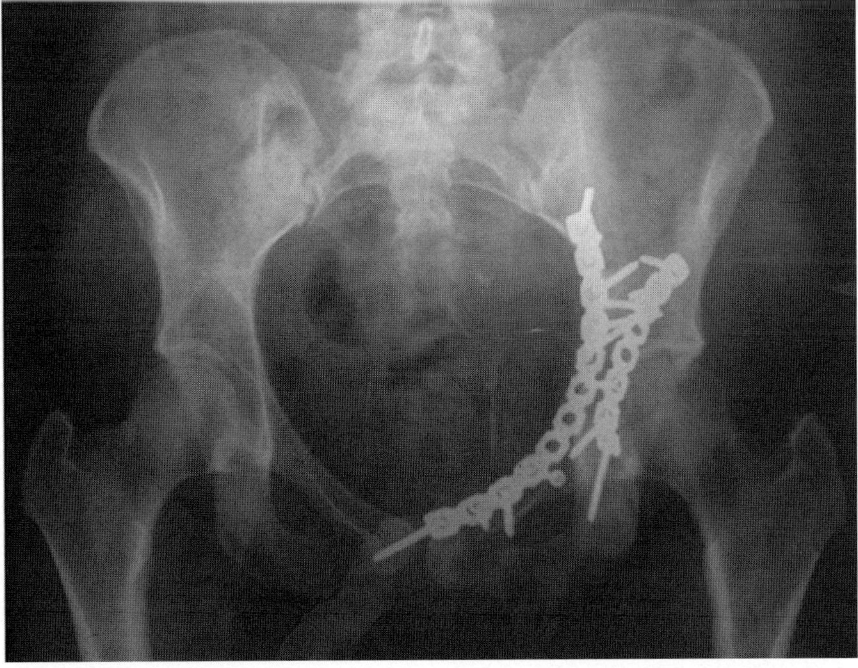

(D)

Figure 8 (*Continued*) (**C**, **D**) While such fractures frequently are approached from the posterior aspect first, this fracture was treated with an anterior approach first, with distraction of the anterior limb and treatment of the impacted dome (elevation and grafting), followed by subarticular screw stabilization (*gray arrow*), and then by an anterior plate. Note multiple unfilled screw holes in the middle of the anterior plate. The anterior screw placement is such that it does not interfere with the second stage, which is posterior column fixation using a standard posterior plate.

posterior approach, the fracture reduction can be continued even with the anterior column screw in place. The guidewire is passed back through the cannulated screw and then the screw is backed out proximal to the fracture line. The anterior screw does not need to be entirely removed. With just the guidewire past the fracture line, there is enough wiggle room to improve the overall reduction. This facilitates reduction of the transverse fracture from the posterior aspect without losing the direction for the anterior column screw. Once the reduction is satisfactory, the cannulated screw is readvanced over the guidewire, and "front and back" fixation is achieved.

In cases where there is a majority of anterior involvement and displacement (and with absence of posterior pathology such as a posterior wall), it may be suitable to approach the fracture from an anterior approach. Also, with recent advances in technique and the use of a modified Stoppa or a "subinguinal" window of the ilioinguinal approach, the posterior column can be addressed from the front and stabilized from "inside-out." In this context, the standard ilioinguinal approach is utilized for the majority of the fracture treatment, but most of the work is done via the lateral and medial windows. From the medial window, the surgeon goes to the opposite side of the table and works under the muscle and vascular bundle and in front of the bladder. With this approach, the entirety of the quadrilateral surface can be directly seen and plated, and the posterior column can be manipulated directly into place. As in the posterior approach, provisional fixation is usually into the sciatic buttress, but in this case, the screws are placed inside out. Furthermore, direct plating of the posterior column from the inside of the pelvis can be performed. We have found the subinguinal window of the standard ilioinguinal approach to be very utilitarian. In fact, the need for use of the middle window has declined precipitously. The lack of dissection around the vascular and lymphatic trunk appears to be beneficial and at little cost to exposure and fixation. As such, as more reports on this technique are published, it may supplant traditional methods.

Summarily, for fixation of the T-shaped fracture using the anterior approach, there is little previous literature describing methodology. Even Letournel himself claimed it was infrequent in his practice. We recommend beginning with the posterior lesion and moving forward. The posterior column segment can be lifted and rotated into place from the inside of the pelvis. Often a bone hook into the sciatic notch can help pull the posterior column back into position. There are three simple fixation options. The first is a direct inside to out screw into the sciatic buttress. These screws are usually quite strong and provide reasonable provisional fixation. Another option is the standard posterior column screws placed via the lateral window of the ilioinguinal. Finally, for added stability, a quadrilateral plate can be placed, spanning from the greater sciatic angle, across the quadrilateral surface, and towards the ischial or pubic ramus (Chapters 11 and 12, Fig. 9). In fact, some cases that have comminuted quadrilateral surface pieces that cannot be secured with standard plate positions are well secured with this plate. The plate functions as a buttress to prevent protrusions. It can be slightly underbent to provide a lateralizing effect on the fragment. Furthermore, it will not interfere with future hip replacement and represents the medial limit of the acetabulum in cases of arthroplasty. We have found this plate to be very useful (Fig. 10). We have not found the traditionally described "spring" plates to be easy to apply and question the ability of a relatively thin plate to resist the loads of the hip,

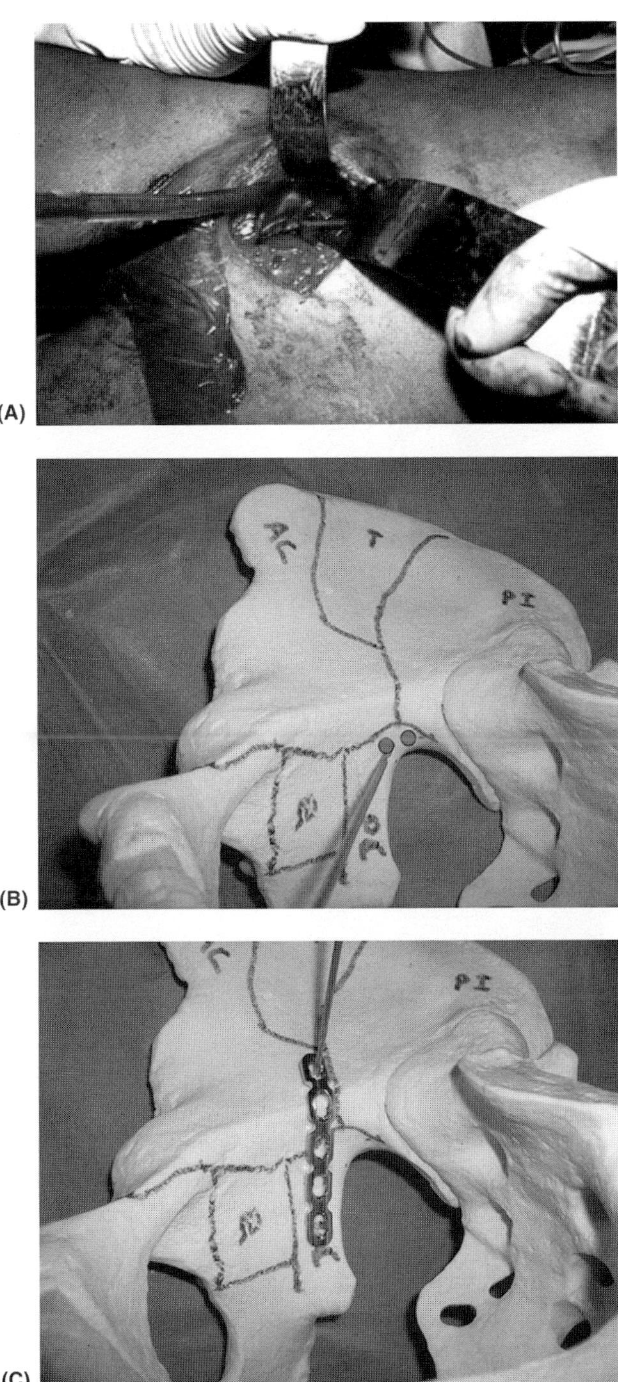

Figure 9 Access to the posterior column and quadrilateral surface from inside the pelvis, using the subinguinal window. (**A**) The medial window of the ilioinguinal or the Pfannensteil is used for access, and the neurovascular structures are "lifted" anteriorly. The bladder is retracted and the obturator nerve and vessels are in view. They can be mobilized and protected during reduction and fixation. Bone model showing location of sciatic buttress screws (**B**). An internal posterior column plate (**C**). (*Continued*)

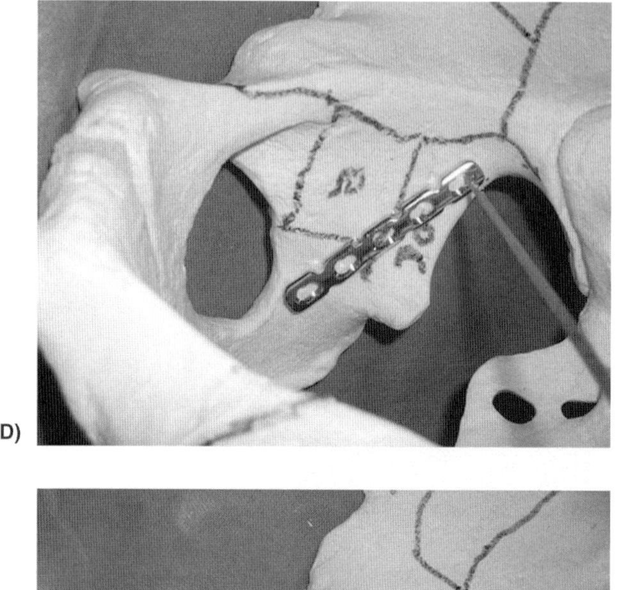
(D)

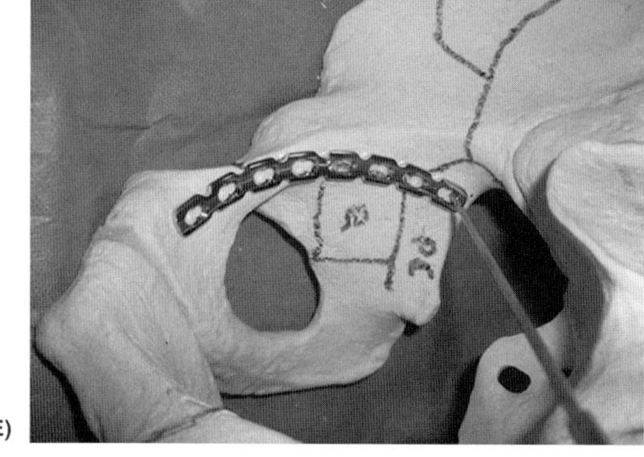
(E)

Figure 9 (*Continued*) A plate spanning the quadrilateral surface to the ischium (**D**) and along the pelvic brim (**E**).

especially when loaded as a cantilever as opposed to the buttressing mode of the plate we describe. Fixation of the anterior segment with this approach is straightforward and can be done with a standard plate along the pelvic brim or in some cases with the use of a retrograde ramus screw.

We emphasize that the choice of approach is determined by the "personality" of the fracture, and T fractures can be very problematic. As Letournel stated himself, while the majority of fractures can be treated via a posterior approach, occasionally a supplemental anterior approach is needed. We concur in that a single approach is not the goal, and, if needed, a second approach should be done to ensure an accurate reduction. Whether one begins with an anterior or posterior approach, the ability to intraoperatively concede that a single approach may not be enough to do the job right is far more admirable than struggling with one approach. Likewise, it is preferable to have two surgical events and two surgical scars instead of one unacceptable treatment.

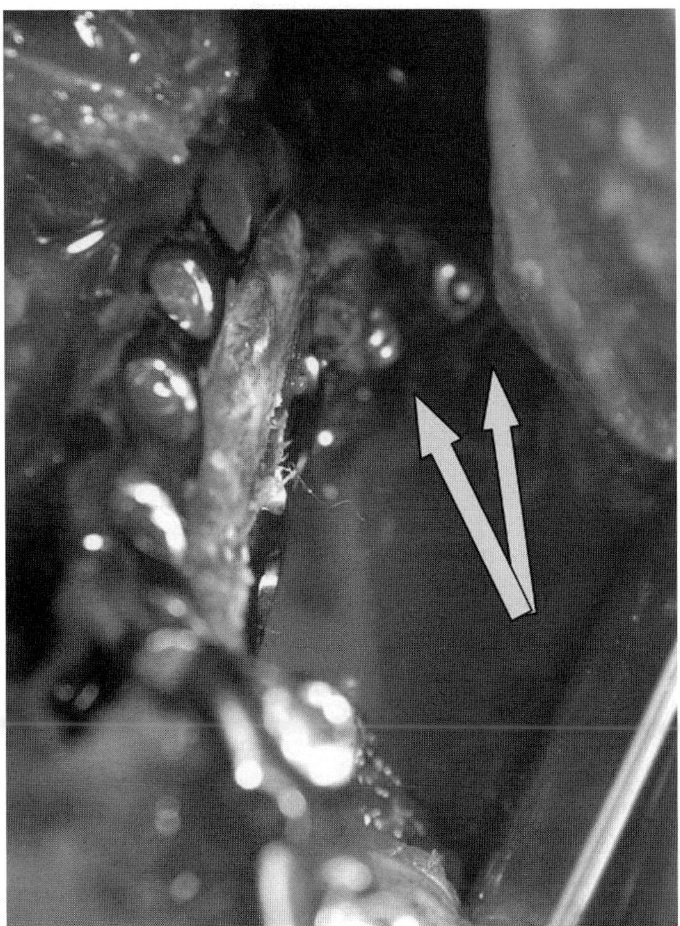

Figure 10 Intraoperative view of internal pelvic brim plate along side standard anterior plate via the subinguinal window of the ilioinguinal (Fig. 9). The internal pelvic brim plate was used to buttress the quadrilateral surface comminution. Note the visualization of the posterior aspect of the plate, which is near the anterior sacro-iliac joint and just above the sciatic notch. The two screws (*arrows*) are placed into the sciatic buttress. The retractor is over the obturator structures, and the bladder is top right of the image.

ANTERIOR COLUMN POSTERIOR HEMITRANSVERSE FRACTURES

While there is a posterior fracture that separates the posterior column and, similarly, a disruption of the anterior column, there must remain a portion of the roof and superior posterior wall that remains attached to the ilium. This is an essential differentiating feature from the both-column fracture pattern. Also, the anterior portion of the fracture has the characteristics of anterior column fractures. In the T fracture, there is a necessary extension into the obturator foramen as well as (some) inferior exit via the ischial ramus (or an equivalent exit such as in "transischial T"). The differentiating component of this fracture pattern (AC/PHT) (lesion) is the recognition of the posterior lesion. Of course, as the configuration of the anterior lesion and posterior lesion vary, there are atypical or transitional fractures that may approach or become either a both-column, or a T-shaped fracture. What is more important to recognize than the "name" of the fracture is the personality or behavior of the fracture. Certainly, some fractures that are "technically" a both-column pattern, may behave more like an anterior hemitransverse, or vice versa.

The majority of these fractures will necessitate an anterior approach because of the involvement of the anterior column. In 2002, Kloen et al. (1) reported their favorable experience in treating 15 patients with a modified ilioinguinal approach, which was combined with a Smith–Petersen anterior approach. An anterior superior iliac spine osteotomy is a component of this modified approach and it greatly enhances access to the anterior wall (Chapter 11, Fig. 4). In simple or high-column fractures, the anterior lesion is relatively straightforward for fixation and reduction. Occasionally, there is the involvement of the anterior or superior–anterior wall, in which case fixation may be difficult and precarious because of the location of the fragment and the lack of adjacent surfaces to use for buttress plating (as done for posterior wall fractures). On occasion, use of small "spring" plates may be used, and in case of superior–anterior fractures, the exposure can be extended to the outer table of the iliac wing (extended ilioinguinal approach or Smith–Peterson) to allow reduction and stabilization. On other occasions, use of small screws placed across the wall and into the pelvic brim or pubic ramus may be needed. Frequently, the anterior wall fragment will be relatively well contained underneath the plate used to span the anterior column, and fixation would consist of reduction and temporary Kirschner wire (K-wire) stabilization, followed by plate placement. Sometimes, a screw can be placed through the plate and across the inner corner of the wall-pelvic brim to secure the wall under the plate. Care must be taken to ensure that hardware is not intra-articular (Figs. 11 and 12, and Chapter 11, Figs. 5 and 6). If the surgeons consider the fracture prognosis to be poor, then anticipation of the inevitable hip arthroplasty should guide placement of hardware to avoid problems of interference during that subsequent procedure.

For fixation of the posterior lesion, again we find that the use of the subinguinal window of the ilioinguinal approach provides excellent visualization of this fragment. If there is little involvement of the quadrilateral surface or if there is little displacement of this fragment, stabilization with long posterior column screws may be performed through the plate. If the plate is not optimally positioned, or if fixation of the posterior fragment is desired before plate application, the screw can still be placed but outside the plate itself. The ideal starting point is posteriorly in the inominate bone, approximately 2 to 3 cm anterior to the sacroiliac joint and 2 to 3 cm lateral from the pelvic brim (Fig. 13). Digital palpation from the lateral window, or direct visualization from the subinguinal window can verify the direction of the drill along the posterior column. This direction is always more distally directed than posteriorly due to the orientation of the column in the supine position. One will find his or her hand on the drill leaning more towards the patient's head and less vertical in orientation. The patient's body habitus is often the biggest detriment to proper screw placement. Likewise, as discussed previously, the posterior fragment can be manipulated and held via the subinguinal window, with provisional fixation using sciatic angle or inside-out screws, or with use of the ischial column screws placed percutaneously from below (see Chapter 6).

(Text continued on page 252.)

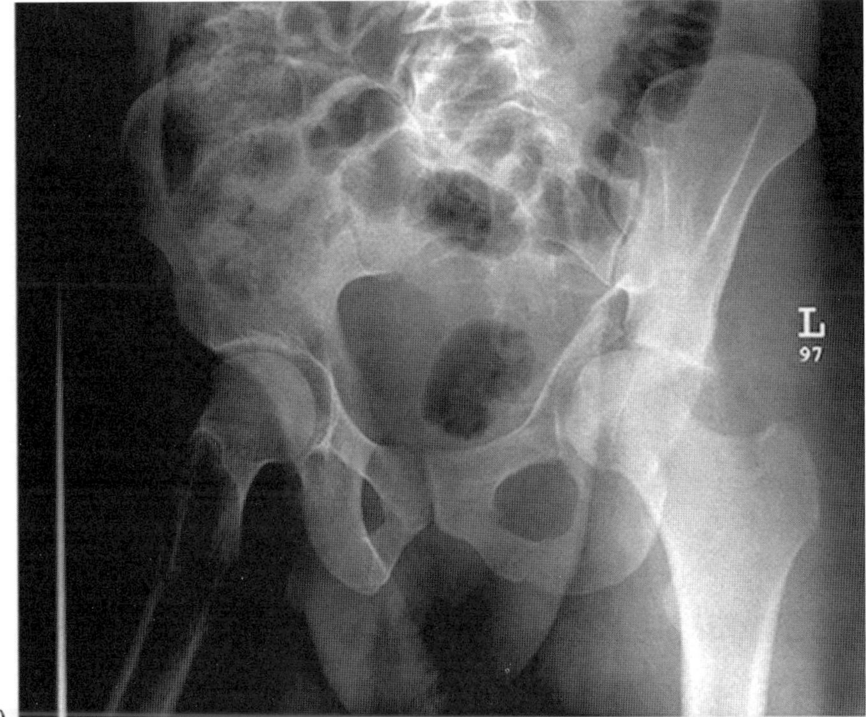

(A)

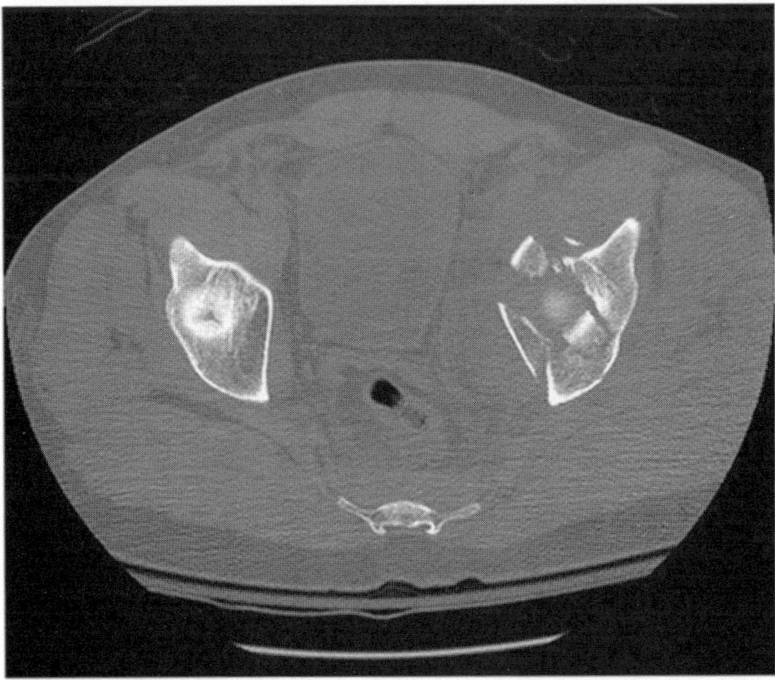

(B)

Figure 11 Obturator oblique radiograph (**A**) and axial CT scan (**B**) reveal low anterior hemitransverse fracture with dome impaction. The anterior wall was opened to allow treatment of the dome lesion, followed by a subarticular buttress screw overlying the plate (**D**). *(Continued)*

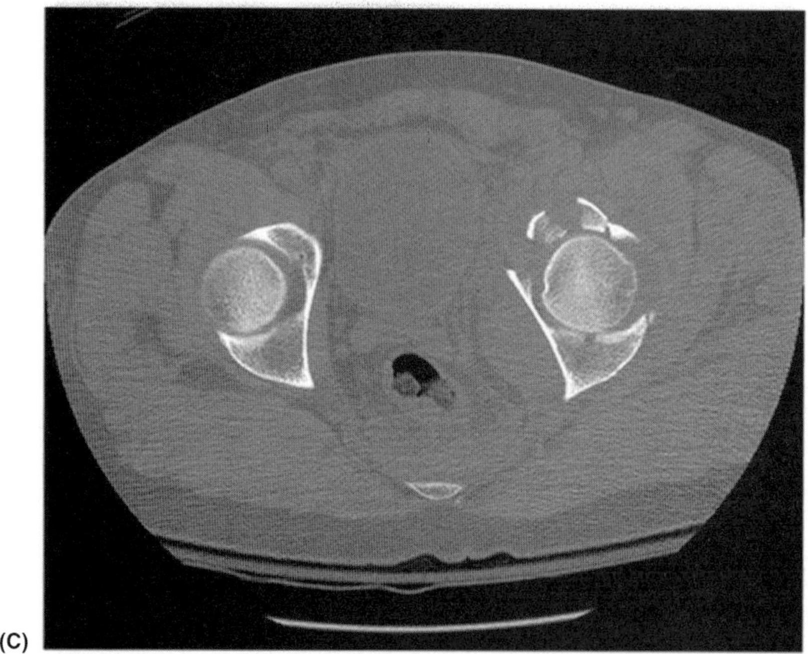

(C)

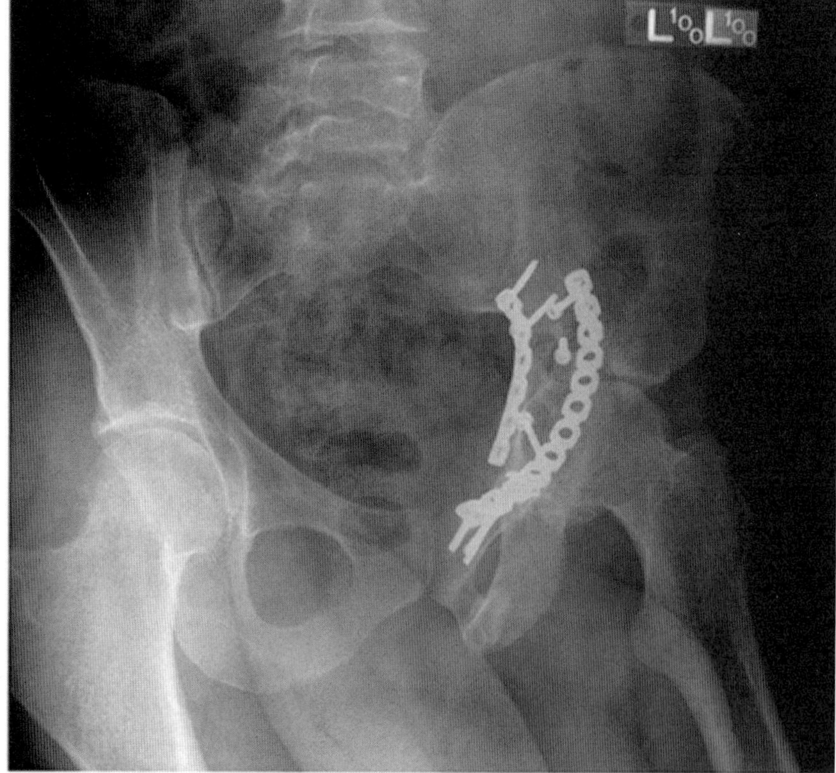

(D)

Figure 11 (*Continued*) Note the incomplete posterior lesion (**C**) treated with an internal push plate (**D**).

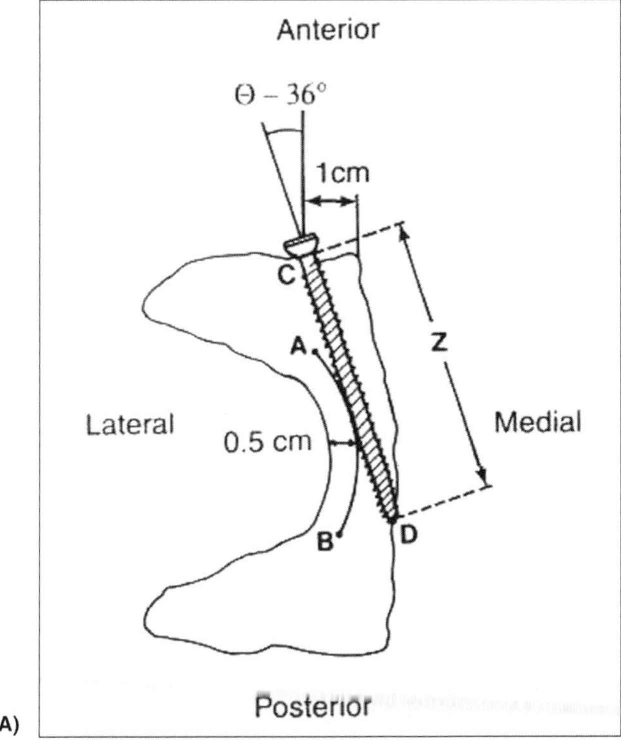

(A)

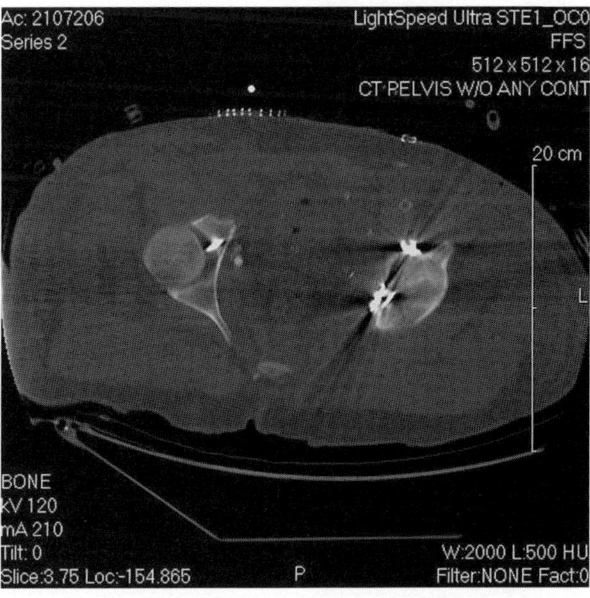

(B)

Figure 12 (**A**) Schematic diagram demonstrating screw placement around the iliopectineal eminence. Care must be taken to prevent intra-articular screw placement. (**B**) CT scan of intra-articular screw placement into the right acetabulum, which null and void any chance of successful outcome. This screw should be revised.

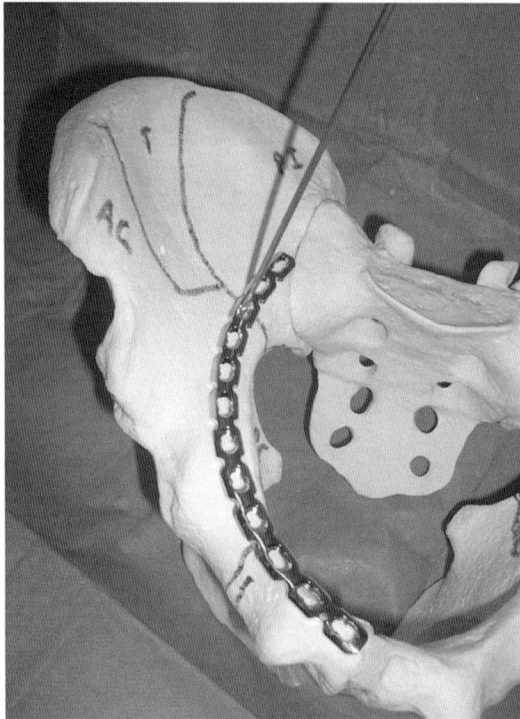

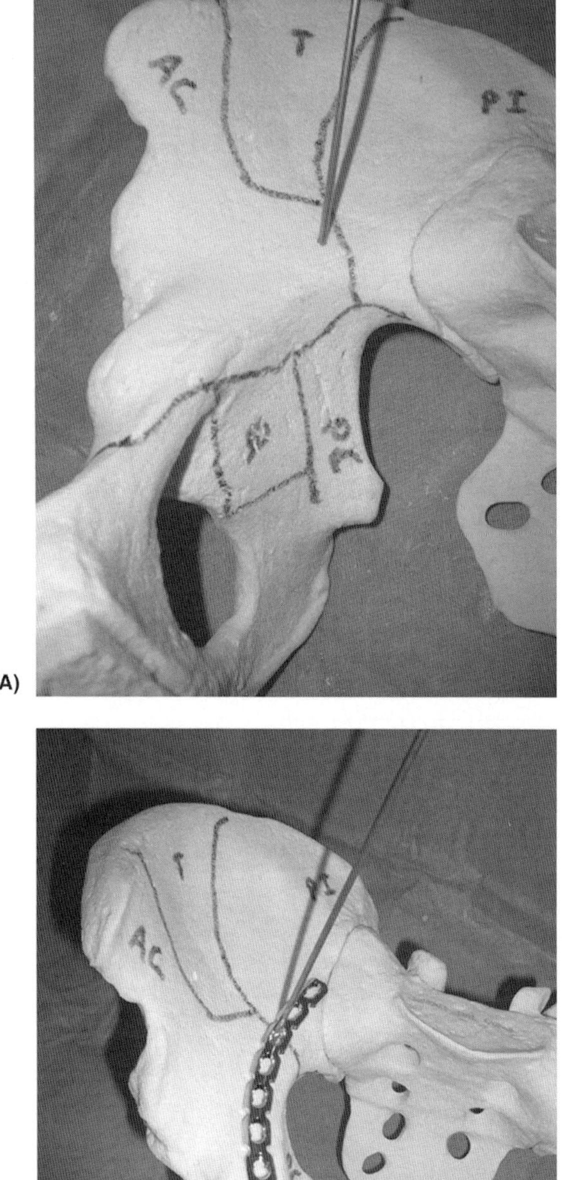

Figure 13 Bone models and radiograph of the posterior column screw. The screw can be placed independently (**A**) or through a plate (**B**). (*Continued*)

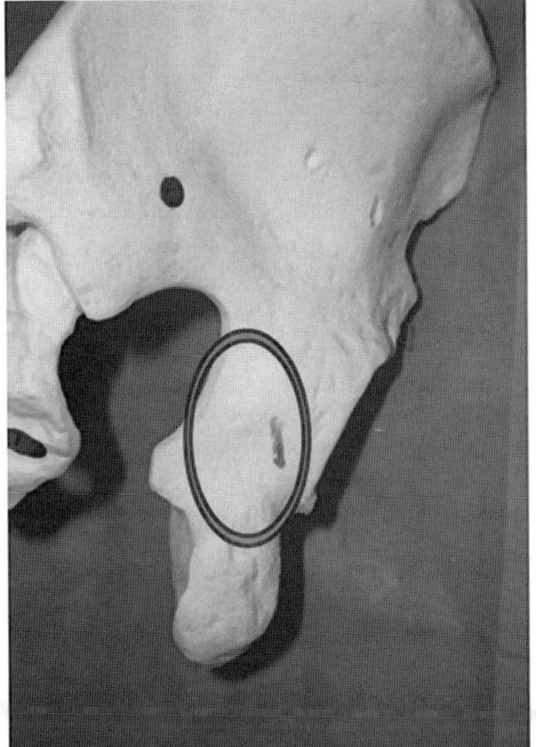

(C)

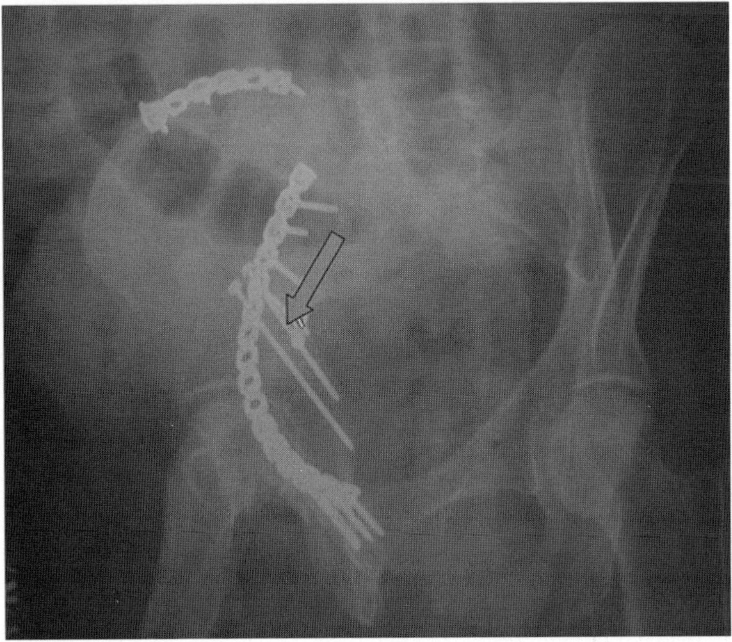

(D)

Figure 13 (*Continued*) The screw exits in the region just behind the posterior wall (**C**). Iliac oblique view of screws (**D**).

BOTH-COLUMN FRACTURES

These fractures can have a variety of differing personalities and are distinguished by the lack of any articular attachment to the intact posterior ilium. Unlike the T and anterior hemitransverse fractures, there is no intact remnant of the dome under which the femoral head can be placed. Most of these fractures can be treated using some variant of the ilioinguinal approach, although some patterns will need either an extended iliofemoral or a sequential front and back approach. It is the exception that a posterior approach can be used for such fractures.

In Letournel's and Tile's classic textbooks, they emphasize the sequence and goals of surgical tactic, stating that the iliac wing and anterior column require accurate reduction. Occasionally, with incomplete fractures or plastic deformation, the fracture through the wing has to be completed to allow suitable reduction. To facilitate this reduction, the displacement of the femoral head into the pelvis needs to be corrected. The head needs to be maintained (with traction) in its approximate normal position to allow a suitable reduction of the anterior column. While not always clearly stated, we believe that most paradigms of reduction and fixation are based on the tenet of beginning from the back (posteriorly) and moving forward (anteriorly). This does not mean beginning with the posterior column, which is usually addressed in a subsequent part of the procedure, but beginning with the posterior aspect of the iliac components and moving forward. Two potential problems well described by Letournel are the triangular fragment of the crest and a small comminuted fragment of the brim (Fig. 14). These fragments can be useful in gauging the reduction and can be fixed with either simple screws or curved plates. For the crest, we have found that placing this plate along the inner cortex of the crest facilitates plate contouring and allows small flexural adjustments to the curvature of the iliac wing while limiting the risk of subcutaneous plate irritation (Fig. 15). The cases with a separate comminuted fragment of pelvic brim can make reduction of the anterior column to the intact iliac segment difficult. In these cases, provisional fixation of this piece to the posterior segment (the keystone of reconstruction) with a simple K-wire can facilitate the subsequent reduction and fixation of the anterior column. In cases where there is a separate fracture extension of the anterior column into the anterior interspinous notch area, a short vertically oriented plate or intraosseous screw can stabilize the anterior column into one piece before proceeding with subsequent parts. After the anterior column has been restored to the posterior iliac segment, the posterior column fragment is addressed. It is necessary to reiterate that during anterior column fixation, care should be taken not to place screws that interfere with posterior column reduction. Again, we have found that the subinguinal window allows excellent visualization of this fragment. Whether a bone hook, ball spike, pelvic clamp, or tenaculum is used, the reduction is obtained and provisionally maintained in whatever fashion possible, typically 2-mm K-wires. Then definitive stabilization with posterior column screws, around or through the plate, or via direct column plating from the inside of the pelvis. Occasionally, if the quality of the bone is adequate and the fracture configuration permits, the fracture can be stabilized by a sequence of well-placed lag screws. If the screws are placed divergently, they may add to the stability of the fixation. Knowledge of the appropriate windows and locations of these screws have

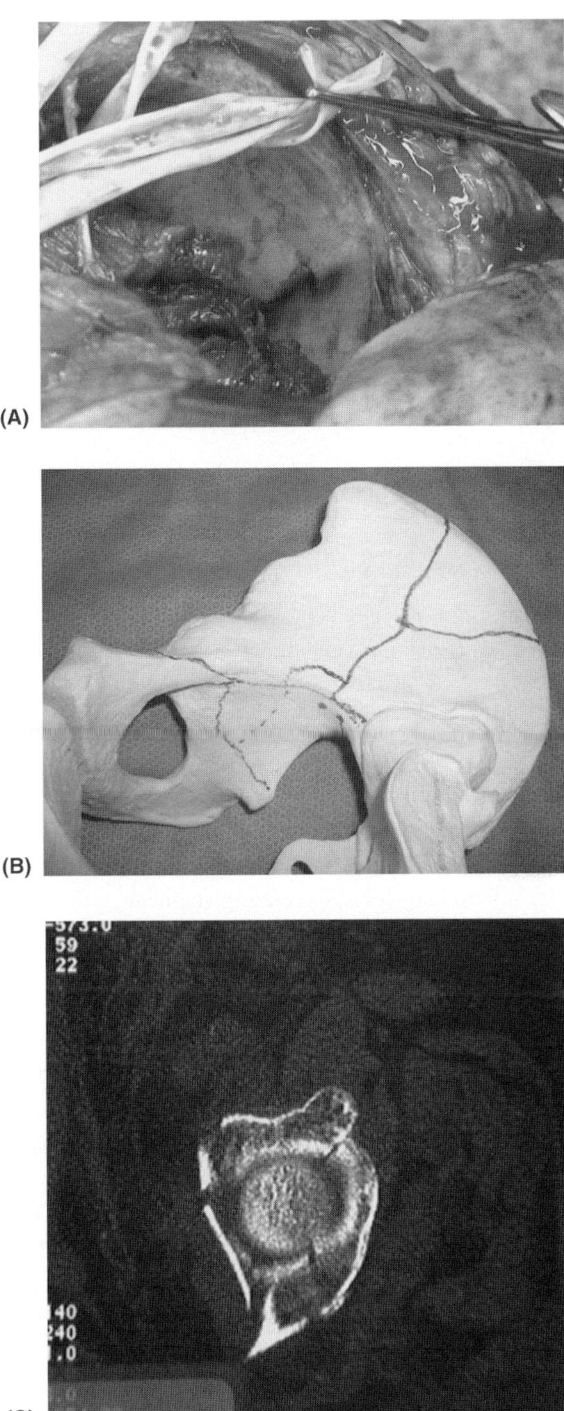

Figure 14 (**A**) A both-column fracture with an incomplete triangular fracture with plastic deformation of the iliac wing. This will require completion of the iliac wing fracture to facilitate reduction of the other components of the fracture. There is frequently this triangular fragment of the wing with a variable brim fragment (**B**). We have found that in more osteoporotic bone, the quadrilateral surface may have more involvement (**C**), possibly due to being osteoporotic.

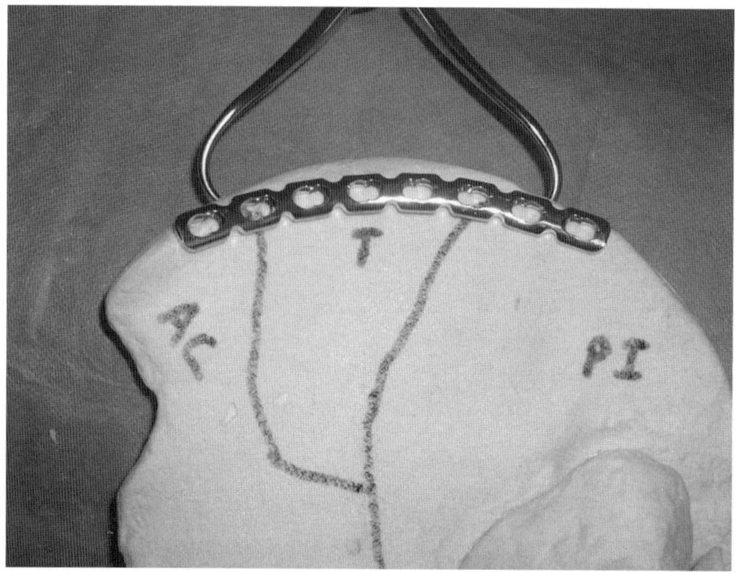

Figure 15 Bone model showing internally placed iliac crest plate for both-column fracture. This plate position (vs. hardware along the top of the iliac crest) limits the risk of subcutaneous plate irritation.

been identified previously and include the anterior column screw, the LC-II screw, the crest screw, retrograde ramus screw, posterior column screw, and the ischial screw. Again, the authors recommend putting a plastic saw bone pelvic model into a clear plastic bag (sterile) for intraoperative referencing for safe screw placement.

Some complex fractures may have an associated anterior–superior wall fracture, or undisplaced posterior wall fractures. In these cases, an extended ilioinguinal approach can be used to expose the outer surface of the iliac wing. For the superior fracture, direct fixation of the superior wall fracture is possible (Fig. 16). In other cases, where there may be a minimally displaced posterior lesion, a spring-type buttress plate can be placed submuscularly to provide support to the posterior lesion without the need for a formal posterior exposure. The alternative would be to utilize an extended iliofemoral approach. However, in the absence of a need for reduction, we feel that the extended ilioinguinal approach with the submuscular plate suffices and avoids the morbidity of the extended iliofemoral approach (Fig. 17).

In some cases, there has been so much comminution that a systematic reduction and stabilization is very difficult. In these cases, we believe that the surgeon has two reasonable choices. The first choice is to ensure the best possible reduction of the acetabular joint surface and then to provide adequate reduction and stabilization of the remaining nonarticular segments. While not an attractive radiograph, the primary goal is accomplished, and slight imperfections of the iliac wing are well tolerated. Bone grafting may be necessary for bone loss or gaps. In other circumstances, and as described by Letournel himself, secondary congruence may be obtained and, while not optimal, it is better than step-offs or gaps.

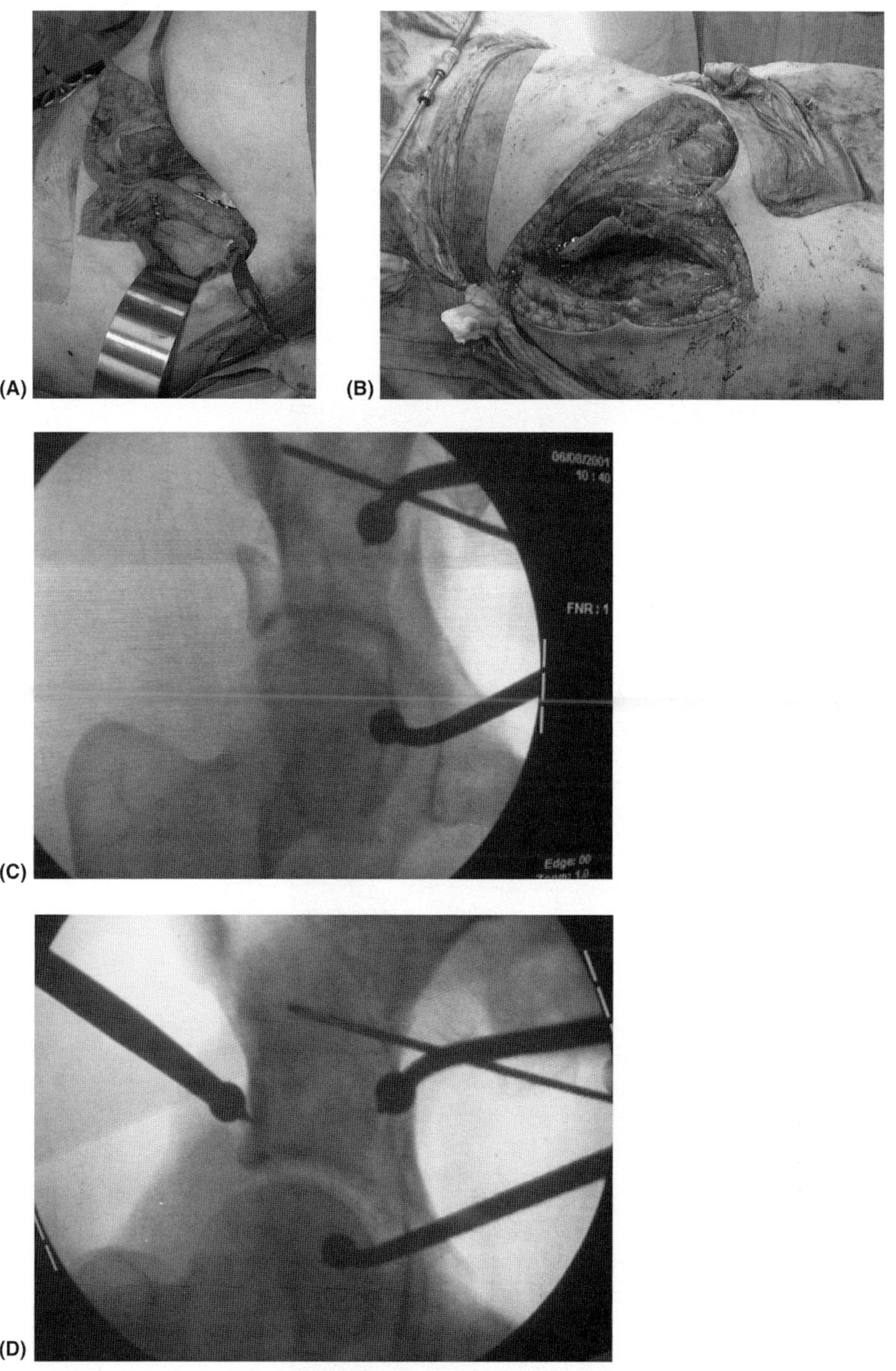

Figure 16 (**A**) Operative view of a left extended ilioinguinal approach. Note the vertically oriented plate on the outer cortex. (**B**) A right extended ilioinguinal approach for a superior wall fracture associated with a both-column fracture and sacro-iliac disruption. (**C**) Intraoperative fluoroscopic view of displaced fragment. (**D**) Reduction with ball spike pusher followed by screw fixation (**E**). (*Continued*)

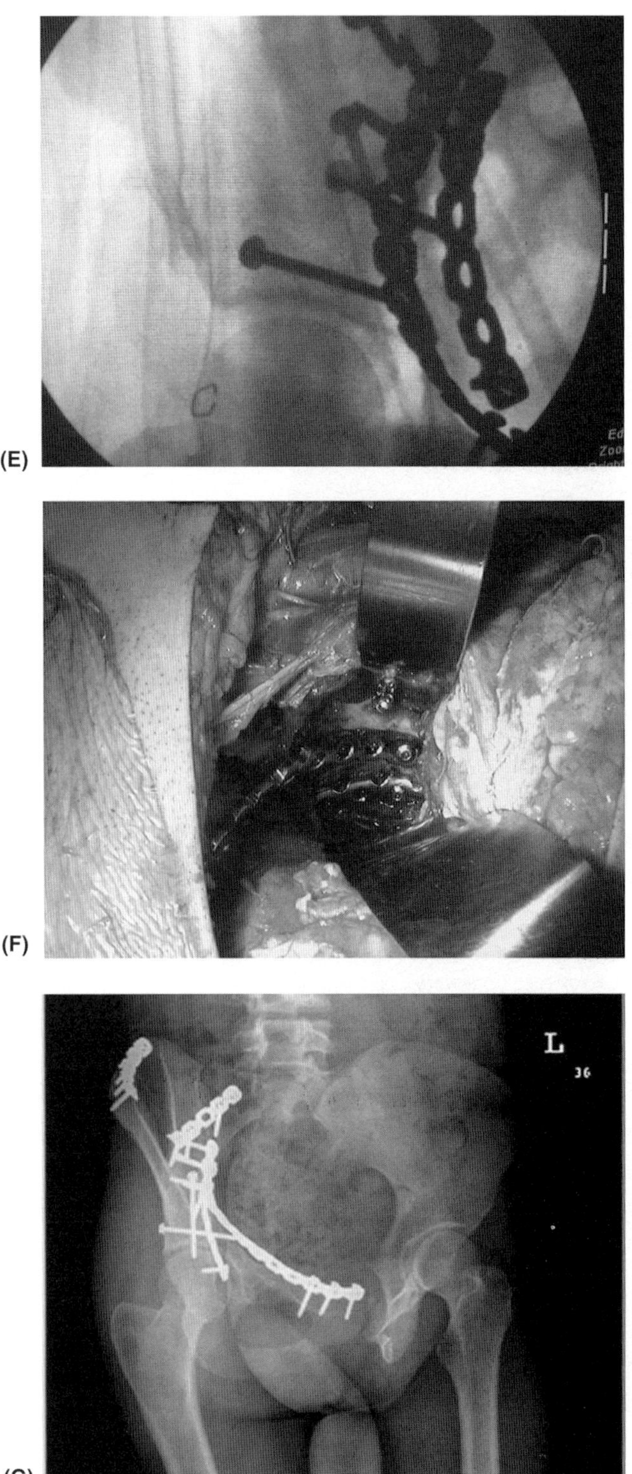

Figure 16 (*Continued*) The same patient showing the internal pelvis and the quadrilateral plate (**F**). Notice elevation of the vessel and nerve envelopes can show the pelvic brim. (**G**) Radiograph of fixation at two years.

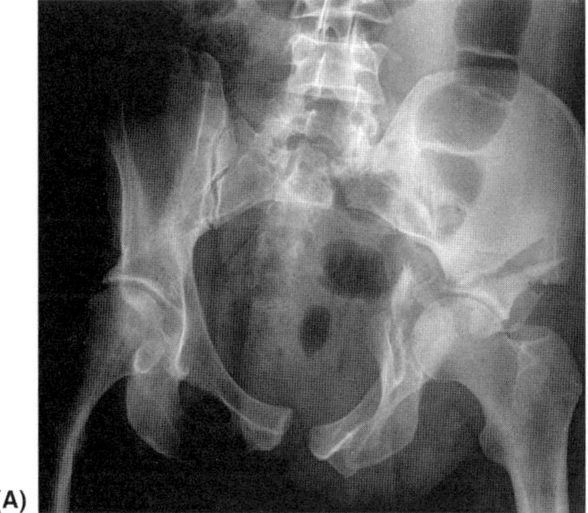

(A)

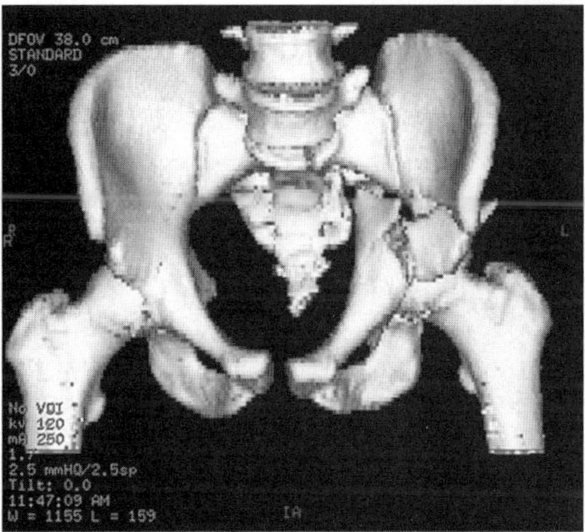

(B)

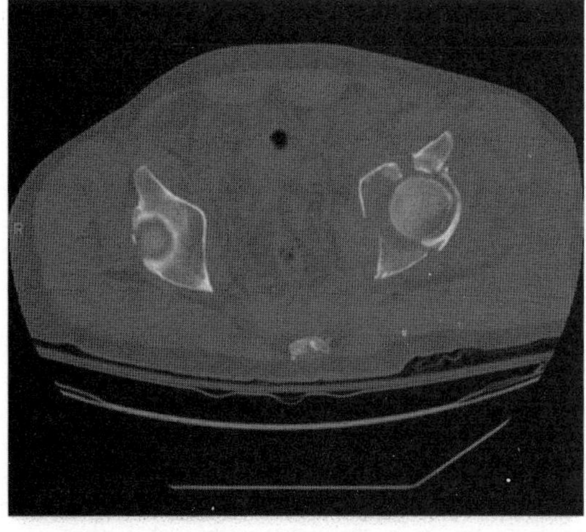

(C)

Figure 17 (**A**) A complex both-column with both anterior wall and posterior wall fractures, along with a pelvic ring disruption. (**B**) Three-dimensional reconstruction of fracture. (**C**) Axial CT view of fracture at the level of the dome. *(Continued)*

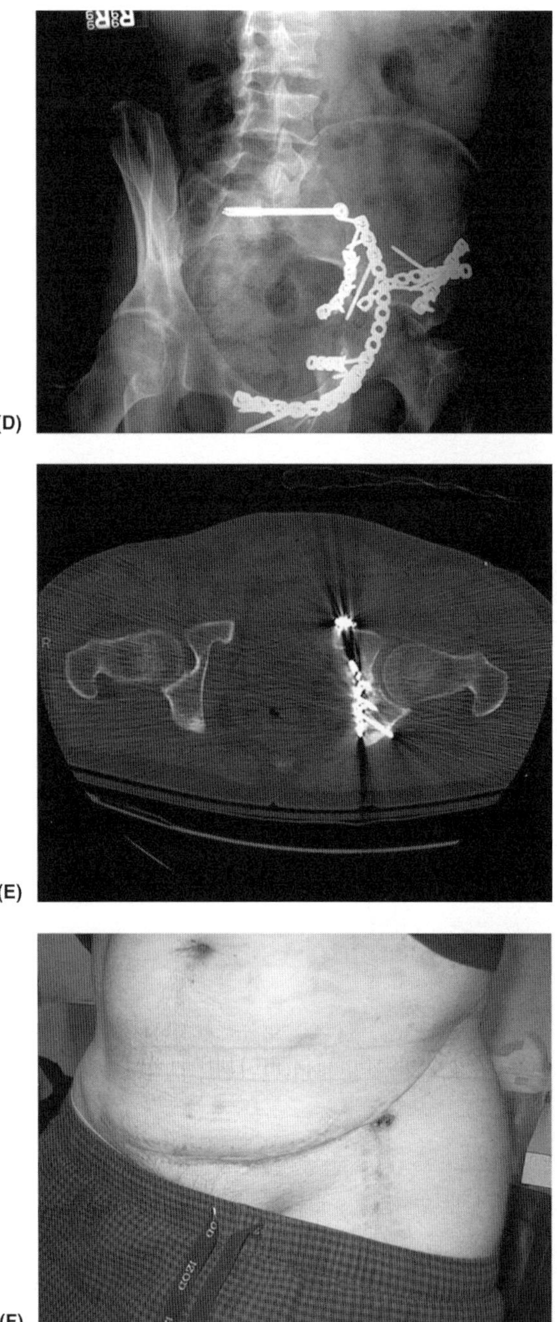

(D)

(E)

(F)

Figure 17 (*Continued*) (**D**) This reconstruction demonstrates several of the operative tactics. The internal posterior column plate as well as the internal ischial plate are depicted. There is a vertical buttress plate used along the inner table between the iliac spines for the anterior wall and a submuscular plate on the outer table utilized for the posterior wall. The pelvic disruption was addressed with the same anterior plate used for the acetabulum as well as a sacro-iliac screw. (**E**) A postoperative CT demonstrating the trajectory of the sciatic buttress screw used from inside-out. This screw was described in Figure 9. In this case, the screw is through a plate. (**F**) The cutaneous result. There is definitely a risk of skin edge necrosis at the trifurcation of the incision.

SPECIAL CIRCUMSTANCES—OSTEOPENIA

We have found that the geriatric acetabulum fracture poses distinct challenges, as the surgeon is faced with a fracture that is generally more comminuted, in weaker bone, and in a patient with less ability to tolerate large reconstructive procedures. In some cases, where surgery was forbidden for medical reasons, we have found a remarkable resiliency of the elderly population to accommodate a stiff and arthritic hip joint. Albeit, they may need an elective arthroplasty, but if "bone stock" is sufficient, the arthroplasty has a reasonable chance of survival. Thus, in this population, we are less concerned with perfection and instead attempt to get the best possible reduction with the least biologic and physiologic cost. Included in this paradigm is reserving a surgical approach (e.g., a posterior approach) for the arthroplasty procedure. One could argue that exposure of native tissue during an arthroplasty procedure and not scarred tissue in theory can minimize the complications of arthroplasty. These complications include but are not limited to infection and dislocations. Furthermore, removal of several column screws versus removal of a long plate with screws is less morbid during conversion to an arthroplasty. Bone stock operations are well described and this may be an excellent indication for the limited open reductions and percutaneous methods outlined and discussed elsewhere in this text. Nonetheless, the population that is aging is maintaining better medical physiology but not necessarily better bone health. Thus, an active 75-year-old who plays tennis and golf may be particularly challenging for decision making. We have classified such patients based on physiology rather than chronology and fully inform the patient on options. An alternative to bone stock preservation is immediate fixation and arthroplasty, which has been well described by Mears et al. In such cases, immediate fixation of the acetabular "foundation" followed by arthroplasty has yielded reasonable results. Considering the nature of such situations, the trauma surgeon either needs to become versed with joint replacement (what we practice) or partner with a another surgeon for such procedures.

SPECIAL CIRCUMSTANCES—CONCOMITANT PELVIC RING DISRUPTION

In cases of acetabular fractures with concomitant pelvic ring disruptions (The Tile C3 injury), reduction and fixation become more difficult because the intact posterior iliac fragment, the keystone of acetabular reconstruction, has been compromised. In this case, we believe there are two useful options. In the first, the posterior segment is still used as the keystone to restore the essential acetabular lesion, and then the entire restored hemipelvis is reduced and stabilized to the remaining sacrum. In these cases, we may add additional fixation to the acetabular reconstruction to protect against the reduction maneuvers of reducing the hemipelvis. In the second paradigm, the tenet of posterior to anterior fixation is followed. Depending on the nature of the pelvic ring disruption, it can be combined with the acetabular fixation for a more elegant tactic. For example, the posterior iliac segment is accurately reduced and fixed to the sacrum via anterior sacroiliac plates or with iliosacral screws. Once the sacroiliac joint is reduced and stabilized, the reduction proceeds anterior to the acetabulum and finally to the

(A)

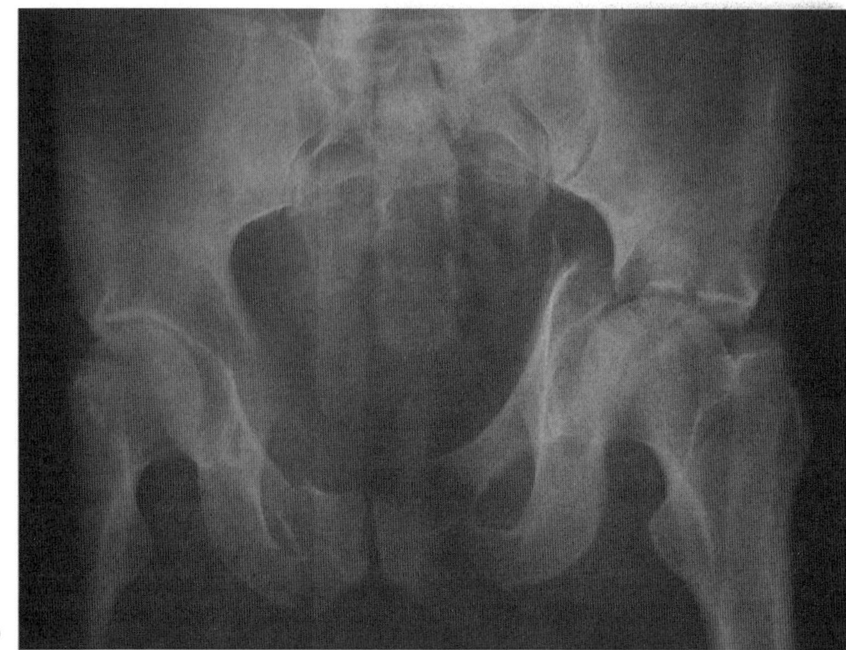

(B)

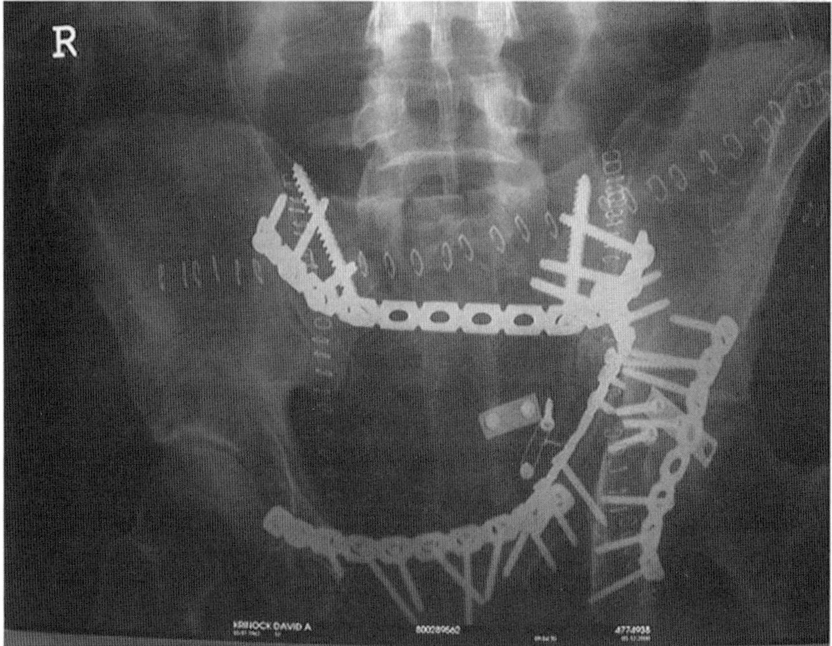

Figure 18 A severe pelvic/acetabular disruption with impaction of the dome, and fractures of the sacrum. (**A**) Injury radiographs and (**B**) fixation with a tension band plate and multiple tactics for the acetabulum and anterior ring. The impacted dome fragment is held up with a single subchondral screw. The pelvic brim plate sits on the inner wall of the pelvis, and small fragment fixation was used for an oblique sacral fracture. We have found the tension band plate to be very useful, providing excellent stability, and with few soft tissue complications when the incisions described by Matta are used. Regarding fixation, we would currently use less screws in each segment.

anterior ring disruption. Some advocate the use of the extended iliofemoral approach for this problem, which provides excellent access to most pieces. We have not found this to be necessary and treat each pelvic-acetabular combination with careful preoperative planning. We assess the different methods of fixation for each injury separately, and then try to determine an elegant operative tactic. Occasionally, a preferred method of fixation has to be altered to facilitate the overall tactic. An example would be an acetabular fracture with sacro-iliac disruption. If this is performed in the prone position, anterior sacro-iliac plating would require separate positioning and a separate approach. Instead, a sacro-iliac screw may be more elegant. Similarly, a surgeon who routinely prefers sacro-iliac screws may opt to plate the anterior sacro-iliac disruption if they are already performing an anterior approach. This would also provide an opportunity to assess the sacro-iliac cartilage, and if indicated perform a primary arthrodesis with bone grafting.

In other circumstances, the posterior lesion must be addressed as a separate procedure. In severe cases, we prefer the use of a posterior tension band plate, which allows for some flexibility during the subsequent parts of treatment. This plate is placed with the patient prone, using the incisions described by Matta. Care should be taken to avoid placement of the screws into areas that would interfere with the acetabular fixation (Fig. 18). Again, depending on the nature of the fracture, the posterior lesion can be addressed first or, occasionally, the acetabular fracture addressed first. These lesions are so severe, and so relatively rare, there is little objective literature to guide the surgeon, and one must rely on judgment, experience, and invoke the principles of pelvic/acetabular surgery. There are Web sites and list servs that allow sharing of ideas and solicitation of suggestions.

Earlier in this chapter we stated that a single approach for an acetabular fracture is not the goal. Likewise for concomitant pelvis and acetabular fractures that if needed, a second approach should be done to ensure an accurate reduction. Whether one begins with an anterior or posterior approach, the ability to intraoperatively concede that a single approach may not be enough to do the job right is far more admirable than struggling with one approach. It is preferable to have two surgical events and two surgical scars instead of one unacceptable treatment.

SUMMARY

Associated patterns of acetabular fractures can be quite challenging and require extensive experience and dedication to ongoing education. There are many controversies and, unlike what has been established for femoral diaphyseal fracture fixation, there is little consensus on the treatment of many acetabular fractures. But, what is known and accepted is that the principles of accurate reduction and fixation remain. These fractures represent some of the most complex surgeries in orthopedics and distinguish the occasional fracture surgeon from the dedicated traumatologist. In fact, most people seeking a career in trauma feel obliged to learn this surgery, and it is a requirement of the American College of Surgeons to have an onsite surgeon proficient with such fractures. This chapter attempts to help guide surgeons interested in such fractures with methods and techniques we have found useful.

REFERENCES

1. Kloen P, Siebenrock KA, Ganz R. Modification of the ilioinguinal approach. J Orthop Trauma 2002; Sep 16(8):586–593.
2. Letournel E, Joudet R. Fractures of the Acetabulum. Berlin: Springer-Verlag, 1993.

13

Acetabular Reconstruction: The Geriatric Patient

Dolfi Herscovici
Department of Orthopaedic Traumatology, University of South Florida, Tampa, Florida, U.S.A.

INTRODUCTION

The population of elderly people in the United States is growing and is expected to continue rising over the next few decades. In 1900, the combination of harsh living conditions, high rates of infectious diseases, and inadequate or insufficient medical care resulted in life expectancies of only 47.3 years. This increased to 68.2 years by 1950, and, with improvements in the health care system, the ensuing 50 years continued to produce greater life spans. During the 2000 census, an estimated 282 million people were identified living in the United States. Almost 12.5% were comprised of patients aged 65 and older with life expectancies averaging 76.9 years (1). With extrapolation, it is estimated that by the year 2030 the population will be close to 350 million people, 19.6% of which will be comprised of people aged 65 years and older, with life expectancies rising to 83.1 years for women and 75.0 years for men (2,3). This increase in life expectancy is a direct result of better health care, accessibility to the medical community, and an increase in the health consciousness of the general population. For the elderly, this has produced more active lifestyles, which has been demonstrated by greater numbers continuing to work after retirement or participating in sporting or recreational activities previously thought to be the domain of younger patients.

However, taking care of the elderly is expensive because it places increased demands on the public health care system and social and medical services. Studies have reported the health care cost per capita of people ≥65 years of age is three to five times greater than people <65 years old (4), but even for people over 65 costs can vary. A 1999 national cross-sectional analysis of Medicare recipients found that 82% had at least one chronic condition and that 65% had two or more chronic conditions (5). In addition, those recipients who had four or more chronic conditions were 99 times more likely to be admitted for treatment, for an average of $13,973 per admission, than patients without any chronic conditions (4–6). That same year, the management of fractures in the elderly cost Medicare more than $8 billion, and were responsible for 67% of the total injury claims, but occurred only in 1 in 17 aged beneficiaries (7). Therefore, although living longer, the cost of taking care of the elderly cannot be understated—it can be very expensive. What does this mean to the orthopedic community as far as injuries to the acetabulum in the elderly are concerned? It means that the care provided must be as aggressive as that given to younger patients in spite of their bony pathology and associated medical comorbidities.

ANATOMY AND EPIDEMIOLOGY

Anatomy

The pelvis is formed by the sacrum and two innominate bones. The acetabulum lies within the innominate bone and forms the "socket" that allows articulation with the femoral head. It is formed by the three ossification centers of the innominate bone—the ilium, the ischium, and the pubis—and is divided into anterior and posterior columns (8). The posterior column is composed superiorly by the ilium and inferiorly by the ischium and extends from an area just below the greater sciatic notch past the ischial tuberosity. In cross-section it is triangular in shape and contains the posterior half of the joint, the posterior rim, the ischial spine, and all of the ischial tuberosity. The anterior column consists of the anterior half of the ilium and extends to the pubic symphysis. It contains the anterior border of the iliac wing, the pelvic brim (superior pubic rami), and the anterior half of the acetabulum. The columns unite at an area above the level of the mid-point of the anterior column and help to form the anatomical roof. Within the inferior region of the acetabulum is an area known as the acetabular or cotyloid fossa. This is a recessed structure that is part of the quadrilateral plate and contains the origin of the ligamentum teres. Surrounding the bony structure of the acetabulum is a fibrocartilaginous labrum crossed inferiorly by the transverse acetabular ligament.

The blood supply to the acetabulum is rich and is due to branches of the internal iliac artery (9) (Fig. 1A and B). Inferomedially, the posterior branch of the obturator artery supplies the cotyloid fossa. Superiorly, the deep inferior branch of the superior gluteal artery supplies the superior portion and posterior rim of the acetabulum. Inferolaterally, the inferior gluteal artery supplies the inferior and posterior portions of the acetabular rim and part of the ischium (9,10). The venous return from the pelvis and acetabulum parallels the arterial supply.

Epidemiology

The epidemiology of fractures to the acetabulum is difficult to accurately identify. Although these are serious injuries resulting from high-energy trauma, in general they are uncommon injuries. Overall, fractures of the pelvis make up 0.3% to 6% of all fractures, with 44% of these occurring as either isolated fractures of the acetabulum or as combined acetabulum and pelvic ring injuries (11–13). In the elderly, especially in those patients with osteoporosis or osteopenia, moderate or low-energy injuries can also produce acetabular fractures and may need to be distinguished from patients presenting with pelvic or periacetabular pain due to insufficiency fractures (14,15). In addition, fractures to the acetabulum may be missed due to an expectation of a hip fracture resulting from a moderate or low-energy injury (16,17). In the elderly, the incidence of proximal femur, pelvic, and acetabular fractures has been expressed by the ratio 60:10:1 (11) translating into approximately 240,000 proximal femur, 40,000 pelvic, and 4000 acetabular fractures per annum for the elderly population in the United States (18). In a recent study, at a level one trauma center over a 13-year period, 1934 acetabular fractures were identified, of which 421 (22%) were in patients who were at least 57 years of age (19). Therefore, even though these are uncommon injuries in the elderly, vigilance needs to be maintained when evaluating patients who present with hip pain.

RADIOLOGY AND CLASSIFICATION

For patients presenting to the emergency department complaining of pain in the pelvic region, the initial X ray of the pelvis should be the anteroposterior radiograph. This is a good screening tool to detect acetabular fractures and should also be inspected for any dislocations of the hip or the sacroiliac joints, widening of the pubic symphysis, and for any fractures involving the pelvic bones, the sacrum, or the proximal femur.

Evaluation of the anteroposterior radiograph (Fig. 2A and B) should yield six major landmarks of the acetabulum. These landmarks are important because they allow for differentiation of the columns and components of the acetabulum, and consist of the ilio-pectineal line, the ilio-ischial line, the radiographic U or teardrop, the anterior and posterior walls, and the roof or "dome" of the acetabulum (13,20). The ilio-pectineal line represents the pelvic brim or border of the anterior column, while the ilio-ischial

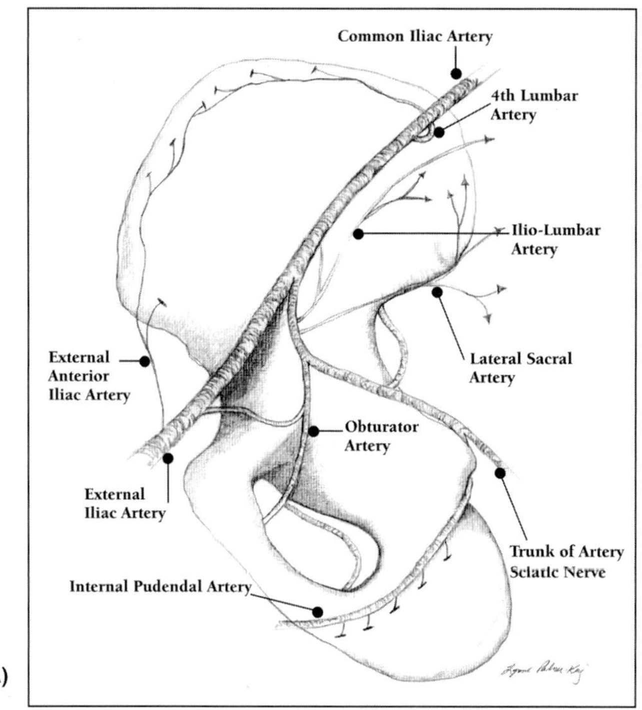

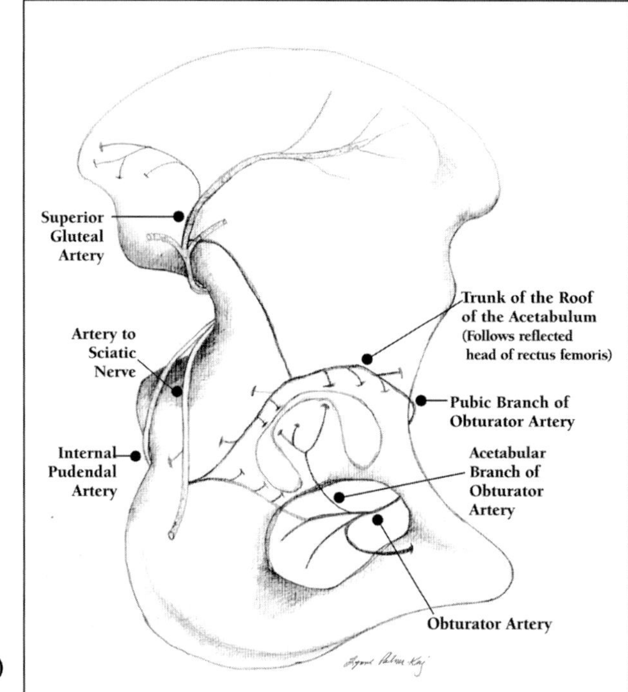

Figure 1 (**A**) Blood supply of the pelvis and acetabulum demonstrating the internal vessels. (**B**) Blood supply demonstrating the external vessels of the pelvis and acetabulum.

line depicts the posterior column. The radiographic U or teardrop has a medial and lateral limb. The lateral limb represents the inferior aspect of the anterior wall, while the obturator canal and the anteroinferior portion of the quadrilateral plate form the medial limb. The roof is a radiographic marker depicting the narrow portion of the subchondral bone of the superior acetabulum, and the walls each correspond to their respective columns.

If fractures of the acetabulum are evident on the anteroposterior pelvic radiograph, further evaluations are warranted. These consist of obturator and iliac oblique views, as described by Judet et al. (20). The iliac oblique view (Fig. 3A and B) is obtained by rolling the patient into 45 degrees of external rotation, elevating the uninjured side. The beam is centered on the pubic symphysis so that both acetabuli can be visualized. This view shows the iliac wing in its largest dimension, and allows visualization of all of the posterior column and the anterior wall. The obturator oblique view (Fig. 4A and B) rolls the patient into 45 degrees of internal rotation, elevating the injured side. Using this view shows the obturator foramen in its largest dimension, and allows visualization of the anterior column, the posterior wall, and a section of the iliac wing. In addition to identifying the location of the fracture, careful evaluation of these acetabular views will also help to determine whether or not the fractures have occurred within the weight bearing area (dome) of the acetabulum (21).

If a fracture is identified, computed tomography (CT) is useful for providing additional information (22,23) (Fig. 5A). The scanning is typically performed at 2–3 mm intervals and allows for two-dimensional visualization of the acetabulum in the axial plane. These views help to: identify fractured fragments and determine whether rotation has occurred (24,25), identify any loose intraarticular fragment, discover marginal impaction of the articular surface or fractures of the femoral head (26), evaluate the posterior pelvic ring, help to detect occult fracture lines, help to estimate the size and comminution of fractures of the anterior and posterior walls (25), and assesses the surrounding soft tissues. In addition, when used in conjunction with the plain films, it also helps to determine whether the fracture extends into the weight-bearing dome of the acetabulum (27). When reformatted, these two-dimensional views allow for a three-dimensional reconstruction of the pelvis and the acetabular fracture (28) (Fig. 5B). Although reformatting is time-consuming and software dependent, the views obtained may be helpful prior to application of any internal fixation.

Classification

Before attempting to classify any fracture, it is essential that an accurate radiographic diagnosis be obtained to understand the fracture pathology and how best to manage it. It is important to remember, however, that not all complaints of pelvic pain are derived from a traumatic event. When trying to differentiate pelvic pain in elderly patients, insufficiency or stress fractures should be considered. These usually present as nondisplaced fractures, may have normal appearing X rays, and may occur not only from high-energy trauma (29) but also from low-energy trauma, such as a fall from a standing height (30,31). In addition, the diagnosis has also been made in patients who present with rheumatological disorders (32,33), Crohn's disease (30), vitamin or mineral deficiencies (34), and osteoporosis (14,15,31,35–38). These fractures can occur

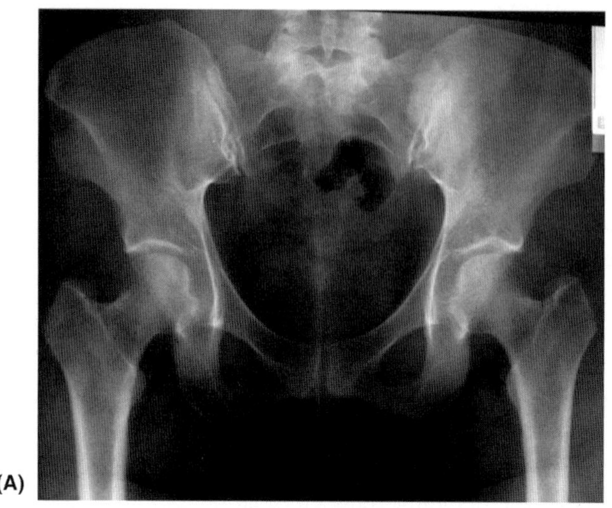

(A)

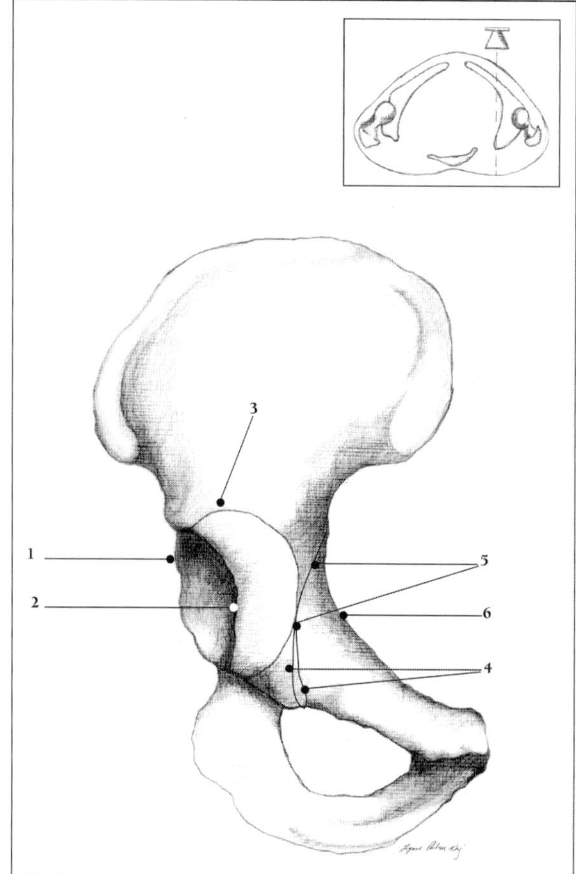

(B)

Figure 2 (**A**) Antero-posterior (AP) radiographic view of the pelvis. (**B**) AP drawing of the pelvis outlining the six landmarks of the acetabulum: *1*, posterior wall; *2*, anterior wall; *3*, roof; *4*, teardrop; *5*, ilioischial line; *6*, iliopectineal line.

(A)

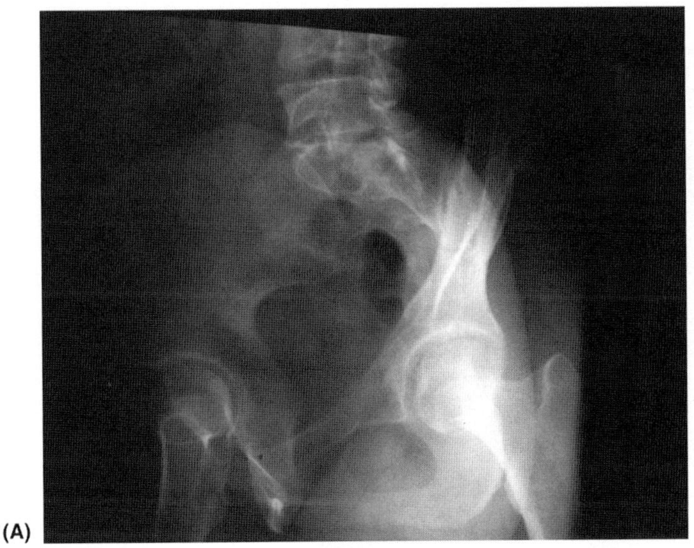

(B)

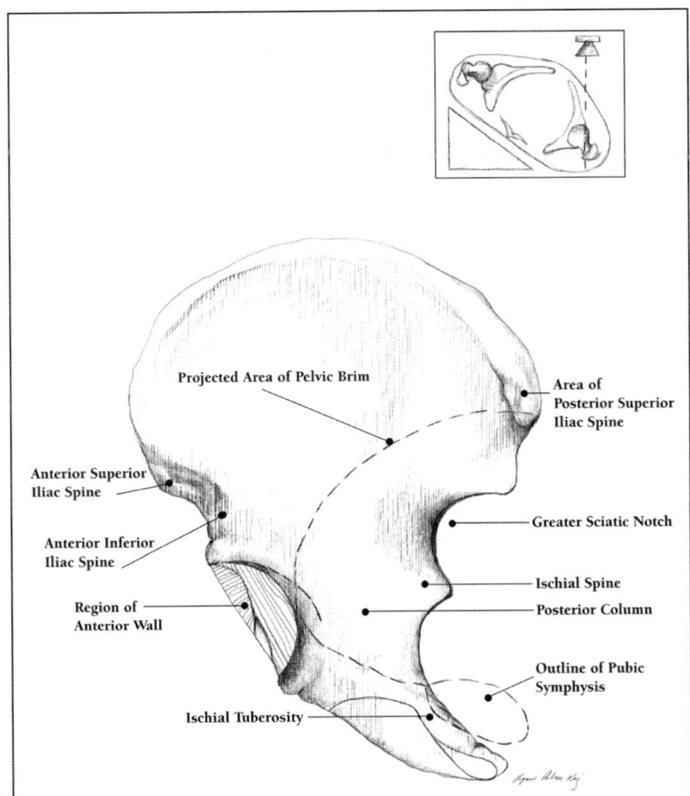

Figure 3 (**A**) Radiograph demonstrating an iliac oblique view of the acetabulum. (**B**) Drawing describing the anatomic structures of an iliac oblique view.

(A)

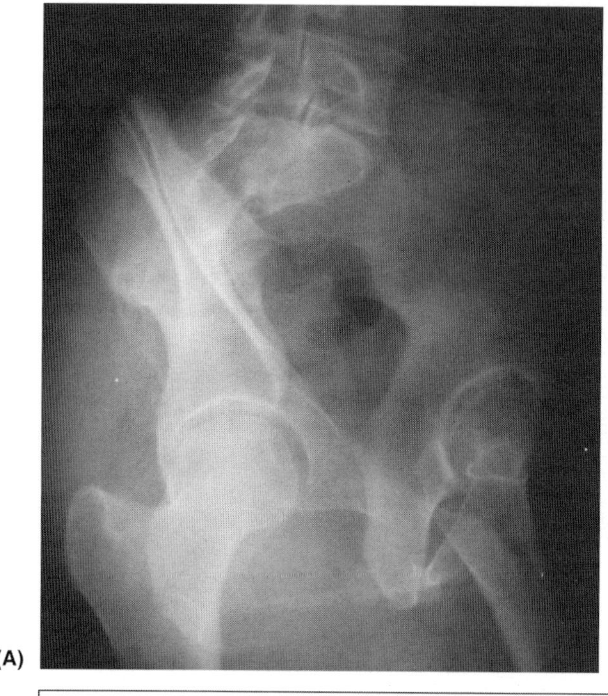

(B)

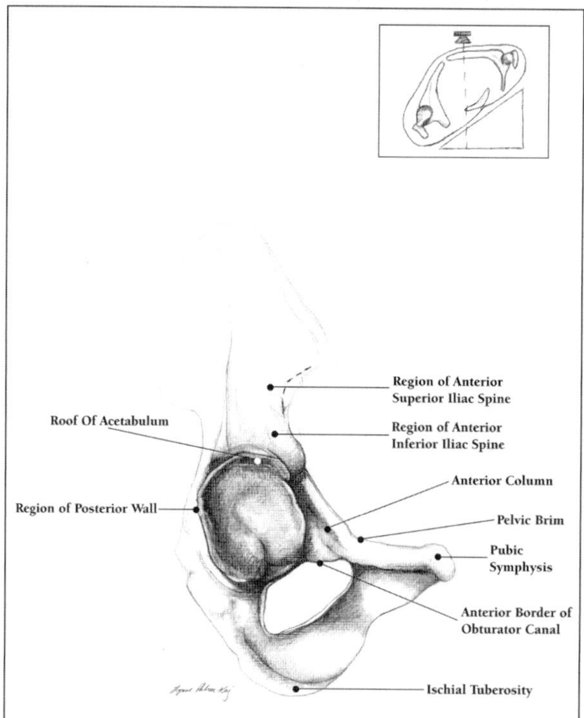

Figure 4 (**A**) Radiograph demonstrating the obturator oblique view of the acetabulum. (**B**) Drawing describing the anatomic structures of the obturator oblique view.

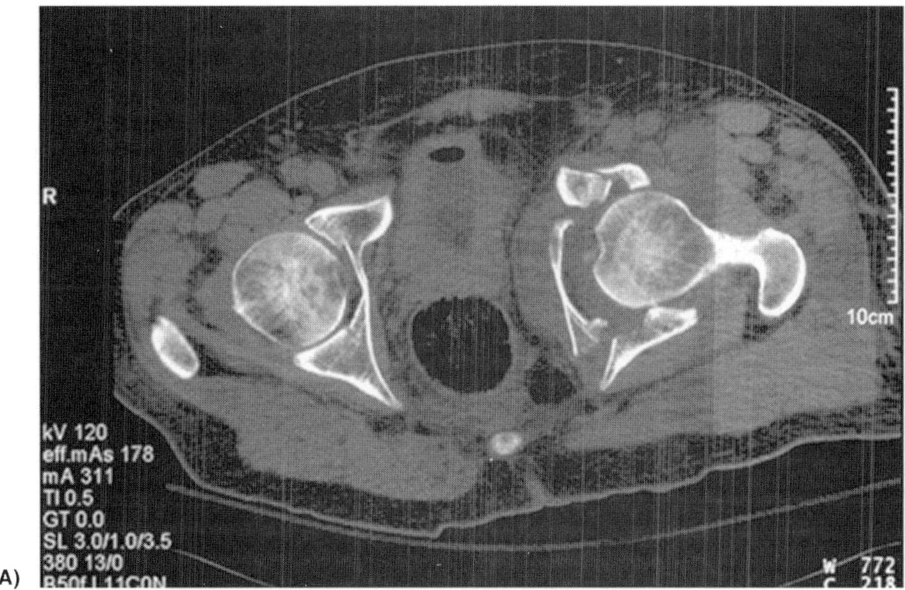

(A)

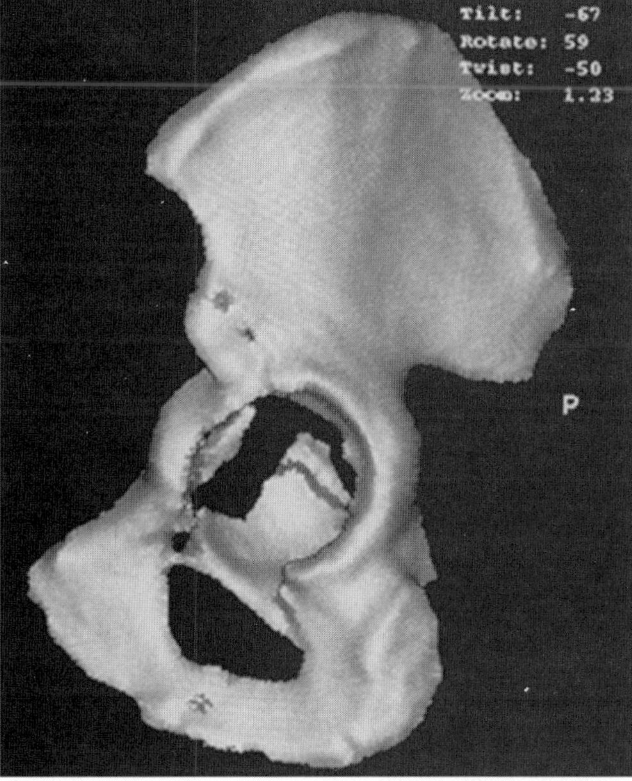

(B)

Figure 5 (**A**) Two-dimensional CT scan of an acetabular fracture. Note the marked amount of comminution. (**B**) Three-dimensional reconstruction of the same patient. Notice that the femoral head is uncovered and protruding through the acetabulum. The use of the three-dimensional view may help in deciding which surgical approach to use.

anywhere about the acetabulum but are most frequently identified in the supra-acetabular region. If suspicion arises, especially in patients who present with complaints of atraumatic hip pain, magnetic resonance imaging (MRI) is a useful tool for diagnosing these fractures (15,39,40).

When trauma does occur, after the radiographic work-up, an attempt should be made to classify these injuries. Historically, some authors have proposed different classification of acetabular fractures (41–43), but by far the most widely used system is the one proposed by Letournel. This classification is based upon the radiographic analysis of the fracture using the anteroposterior and Judet views of the pelvis (8,20,44). Letournel's concept was that the fractures should be identified as those involving only the posterior column, only the anterior column, or those involving both columns. He proposed dividing these fractures into two major groups: elementary or simple types and associated types. There are five simple types and, with the exception of the transverse fracture, involve either a single portion or all of one column. These consist of fractures of the posterior wall, posterior column, anterior wall, anterior column and a transverse fracture. The associated types involve two or more portions or columns. There are also five types and these consist of fractures involving the posterior column and posterior wall, transverse and posterior wall, anterior column and posterior hemitransverse, T-fractures and both column fractures (8).

Attempting to classify acetabular fractures in the elderly may be difficult to achieve. This is due to the fact that although some studies of the elderly have discussed involvement of the anterior column or the anterior wall as frequent presentations, there is no overwhelming pattern that is more common in these patients (31,45). This is due to the fact that the fracture patterns discussed by Letournel require some provocative force be exerted on relatively normal bone. In contrast, the elderly frequently sustain acetabular fractures that occur through osteoporotic bone, which can be produced after moderate or minor falls, resulting in comminuted fractures that may not be classifiable with associated impaction of the femoral head and the acetabulum (11,46) (Fig. 6A, B). Therefore, even after careful radiologic evaluation, acetabular fractures in the elderly may not be clearly defined or easily classifiable. This should suggest that there is some obvious pathology of the pelvis and acetabulum.

TREATMENT OF ACETABULAR INJURIES

The goals of managing patients with acetabular fractures are to restore the congruity of the articular surface, minimize pain, and improve long-term function (47). In the elderly, special considerations should be given to those presenting with significant medical problems, osteopenic bone, and patients who also present with concurrent femoral head fractures or those who also present with moderate or severe arthritis of the hip joint. These orthopedic comorbid factors may result in a treatment that may need to be tailored to the specific needs of that patient.

Initial Management

The initial care of any elderly patient presenting with an acetabular fracture resulting from high-energy trauma should be the same as with any critically injured trauma

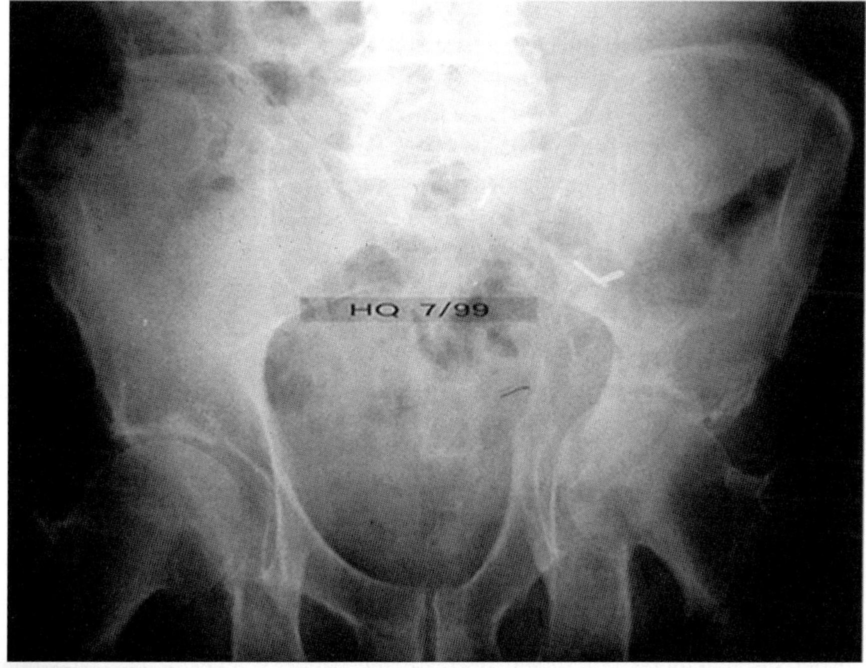

(A)

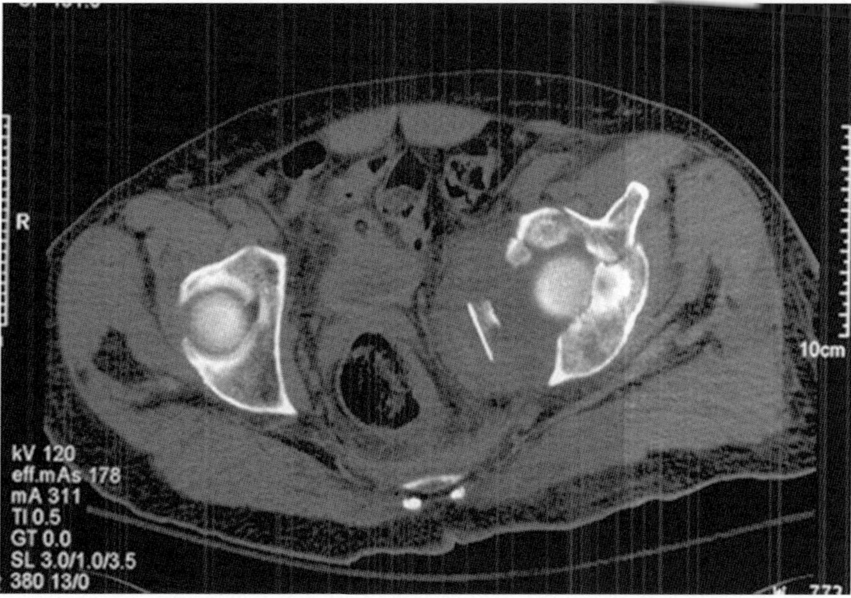

(B)

Figure 6 (**A**) Antero-posterior (AP) radiograph of the pelvis in a 79-year-old female who sustained an acetabular fracture after tripping on a rug in her home. Notice the femoral head protrusion along with a disruption of most of the bony landmarks of the acetabulum. (**B**) CT scan demonstrating impaction and significant displacement of the acetabular fragments.

patient. This requires a team effort involving general surgery, neurosurgery, urology, and orthopedic surgery, all directed at assessing the patient's injuries. The initial history should include the mechanism of injury, their current medications, any existing medical problems, and whether they were independent or limited ambulators prior to their injury. During the orthopedic physical examination, an effort should be made to "touch all the bones," while avoiding the temptation to focus on obvious injuries. The spine should be inspected and palpated and the pelvis should be stressed looking for any instability. The examination should also include a thorough neurologic and vascular examination and an attempt should be made to look for any wounds, contusions, or hemorrhage along the flank, buttocks, or perineum (48). To complete the examination, the rectum and vagina should also be evaluated for any tears. In males, a high riding prostate or any other abnormality should be identified. After examining these patients, they should, if necessary, be aggressively resuscitated using Advanced Trauma Life Support (ATLS) protocols (49).

The initial orthopedic care for these patients should consist of correcting any deformity, promptly reducing any obvious dislocations, especially of the hip since this may decrease the incidence of femoral head osteonecrosis (50), applying sterile dressings to all wounds, and splinting all injuries until formal treatment can be performed. For displaced acetabular fractures, the application of skeletal traction through a small diameter distal femoral pin should decrease the patient's level of pain and improve alignment of the fracture. In addition to providing some comfort to the patient, the traction may also prevent further abrasions to the cartilage of the femoral head on the raw bony acetabular fragments. Skin traction is ineffective and traction applied through a trochanteric pin is contraindicated due to its ineffectiveness and high rates of infection. However, because a large number of elderly patients can present with isolated acetabular fractures resulting from a low-energy falls (19), a different algorithm may be needed for the initial care of these patients.

For those patients presenting with isolated fractures of the acetabulum occurring from low-energy injuries, the initial assessment and treatment should include all that has been previously discussed. In addition, since these fractures are not an emergency, with surgery usually delayed for four to seven days, medical consultations should be obtained prior to surgery to evaluate for any pre-existing or unidentified medical problems. Hopefully, by preoperatively stabilizing any comorbid condition, morbidity and mortality rates can be decreased. Once all the work-ups and evaluations have been completed, a decision should be made as how to best manage the acetabular fracture. In the elderly, treatment of these injuries falls broadly into conservative or nonoperative care, primary or acute total hip arthroplasty, delayed total hip arthroplasty, open reduction internal fixation, or combined hip surgery.

Nonoperative Management

Those patients presenting with stable, concentrically reduced fractures not involving the weight-bearing dome (27) can be considered candidates for nonoperative treatment (51). These may include insufficiency fractures, all nondisplaced fractures, minimally displaced acetabular fractures classified with less than 2 mm of joint displacement (52), displaced low anterior column, low transverse, or low T-fractures, as long as the fracture is stable and the joint remains congruent, both-column fractures where secondary congruence has been obtained between the femoral head and the acetabular components (8,52), fractures of the acetabular walls where stability of the hip can be maintained, and in patients presenting with significant medical instability precluding any surgical intervention. If concern exists that these are unstable fractures or that displacement may occur over time, then dynamic fluoroscopic stress views of the patient under general anesthesia (53) or weekly radiographs of the acetabulum may be used to identify those fractures at risk.

The nonoperative treatment of these patients consists of bed rest, eventual mobilization of the joint, and gait training. In the elderly, bed rest may be indicated for symptomatic relief. If motion of hip is to be limited, a knee immobilizer may be used for two to three weeks to prevent flexion of the hip. Mobilization of the joint should be started as soon as symptoms allow. Unless there is a concern regarding congruency, radiographs should be taken at four- to six-week intervals for the first three months. At approximately 12 weeks, partial weight bearing can be started and gradually progressed to full weight bearing as tolerated. Caution should be used in those patients demonstrating significant osteoporosis so that these patients may be advanced more slowly, requiring an additional four to six weeks to reach full weight bearing. In those patients requiring traction to maintain congruency of the hip, traction may be needed for up to 12 weeks (54).

The results using nonoperative treatment have varied. In those fractures presenting as either nondisplaced injuries, not involving the superior dome, or where joint congruency and stability have been maintained, 75 to 92% have demonstrated good or excellent results in mostly young, trauma patients (43,53). However, in those patients with displaced fractures of the dome or injuries that involve either the posterior column or wall, poor clinical outcomes have been reported in 67 to 75% of patients (43). Unfortunately, most acetabular studies are not stratified into elderly and nonelderly patients so that the results obtained usually discuss all patients rather than any specific group of individuals. In those few studies evaluating the elderly, however, poor results have been recorded in at least 30% of patients treated conservatively (31). Factors noted to increase the rates of failure in the elderly have included osteoporosis, femoral head fractures, inappropriate traction, and early weight bearing. Therefore, in patients presenting with stable patterns or medical instability precluding any operative intervention, nonoperative treatment may be indicated. In patients who present with unstable injuries and in whom no contraindications to surgery exist, operative intervention may improve functional outcomes.

Operative Management

Traditional methods for managing displaced acetabular fractures in the elderly consist of open reduction internal fixation (45), delayed total hip arthroplasty (55–64) or primary or acute total hip arthroplasty (62,65–69). An attractive alternative may be the use of combinations of surgeries to obtain good outcomes.

Open Reduction Internal Fixation

That there are various surgical approaches for the management of acetabular fractures in the elderly is not unexpected given the differences in the strength and structure of their bones, their physical needs and expectations, the fracture patterns of their injuries, their comorbidities, and the experience and skills of the treating surgeon. Without performing an exhaustive review of the literature, most surgeons providing routine care to the elderly intuitively know that there is a significant difference in treating patients who present after high-energy injuries versus those presenting after a low-energy injury. In the former, the bone stock of the acetabulum may be similar to that seen in younger patients so that the use of established open reduction techniques to fix the acetabulum may be used. In these patients successful outcomes can be expected to be similar to those reported for younger patients (45). It should be noted however that post-traumatic arthritis has been reported in up to 30% of all patients due to imperfect reductions, chondrolysis of the cartilage from the initial trauma, osteochondral defects, or the development of vascular necrosis of the head or acetabulum (44,64,70–72,73) (Fig. 7 A–D), all of which will affect outcomes.

In those patients sustaining fractures from low-energy traumas, age-related bone loss or bone loss occurring secondary to osteoporosis will result in diminished bone stock. This is seen at the microstructural level, resulting in a reduction in the bone mineral density and a change in the trabecular orientation of the bone. Studies have demonstrated that these structural changes narrow the tolerable loading directions of the bone, increasing the risk of a fracture (74,75). In addition, these patients may also have already have pre-existing arthritis of the hip so that the additional insult of an acetabular fracture may produce displaced, unrecognizable fracture patterns with severe comminution, erosion of the articular surfaces, and associated fractures of the femoral head (65,73) (Fig. 8A–F). The combination of the four factors of osteoporosis, comminution, associated head fractures, and arthritis may ultimately produce bone that does not allow any anchorage of the fixation devices, or ultimately results in loosening and failure of the applied fixation or collapse of the hip joint.

When evaluating outcomes by age, using traditional surgical approaches and techniques, studies have demonstrated that the numbers of anatomic reductions and the ability to obtain a successful outcome decreases with advancing age (8,70,76). Therefore, an alternative to standard approaches should be considered. One alternative may be the use of minimally invasive or percutaneous approaches for the management of these injuries (46,77–83). Since the goal may not be an absolute anatomic reduction of the joint, this approach may allow for a rapid relief from the pain of the fracture and allow early mobilization of the patient. However, these are difficult techniques to learn, may require specialized instruments to obtain the reduction, have potentially life-threatening complications if the screws are misplaced, and may work best with minimally displaced or unstable but congruent fractures. Because some malalignment of the joint may persist, one needs to remember that even though small incisions or percutaneous screw placements are used, significant post-traumatic arthritis or avascular necrosis of the femoral head may still occur similar to those seen after open techniques (46,70,76,78).

Therefore, prior to using open reduction internal fixation or percutaneous techniques to repair the fracture in an elderly patient, it is important to differentiate fractures occurring from high- or low-energy mechanisms of injury. If after the radiologic evaluation pre-existing arthritis of the hip is identified, fractures are not easily classifiable, demonstrate associated femoral head fractures, or present with severe displacement of the fragments, then other surgical options should be considered for use in the management of these patients. If the decision is made to fix the fracture, then one should remember that, regardless of the fixation technique, posttraumatic arthritis may develop in up to 30% of these patients.

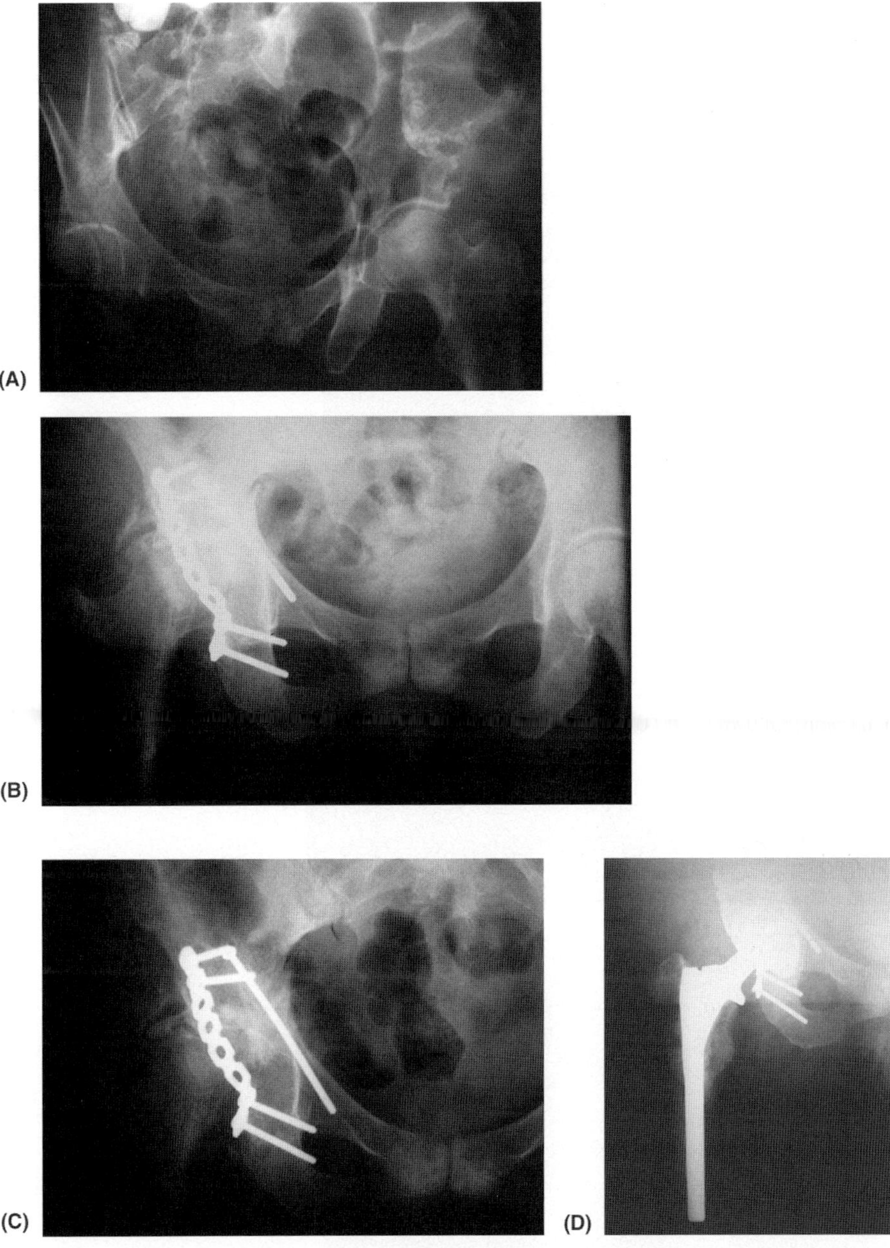

Figure 7 (**A**) Antero-posterior (AP) radiograph of a 69-year-old female who fell from a standing height. The fall produced an acetabular fracture along with a posterior hip dislocation on the right side. (**B**) AP radiograph three months after fixation. The joint space has become narrowed and the femoral head is starting to lose its spherical shape. (**C**) At nine months, the femoral head has collapsed as a result of avascular necrosis. In addition, some the areas of the acetabulum have also developed some avascularity, resulting in severe posttraumatic arthritis of the hip joint. (**D**) Salvage achieved through the use of a total hip arthroplasty performed at 15 months postinjury.

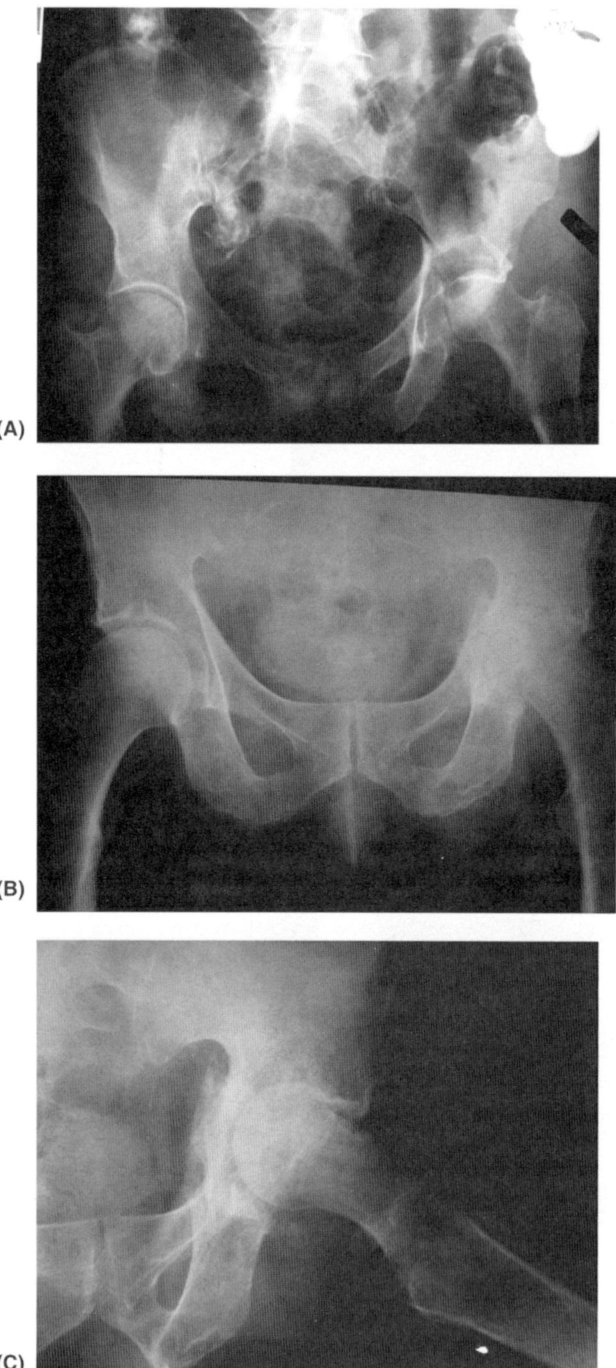

Figure 8 (**A**) Antero-posterior (AP) radiograph of the pelvis in a 71-year-old male who sustained a fracture of the acetabulum and a posterior dislocation of the hip as a result of a motor vehicle accident. (**B**) AP view after reduction of the hip dislocation. Note the impaction of the joint, as the femoral head appears to be penetrating through the acetabulum. (**C**) Lateral view of the hip joint after the closed reduction of the dislocation. Note the impaction of the femoral head superiorly, at the roof of the acetabulum. (*Continued*)

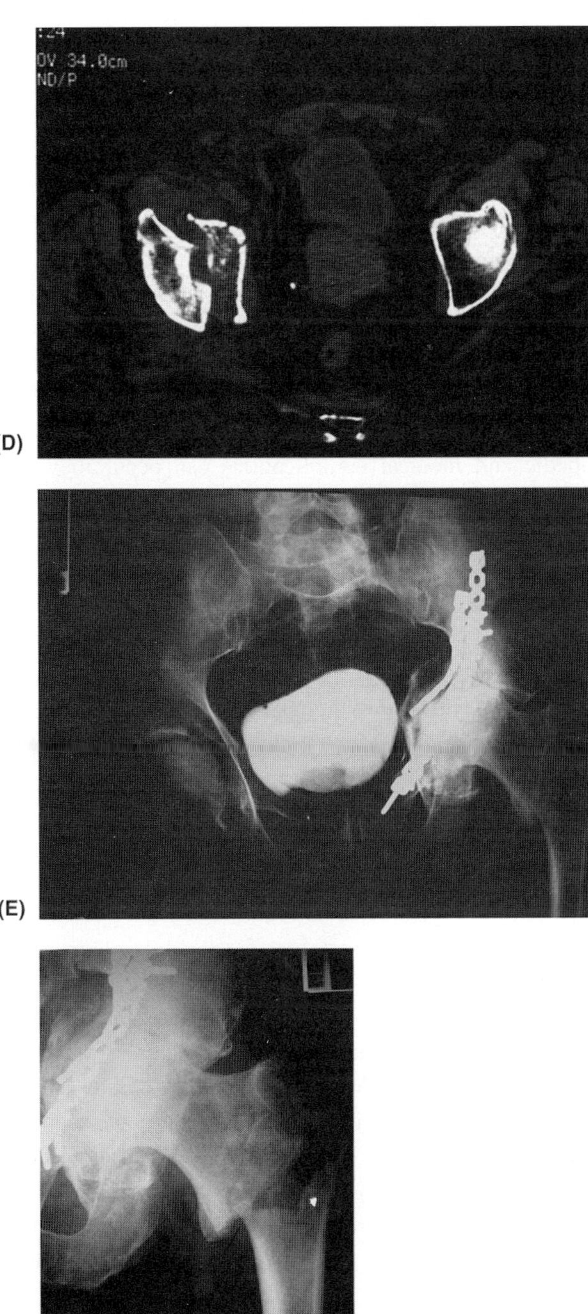

Figure 8 (*Continued*) (**D**) Two-dimensional CT scan demonstrating comminution of the weight-bearing dome of the acetabulum. (**E**) Fixation was performed to provide stability to the acetabulum. At three months postfixation, notice that there is continued protrusion of the femoral head. (**F**) Subsequent degeneration of the hip joint produced a femoral head and neck that became locked within the acetabulum, allowing no motion of the hip joint. Eventually the patient sustained a low-energy injury, which produced an ipsilateral subtrochanteric femur fracture. Salvage was with a calcar total hip replacement.

Delayed Total Hip Arthroplasty

In those patients who have significant osteoporosis, comminution, arthritis, associated femoral head fractures, or significant medical comorbidities that preclude the use of any early orthopedic surgical intervention, some surgeons may elect to initially treat the patient with the use of bedrest or traction followed by late arthroplasty. Unfortunately prolonged immobilization, with or without traction, may result in significant complications including the development of deep vein thrombosis, decubitus ulcers, pulmonary problems, and joint stiffness. Orthopedic complications resulting from the nonoperative treatment of these patients may include the development of significant osteoporosis, loss of bone stock, severe pelvic deformities, the development of posttraumatic arthritis of the hip, and the potential development of avascular necrosis of the femoral head and acetabulum (60,63,71,84).

Knowing that these orthopedic and medical complications can occur may persuade surgeons to perform an open reduction of the fracture in an attempt to minimize late complications. Unfortunately, as just described, the fixation may fail or be inadequate, resulting in collapse of the joint, producing a malunion or nonunion of the acetabulum, contributing to disuse osteoporosis, producing heterotopic bone, and resulting in the development soft tissue contractures about the hip joint (60,72). Therefore, if late arthroplasty is to be considered as the treatment for these patients, it should be reserved as salvage for those who have developed symptomatic posttraumatic arthritis of the hip and have failed an attempt at conservative care (Fig. 9A–C). Regardless of conflicting reports as to whether cemented or cementless arthroplasties are better for these patients, some things are certain. Operative times, blood loss, transfusion requirements will be increased, and the difficulty in performing a total hip arthroplasty is expected to be greater for these patients than those treated with arthroplasties for nontraumatic arthritis of the hip (57,58,60).

In performing a late arthroplasty, it is important that a thorough preoperative assessment and planning of the procedure are performed. Preoperative assessments should include obtaining medical clearance for any underlying medical comorbidities, potential vascular work-ups if concern exists regarding the vascular status of the extremity, along with the predonation of autologous blood. Radiographic studies should include standard anteroposterior and lateral views of the hip in addition to anteroposterior, obturator, and iliac oblique views of the pelvis. Two- and three-dimensional computed tomographic (CT) scans of the acetabulum may be helpful in assessing bone loss, heterotopic bone, and the pathology of the acetabulum. In the presence of previous fixation, however, some scatter of the scans may result in difficulty in adequately evaluating the acetabulum. Component selection is at the discretion of the surgeon, but implants and instrumentations used to reduce and fix an acetabular fracture should also be available. If bone graft is to be used, and the patient's femoral head is considered inadequate due to the size of the defect, an allograft should be made available.

Although some studies have demonstrated good results in patients treated with arthroplasty after an acetabular fracture, it is not surprising that most long-term studies, following operative or nonoperative treatment of acetabular fractures, have demonstrated higher rates of failure than arthroplasties that were performed in patients with nontraumatic arthritis of the hip (55,58,60,61,64,85). Romness and Lewallen (55)

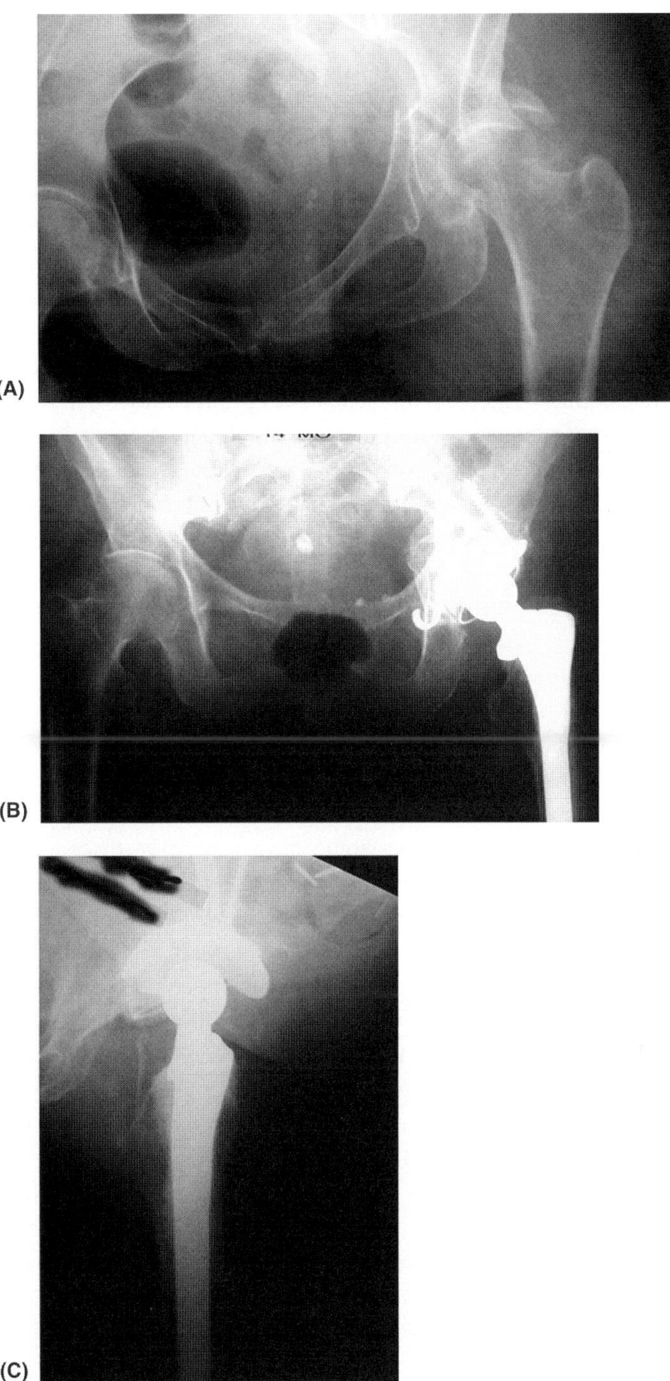

Figure 9 (**A**) Antero-posterior (AP) radiograph in a 77-year-old female who fell at home. The concern was that because of the patient's age and fracture pattern she would not do well with surgery. The initial treating surgeon subsequently managed the patient with nonoperative care. (**B**) At 2 years, the patient had developed severe degeneration of the hip and was referred for treatment options. AP radiograph demonstrating salvage through the use of a total hip arthroplasty using a protrusion cup. (**C**) Lateral view of the total hip arthroplasty.

described a projected 10-year failure rate (revision plus symptomatic loosening without revision) of 39.1%, increasing to 49% if they included all symptomatic or asymptomatic cases of loosening. They also noted that radiographic loosening of the acetabular component (52.9%) was more common than the femoral component (29.4%). Mears (86) also documented high rates of failure, approaching 51% within two years of the initial arthroplasty, with almost 40% of the entire population eventually requiring a revision arthroplasty. Finally the studies by Weber et al. (60) and Harris (61) have also described the difficulties in managing these patients reporting failures approaching 40%. This is significant when one realizes that the frequency for aseptic loosening after 10 years has fallen from 8% of all primary hips in 1979 to 3% by 1985 (87).

Excluding a poorly performed surgery, some factors have been identified as contributing to high failure rates. One is the development of deep infections (87), which may be decreased with the use of preoperative intravenous antibiotics. A second factor is performing arthoplasties in younger, higher demand patients. Failure rates have been reported near 80% when performed in patients younger than 60 years compared to 45% for those individuals over 60 years of age (55). A third factor is performing the procedure on male patients who already have posttraumatic arthritis of the hip. Studies have reported that at two years, men were already at risk for needing a revision, which is theorized to be due to greater activity levels in these individuals (55,87). A fourth cause has been noted to be patients who have large acetabular defects necessitating the use of bone grafts. These may ultimately reabsorb and contribute to radiolucency that develops, specifically around the acetabular component (88). One final factor may be the development of avascular necrosis about the acetabulum (86). Biopsy specimens at the time of arthroplasty have demonstrated avascular necrosis about the central portion of the acetabulum (89), which may be the reason some physicians have discouraged initial open reduction for these patients (92). Looking at these five factors, however, only the first three may be preventable or electively excluded for surgical treatment. So in addition to being difficult surgeries to perform, with potentially high rates of failure, and greater risks for causing neurovascular injuries, producing infections, heterotopic bone, and developing soft tissue contractures, why offer late arthroplasty to any of these patients? Because the other option is to allow patients to continue to live with poorly functioning hips or undergo an arthrodesis. Neither of these alternatives is particularly attractive to patients who are otherwise healthy and may have projected life spans ranging between 15 and 50 years.

Fortunately, not all studies describe such terrible results. Some studies, using actual and projected 10-year survival rates (90), with component survival and no revision or radiographic loosening, have reported rates of success occurring between 78 and 100% (56,57,59,60,91). The question is why these studies have reported lower rates of failure than other studies. Some measures have been identified that help reduce the risk of later revisions. These include improved fixation, advanced surgical techniques, and better implants (87). Studies have shown that using preventative measures have decreased the risk of deep infections. These have included using prophylactic systemic antibiotic therapy, gentamycin containing cement, laminar airflow, and the use of exhaust gowns (87). Studies have also shown that by using third generation cementing techniques, consisting of retrograde filling, cleaning by pulse lavage, distal plugging, and pressurization by means of a proximal seal, the risk of osteolysis can be decreased

(93,94). Incorporating these steps has been shown to reduce the risk for a revision by approximately 25% (87). Interestingly, one other factor has been shown to improve the rates of success, the use of cementless techniques (56,57,59,60,91). The common denominator for high 10-year survival in these studies appears to be cementless application of the implants. This may be due to the implants having a collared along with a matte surface, but is more likely due to improved design and instrumentation of the implants along with careful bone bed preparation.

Therefore, it appears that with modern designs, especially for instrumentation and techniques, improved rates of survival can occur using late arthroplasy in patients who develop post-traumatic arthritis of the hip after a fracture of the acetabulum. However, one should realize that there are significant risks and difficulties in performing an arthroplasty in these patients, and that the overall rates of success are still lower than those procedures performed in patients for primary arthritis of the hip (55,58,95).

Acute Total Hip Arthroplasty

With concerns about potential failures of fixation or that a "wait and see" attitude in a displaced acetabular injury will produce significant morbidity to that patient, the options for treatment of acetabular fractures in the elderly become limited. The use of an acute arthroplasty for these patients may result in failure due to the development of pelvic nonunions, or insufficient bone stock resulting in loosening of the implants. In addition to these problems and concerns for failures from late arthroplasties, including the potential need for revisions or the use of multiple procedures performed through compromised tissues, investigations have resulted in the development of therapeutic alternatives for the management of these patients.

A suggested option is to combine procedures in an attempt to improve function and decrease morbidity. A combined approach, consisting of stabilization of the acetabular fracture along with immediate application of a total hip arthroplasty, has certain advantages (9,19,64,65,96). First, fixing the acetabular fracture stability to the pelvis allows a solid base to be built for the placement of a total hip. Second, fixing the fracture may help prevent the development of severe deformity of the pelvis and avoid the development of a nonunion. Last, it should be remembered that, since the goal is a rigid and stable fixation of the fracture, an anatomic reduction of the acetabulum is not necessary for success of this technique. Once the acetabular fracture has been stabilized, then the application of an acute arthroplasty of the hip can be performed (Fig. 10A–F). A combined approach, however, is not recommended for all elderly patients. Indeed, most elderly patients with acetabular fractures either present with nondisplaced injuries requiring nonoperative management, or with displaced fractures, who also possess excellent bone stock, for whom fixation using standard open reduction techniques produces satisfactory results (19,45). It is primarily recommended for acetabular fractures in the elderly who have also have arthritis of the hip joint, significant osteoporosis producing fractures that are not classifiable radiographically, those injuries resulting from low-energy mechanisms that produce marked displacement of the columns involving the weight-bearing dome, and in patients who present with associated fractures of the femoral head.

(A)

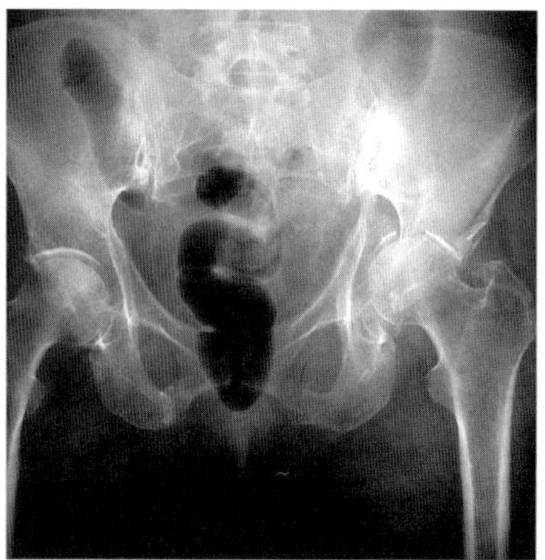

(B)

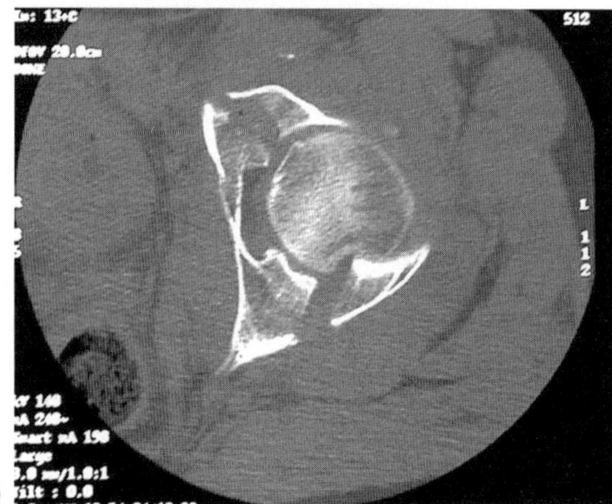

(C)

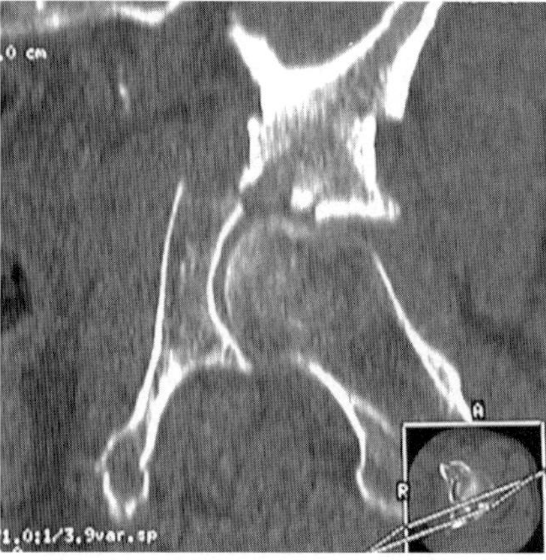

Figure 10 (**A**) Antero-posterior (AP) radiograph of a 73-year-old male who sustained an acetabular fracture after a motor vehicle accident. Notice the impaction of the roof and the medial displacement of the anterior and posterior columns. (**B**) Two-dimensional CT scans demonstrating displacement of the weight-bearing surface of the dome along with impaction of the femoral head. Notice that the acetabular fragment appears to be impinging on the femoral head. (**C**) CT reconstruction showing impaction of the joint along with flattening of the superior region of the femoral head. (*Continued*)

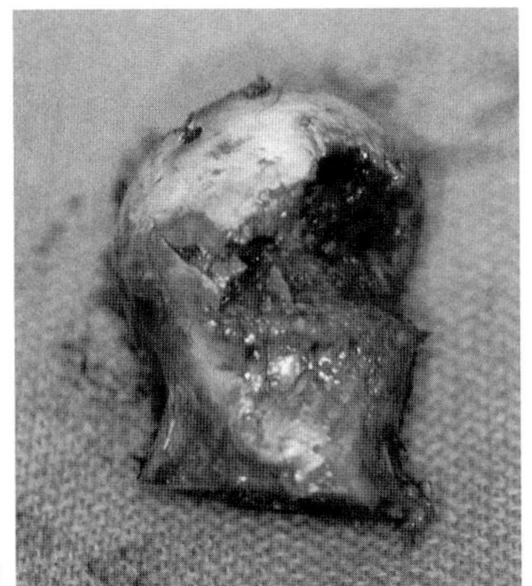

(D)

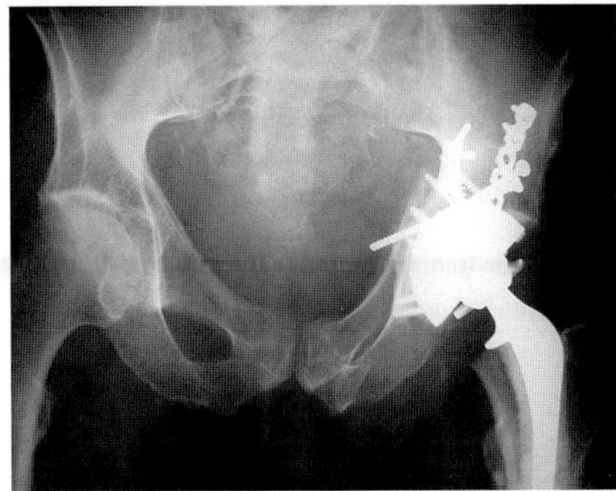

(E)

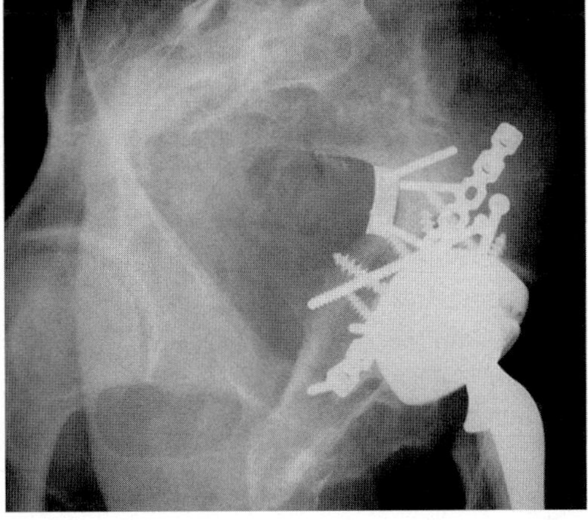

(F)

Figure 10 (*Continued*) (**D**) Anatomic specimen at the time of surgery demonstrating significant impaction of the femoral head. (**E**) AP radiograph of the pelvis after completion of a combined hip technique. Notice that anatomic fixation of the joint was not attempted but, rather, the goal of stable fixation of both columns was achieved, allowing for the placement of a total hip arthroplasty. (**F**) An iliac oblique view of the pelvis after the use of a combined hip technique.

Results using a combined technique have reported a 100% union rate of the acetabular fractures, using either a posterior, anterior, or extended approach, between 6 and 12 weeks. At follow-up, using Harris hip scores (61), patients have averaged 80 points, there have been no reports of sciatic nerve injuries, failures of fixation, or deep wound infections, and the majority of patients have been able to ambulate either without support or require the use of a cane for long distances (19,65). Although lengths of surgery, blood loss, transfusion requirements, and lengths of stay were greater than for primary total hip surgeries, they appear to be consistent for those patients undergoing a total hip arthroplasty after an acetabular fracture (57,60). Orthopedic complications, consisting of the development of heterotopic bone, hip dislocations, osteolysis, and failure of the arthroplasty have all been reported, but not seen at noticeable levels when using either late arthroplasties, open reduction techniques, or nonoperative treatment of these patients.

It should be remembered however that there are few studies using a combined technique and, although it presents an attractive alternative for the management for these patients, there is concern that these patients may require substantial medical work-ups prior to surgery. There is also concern that the surgeries may be difficult to perform, resulting in higher rates of complications due to an unfamiliarity with the surgical approaches or the techniques needed for the management of acetabular fractures. Therefore, prior to using a combined technique, a careful preoperative planning should be undertaken. Surgeons should feel comfortable using open reduction techniques, instrumentation, and approaches as well as the implants and techniques used for the application of a hip arthroplasty. For those surgeons comfortable with both approaches, a combined technique may avoid high rates failure.

SUMMARY

Acetabular fractures in the elderly can be difficult to manage. A careful history and physical examination should be performed to determine the mechanism of injury along with the presence of any medical comorbidities. Radiologic studies, consisting of plain radiographs and CT scans, should then be used to assess the fracture pattern and to determine if there are any associated injuries to the hip joint. Patients can be treated nonoperatively if they present with: stable, concentrically reduced fractures not involving the weight-bearing dome; a nondisplaced fracture; minimally displaced acetabular fractures with less than 2 mm of joint displacement; a displaced low anterior column, low transverse, or low T-fracture; both-column fractures where secondary congruence has been obtained between the femoral head and the acetabulum (8,52); or fractures of the acetabular walls where stability of the hip can be maintained.

For patients who present with displaced acetabular fractures with good bone stock, a viable treatment option is the use of an open reduction internal fixation technique. For those patients with displaced fractures who also have arthritis of the hip joint, significant osteoporosis producing fractures that are not classifiable, injuries resulting from low-energy mechanisms with marked displacement of the columns extending into the weight-bearing dome, or in patients who present with associated fractures of the femoral head, the treatment options include late arthroplasty of the hip or the use of a combined technique. In both latter options, surgeons should feel comfortable using open reduction techniques, instrumentation, and approaches as well as the implants and techniques used for the application of a hip arthroplasty.

ACKNOWLEDGMENT

The author wishes to thank Ms. Julia M. Scaduto, ARNP, for her help in the preparation of this manuscript.

REFERENCES

1. Minimo AM, Arias E, Kochanek KD, Murphy SL, Smith BL. Final data for 2000. National vital statistics report. Vol. 15. No 12. Hyattsville, Maryland: National Center for Health Statistics, 2002, available at http://www.cdc.gov/nchs/fastats/lifepec.htm
2. Schneider EL, Guralnik JM. The aging of America: Impact on health care costs. JAMA 1990; 63:2335–2340.
3. Goulding MR. Public health and aging: Trends in aging-United States and worldwide. JAMA 2003; 289:1371–1373.
4. Levit K, Smith C, Cowan C, Lazenby H, Sensenig A, Catlin A. Trends in U.S. health care spending, 2001. Health Affairs 2003; 22:154–164.
5. Wolff JL, Starfield B, Anderson G. Prevalence, expenditures, and complications of multiple chronic conditions in the elderly. Arch Intern Med 2002; 162:2269–2276.
6. Jacobzone S, Oxley H.'Aging and health care costs. International politics and Society1/2002. Available at http://fesportal.fes.de/Pls/portal30/docs/folder/ipg/ipg1_2002/artjacobzone.htm
7. Bishop CE, Gilden D, Blom J, et al. Medicare spending for injured elders: Are there opportunities for savings? Health Affairs 2002; 21:215–223.
8. Letournel E, Judet R. Fractures of the Acetabulum. 2nd ed. Berlin: Springer-Verlag, 1993:17–361.
9. Howe W Jr, Lacy T, Schwartz RP. A study of the gross anatomy of the arteries supplying the proximal portion of the femur and acetabulum. J Bone Joint Surg 1950; 32A:856–866.
10. Clemente CD. Gray's Anatomy of the Human Body. 13th American ed. Philadelphia: Lea and Febiger, 1985:752–765.
11. Ragnarsson B, Jacobsson B. Epidemiology of pelvic fractures in a Swedish country. Acta Orthop Scand 1992; 63:297–300.
12. Gānsslen A, Pohlemann T, Paul CH, Lobenhoffer PH, Tschernne H.'Epidemiology of Pelvic Ring injuries. Injury 1966; 27(suppl 1):13–20.
13. Melton LJ, Sampson JM, Morrey BF, Ilstrup DM. Epidemiologic features of pelvic fractures. Clin Orthop 1981; 155:43–47.
14. Cooper KL, Beabout JW, McLeod RA. Supraacetabular insufficiency fractures. Radiology 1985; 157:15–17.
15. Otte MT, Helms CA, Fritz RC. MR imaging of supra-acetabular insufficiency fractures. Skeletal Radiol 1997; 26:279–283.
16. Hedlund R, Lindgren U, Ahlbom A. Age and sex specific incidence of femoral neck and trochanteric fractures. Clin Orthop 1987; 222:132–139.
17. Gallagher JC, Melton LJ, Riggs BL, Bergtrath E. Epidemiology of fractures of the proximal femur in Rochester Minnesota. Clin Orthop 1980; 150:163–167.
18. Koval KJ, Skovran ML, Polatsch D, Aharonoff GB, Zuckerman JD. Dependency after hip fracture in geriatric patients: a study of predictive factors. J Orthop Trauma 1996; 10: 531–535.

19. Herscovici D, Bohlhofner BR, Lindvall E, Scaduto JM. The combined hip procedure: open reduction internal fixation with concurrent total hip arthroplasty for the management of acetabular fractures in the elderly. Presented at the 17th Annual Orthopaedic Trauma Association Meeting, San Diego CA, 2001.
20. Judet R, Judet J, Letournel E. Fractures of the Acetabulum classification and surgical approaches for open reduction. Preliminary report. J Bone Joint Surg 1964; 46A:1615–1646.
21. Matta JM, Anderson LM, Epstein HC, Hendricks P. Fractures of the acetabulum. A retrospective analysis. Clin Orthop 1986; 205:230–240.
22. Olsen SA, Maurizi MG, Hassien J, Pear AJ. A review of computerized tomography evaluation of acetabular fractures. Part 2. Contemp Orthop 1991; 23:436–447.
23. Griffiths HJ, Standertskjold-Nordenstany CG, Burke J, Lamont B, Cimmel J. Computed tomography in the management of acetabular fractures. Skeletal Radiol 1984; 11:22–31.
24. Calkins MS, Zych G, Latta L, Borja FJ, Mnaymneh W. Computerized tomography evaluation of stability in posterior fracture dislocations of the hip. Clin Orthop 1988; 227:152–1613.
25. Keith JE, Brashear HR, Guilford WB. Stability of posterior fracture dislocations of the hip: quantatative assessment using computed tomography. J Bone Joint Surg 1988; 70A: 711–714.
26. Brumbak RJ, Holt ES, McBride MS, Poka A, Bathon GH, Burgess AR. Acetabular depression fracture accompanying posterior fracture dislocation of the hip. J Orthop Trauma 1990; 4:42–48.
27. Olsen SA, Matta JM. The computerized tomography subchondral arc: a new method of assessing acetabular articular continuity after fracture. (A preliminary report) J Orthop Trauma 1993; 7:402–413.
28. Gautsch TL, Johnson EE, Seeger LL. The three dimensional stereographic display of 3D reconstructed CT scans of the pelvis and acetabulum. Clin Orthop 1994; 305:138–151.
29. Schachter AK, Roberrts CS, Seligson D. Occult bilateral acetabular fractures associated with high-energy trauma and osteoporosis. J Orthop Trauma 2003; 17: 386–389.
30. Törnkvist H, Schatzker J. Acetabular fractures in the elderly: an easily missed diagnosis. J Orthop Trauma 1993; 3:233–235.
31. Spencer RF. Acetabular fractures in older patients. J Bone Joint Surg 1989; 71B: 774–776.
32. Ozaki D, Shirai Y, Nakayama Y, Uesaka S. A case report of insufficiency fracture of the fossa acetabuli in a patient with rheumatoid arthritis. J Nippon Med Sch 2000; 67:267–270.
33. Lin YM, Tong KM, Lee TS. Isolated supra-acetabular insufficiency fracture: a case report. J Formos Med Assoc 2002; 101:372–375.
34. Chary-Valckenaere I, Pere P, Grignon B, Pourel J, Gaucher A. Supra-acetabular insufficiency fractures: role of fluoride treatment and vitamin D deficiency? Br J Rheumatol 1997; 36:603–605.
35. Timsit MA, Loite F, Touchard P, Dryll A. Acetabular fractures due to bone insufficiency. A case report. Rev Rhum Engl Ed 1996; 63:364–366.
36. Schreiber S. Radiological vignette. Insufficiency fracture of the acetabulum. Clin Rheumatol 1992; 11: 440–442.
37. Lee TS, Tong KM, Ku MC. Insufficiency fracture of the acetabulum: a case report. Zhonghua Yi Xue Za Zhi 1995; 55: 274–277.
38. Rosa MA, Maccauro G, D'Arienzo M. Bilateral acetabular fracture without trauma. Int Orthop 1999; 23:120–121.
39. Grangier C, Garcia J, Howarth NR, Mar R, Rossier P. Role of MRI in the diagnosis of insufficiency fractures of the sacrum and acetabular roof. Skeletal Radiol 1997; 26:517–524.
40. May DA, Purins JL, Smith DK. MR imaging of occult traumatic fractures and muscular injuries of the hip and pelvis in elderly patients. AJR 1996; 166:1075–1078.

41. Cauchoix M, Truchet P. Les fractures articulares dl la hanche (col excepté). Rev Chir Orthop 1951; 37:266–332.
42. Creyssel J, Schnepp J. Contribution à l'étude radiologique des fractures transcotyloidiennes du bassin. J Radiol Electrol Med Nuc 1961a; 42:601–699.
43. Rowe CR, Lowell JD. Prognosis of fractures of the acetabulum. J Bone Joint Surg 1961; 43A: 30–59.
44. Letournel E. Acetabular fractures: classifications and management. Clin Orthop 1980; 151:81–106.
45. Helfet DL, Borrelli J, DiPasquale T, Sanders R. Stabilization of acetabular fractures in elderly patients. J Bone Joint Surg 1992: 74A:7533–7765.
46. Mears DC. Surgical treatment of acetabular fractures in elderly patients with osteoporotic bone. J Am Acad Orthop Surg 1999; 7:1228–1241.
47. Matta JM. Operative treatment of acetabular fractures through the ilioinguinal approach. A ten year prospective. Clin Orthop 1994; 305:10–19.
48. Hak DJ, Olsen SA, Matta JM. Diagnosis and management of closed internal degloving injuries associated with pelvic and acetabular fractures. The Morel-Lavellé lesion. J Trauma 1997; 42:1046–1051.
49. Committee on Trauma, American College of Surgeons, eds. Advanced Trauma Life Support Manual. Chicago: American College of Surgeons, 1993.
50. Roffi RP, Matta JM. Unrecognized posterior dislocation of the hip associated with transverse and T-type fractures of the acetabulum. J Orthop Trauma 1993; 7:23–27.
51. Heeg M, Oostvogel HJM, Klasen HJ. Conservative treatment of acetabular fractures. The role of the weight-bearing dome and anatomic reduction in the ultimate results. J Trauma 1987; 27:555–559.
52. Matta JM. Fractures of the acetabulum: accuracy of reduction and clinical results in patients managed operatively within three weeks of injury. J Bone Joint Surg 1996; 78A:1632–1635.
53. Tornetta P III. Non-operative management of acetabular fractures: the use of dynamic stress views. J Bone Joint Surg 1999; 81B:67–70.
54. Templeman DC, Olsen S, Moed BR, Duwelius P, Matta J. Surgical treatment of acetabular fractures. Inst Course Lect 1999; 48:481–496.
55. Romness DW, Lewallen DG. Total hip arthroplasty after fracture of the acetabulum. J Bone Joint Surg 1990: 72B:761–764.
56. Huo MH, Solberg BD, Zatorski LE, Keggi KJ. Total hip replacements done without cement after acetabular fractures. A 4 to 8 year follow-up study. J Arthroplasty 1999; 14:827–831.
57. Bellabarba C, Berger RA, Bentley CD, et al. Cementless acetabular reconstruction after acetabular fracture. J Bone Joint Surg 2001; 83A: 868–876.
58. Boardman KP, Charnley J. Low-friction arthroplasty after fracture-dislocations of the hip. J Bone Joint Surg 1978; 60B:495–498.
59. Pritchett JW, Bortel DT. Total hip replacement after central fracture dislocation of the acetabulum. Orthop Rev 1991; 20:607–610.
60. Weber M, Berry DJ, Harrisen WS. Total hip arthroplasty after operative treatment of an acetabular fracture. J Bone Joint Surg 1998; 80A:1295–1305.
61. Harris WH. Traumatic arthritis of the hip after dislocation and acetabular fractures: treatment by mold arthroplasty. An end-result study using a new method of result evaluation. J Bone Joint Surg 1969; 51A:737–755.
62. Coventry MB. The treatment of fracture-dislocation of the hip by total hip arthroplasty. J Bone Joint Surg 1974; 56A:1128–1134.
63. Hamilton WG, Born CT, Delong WG. Total hip arthroplasty after surgically treated acetabular fractures. Seminars in Arthroplasty 2001; 12:201–210.

64. Jimenez ML, Tile M, Schenk RS. Total hip replacement after acetabular fracture. Orthop Clin N Am 1997; 28:435–446.
65. Mears DC, Velyvis JH. Acute total hip arthroplasty for selected displaced acetabular fractures. Two to twelve year results. J Bone Joint Surg 2002; 84A:1–9.
66. Jolly MJ, Mears DC. The role of total hip arthroplasty in acetabular fracture management. Operative Tech Orthop 1993; 1:80–102.
67. Westborn A. Central dislocation of the femoral head treated with mold arthroplasty. J Bone Joint Surg 1954; 36A:307–342. .
68. Rowe CR, Lowell JD. Prognosis of fractures of the acetabulum. J Bone Joint Surg 1961; 43A:30–59.
69. Kelly PJ, Lipscomb PR. Primary vitallium mold arthroplasty for posterior dislocation of the hip with fracture of the femoral head. J Bone Joint Surg 1958; 40A:675–680. .
70. Matta JM. Fractures of the acetabulum: accuracy of reduction and clinical results in patients managed operatively within three weeks after injury. J Bone Joint Surg 1996; 78A: 1632–1645.
71. Mayo KA. Open reduction and internal fixation of fractures of the acetabulum. Results in 163 fractures. Clin Orthop 1994; 305:31–37.
72. Ragnarsson B, Mjoberg B. Arthrosis after surgically treated acetabular fractures. A retrospective study of 60 cases. Acta Orthop Scand 1992; 65:511–514.
73. Anglen JO, Burd TA, Hendricks KJ, Harrison P. The "gull" sign. A harbinger of failure for internal fixation of geriatric acetabular fractures. J Orthop Trauma 2003; 17:625–634.
74. Weavers JK, Chalmers J. Cancellous bone: it's strength and changes with aging and an evaluation of some methods for measuring it's mineral content. J Bone Joint Surg 1966; 48A:289–299.
75. Wagner HD, Wein S. On the relationship between the microstructure of bone and it's mechanical stiffness. J Biomech 1992; 25:1311–1320.
76. Mears DC, Velyvis JH, Chang C. Displaced acetabular fractures managed operatively: indicators of outcome. CORR 2003; 407:173–186.
77. Routt MLC Jr, Simonian PT, Grujic L. The retrograde medullary superior ramus screw for the treatment of anterior pelvic ring disruptions: a new technique. J Orthop Trauma 1995; 9:355–44.
78. Starr AJ, Jones AL, Reinert CM, Borer DS. Preliminary results and complications following limited open reduction and percutaneous screw fixation of displaced fractures of the acetabulum. Injury 2001; 32(suppl 1):A45–50.
79. Starr AJ, Reinert CM, Jones AL. Percutaneous fixation of the columns of the acetabulum: A new technique. J Orthop Trauma 1998; 12:51–58.
80. Routt MLC Jr, Barei DP, Schildhauer T. Percutaneous fixation of pelvic and acetabular injuries. Seminars in Arthroplasty 2001; 12:173–184.
81. Crowl AC, Kaher DM. Closed reduction and percutaneous fixation of anterior column acetabular fractures. Comput Aided Surg 2002; 7:169–178.
82. Jacob AL, Suhm N, Kaim A, Regazzoni P, Steinbrich W, Messiner P. Coronal acetabular fractures: the anterior approach in computed tomography-navigated minimally invasive percutaneous fixation. Cardiovasc Intervent Radiol 2000; Oct (5):327–331.
83. Parker PJ, Copeland C. Percutaneous fluoroscopic screw fixation of acetabular fractures. Injury 1997; 28:597–600.
84. Garino J, Whitfield B. Complex acetabular reconstruction in total hip arthroplasty following acetabular fractures. Seminars on Arthroplasty 2001; 12:191–200.
85. Stauffer RN. Ten year follow-up study of total hip replacement. J Bone Joint Surg 1982; 64A:983–990.
86. Mears DC. Avascular necrosis of the acetabulum. Oper Tech Orthop 1997; 7:241–249.

87. Herberts P, Malchow H. How outcome studies have changed total hip arthhroplasty practices in Sweden. Clin Orthop 1997; 344:44–60.
88. Padgett DE, Kull LR, Rosenberg A, Summer DR, Galante JD. Revision of the acetabular component without cement after total hip arthroplasty. Three to six year follow-up. J Bone Joint Surg 1993; 75A:663–673.
89. Mears DC, Ward AJ. Late Results of Total hip Arthroplasty to Manage Post-traumatic Arthritis of Acetabular Fractures. Fractures of the Pelvis and Acetabulum. Pittsburgh, PA: The Third International Consensus, 1996.
90. Kaplan EL, Meier P. Nonparametric estimation from incomplete observations. J Am Statist Assn 1958; 53:457–481.
91. Karpos PAG, Christie MJ. THR following acetabular fracture using cementless acetabular components: 4 to 8 year results. Presented at the Annual Meeting if the American Association of Hip and Knee Surgeons, Dallas, TX, October 1995.
92. Carnesale PG, Stewart MJ, Barnes SN. Acetabular disruption and central fracture-dislocation of the hip. A long term study. J Bone Joint Surg 1975; 57A: 1054–1059.
93. Nivbrantt B, Kärrholm, Önsten I, Carlsson Å, Snorrason F. Migration of porous press fit cups in hip revision arthroplasty. A stereoradiographic 2-year follow-up of 50 hips. J Arthroplasty 1996; 11:390–396.
94. Önsten I, Åkesson K, Besjakov J, Obraut KJ. Migration of the Charnley stem in rheumatoid arthritis and osteoarthritis. A roentgen stereophotogrammetric study. J Bone Joint Surg 1995; 77B: 18–22.
95. Malkin C, Tauber C. Total hip arthroplasty and acetabular bone grafting for unreduced fracture-dislocation of the hip. Clin Orthop 1985; 201:57–59.
96. Mears DC, Shirahama M. Stabilization of an acetabulum fracture with cables for acute total hip aarthroplasty. J Arthrop 1998; 13:104–107.

14

Surgical Treatment of Acetabular Fractures: Delayed Open Reduction and Revision Open Reduction

Steven A. Olson
Division of Orthopaedic Surgery, Duke University Medical Center, Durham, North Carolina, U.S.A.

INTRODUCTION

Surgical treatment of acetabular fractures is a complex undertaking in the acute setting. The complexity is increased with previous open reduction and internal fixation and/or delays in treatment. The decision to undertake late open reduction internal fixation (ORIF) or revision acetabular surgery must be individualized and based on multiple variables, including pattern of deformity, patient age, symptoms, and surgeon experience.

INDICATIONS FOR REVISION OR DELAYED OPEN REDUCTION AND INTERNAL FIXATION

The indications for open reduction and internal fixation on a delayed basis are similar to the indications for acute injuries (1–3). The indications for revision of open reduction and internal fixation include the criteria regarding articular displacement, as well as consideration of the condition of the soft tissues, and location of internal fixation implants (2–4).

Strong indications for open reduction internal fixation in these situations are the following:

1. Articular displacement >5 mm of fractures or malreductions involving the superior acetabulum [within the superior 10 mm of the computed tomography (CT) arc] (5).
2. Loss of congruence (subluxation) of the femoral head with the acetabulum on any of the other three plain radiographic views.
3. Posterior wall fracture associated with hip instability.
4. Incarcerated osteochondral fragment with a nonconcentric reduction of the femoral head.
5. Intra-articular placement of hardware (screws) that can potentially lead to damage of the articular surfaces of either the acetabulum, femoral head, or both.

These indications must take into consideration the experience of the surgeon, the complexity of the injury (fracture pattern and comminution), the condition of the femoral head, and the general status of the patient (1–3). The surgeon contemplating revision open reduction internal fixation of an acetabular fracture or surgical reduction and fixation of an acetabular fracture on a delayed basis (>21 days from injury) should have extensive experience with the acute operative management of acetabular fractures. Just as with an acute acetabular injury, the exact fracture pattern and degree of displacement should be understood preoperatively. The soft tissue envelope about the pelvis should be stable without sign of vascular compromise or infection. The ideal candidate for revision or delayed reduction and fixation has a fracture pattern in which there are large pieces of the articular surface to work with. There should be no obvious bony wear of the femoral head. Occasionally there can be a significant articular surface injury without underlying bony wear that can compromise the long-term outcome. There should be no evidence of avascular necrosis of the femoral head.

Occasionally the implants used for the original fixation may have been placed through an incision that is not optimal for performing the revision open reduction internal fixation. It is often necessary to reuse the original incision in order to be able to remove the initial fixation. Occasionally, however, an alternative incision is indicated. For example, implants placed initially through a Kocher–Langenbeck can often be removed through an extensile lateral approach at time of revision, reduction, and fixation.

CHOICE OF SURGICAL APPROACH FOR DELAYED AND REVISION OPEN REDUCTION

For fracture types isolated to one column, use the appropriate nonextensile approach (1–3). The Kocher–Langenbeck approach is typically used for the isolated posterior wall fracture, isolated posterior column fracture, or the combined posterior column plus posterior wall fracture. The ilioinguinal approach is typically used for revision of the anterior column fracture, the anterior wall fracture, as well as revision of the anterior column and posterior hemitransverse fractures where there is a nondisplaced posterior hemitransverse fracture line.

The associated patterns can occasionally be operated through a nonextensile approach, depending on the delay between initial fixation and revision. Typically, fractures such as a both-column that could be operated through an ilioinguinal primarily, or a transverse plus posterior wall that could be operated through a Kocher–Langenbeck primarily, may be revised through the same single nonextensile approach if operated before substantial soft tissue and bony healing have occurred, typically before 21 days after injury (1–4).

Fractures that involve both the anterior and posterior columns (transverse, T-shaped, transverse plus posterior wall, both-column, and anterior column plus posterior hemitransverse) that are treated either primarily or with revision on a delayed basis >21 days, typically require an extensile lateral surgical approach (1). The extended iliofemoral approach is the author's preference. However, the triradiate approach and the modified extensile T-shaped approach have also been described (4,6). The extensile lateral approach provides the surgeon with the most complete access to the entire articular problem through a single field of view. The extensile iliofemoral approach has been used successfully following the initial use of a Kocher–Langenbeck approach (1,2).

Occasionally, certain fracture types can be operated through a combined Kocher–Langenbeck and ilioinguinal approach. These approaches are typically performed sequentially. Potential indications for sequential approaches would include an anterior column with a posterior hemitransverse fracture type, in which there is significant displacement of both anterior column and posterior column components (2). Also, an infratectal T-shaped fracture with significant components of both the anterior–posterior column may be considered for sequential approaches. Occasionally, it may be necessary to remove hardware or free up the fracture lines via one approach in order to allow reduction and fixation through the other approach.

OPERATIVE TECHNIQUES FOR DELAYED OR REVISION OPEN REDUCTION AND INTERNAL FIXATION

Every effort should be made to preserve soft tissue attachments to all fracture fragments. This includes maintaining capsular attachments to anterior and posterior wall fragments and avoiding complete devascularization of the iliac wing segment during dissection. The initial implants used for fixation should be removed completely, if possible. However, occasionally retaining a small screw or other implant that does not affect the articular reduction is acceptable (2,3).

If the fracture lines are apparent and substantial callus formation has not occurred, the techniques of reduction and fixation are often similar to surgery performed before 21 days from injury. Each fracture fragment requires that the fibrous tissue be debrided, as needed, to allow an anatomic reduction to be performed (2,3). Capsulotomy is often helpful to adequate visualization of the articular surfaces. The fragment surfaces are often irregular and can be more difficult to reduce anatomically.

Multiple attempts at reducing the articular surface may be necessary to achieve the optimal result (1–3). Patience on the part of the operating surgeon is an asset in these situations.

Nonunions of the major fracture lines is not uncommon with or without fixation in displaced acetabular fractures (1–3). The relative thinness of the innominate bone and the quadrilateral surface can result in little bony apposition with moderate fracture displacement, resulting in a nonunion or incomplete union. Thus, the fracture line may be partially healed in a malposition, requiring osteotomy in one column but not the other. The fracture lines may be filled with a fibrous tissue that requires a debridement back to the bleeding bony surface and articular margins (1–3).

The fracture lines may be filled with a combination of both fibrous tissue and heterotopic bone and callus, or callus alone (2,3). Typically, heterotopic bone has a slightly different consistency of the underlying normal bony tissue in the early phases of fracture healing (1,7). However, in the latter phase of fracture remodeling, it is often difficult to determine where the original cortical and articular margins stop and the healing callus begins. When dealing with posterior wall fragments, it is essential that some soft tissue attachment to the capsule be maintained as the fragment is freed from the callus and fibrous tissue. In very late cases, the fracture line can be completely obscured by bony remodeling (1–3). Great care must be used during osteotomy through these fracture lines.

Late revision or loss of reduction may require an intra-articular osteotomy. This should be done with the osteotome directed from the articular surface through the remaining innominate bone. This typically requires an extensile surgical approach to gain adequate access to the articular surface to perform the osteotomy without damaging the femoral head (1–3).

Old deformity of the pelvic ring may contribute to the ability to accurately reduce the acetabulum (1,4,8). This factor should be carefully considered in the preoperative plan. The injury may require reduction of the pelvic ring or osteotomy of the contralateral pubic rami to allow accurate correction of the acetabular component.

RESULTS OF FRACTURES OPERATED MORE THAN 21 DAYS AFTER INJURY

The data indicate acute treatment of acetabular fractures within 21 days of injury may achieve up to 80% good to excellent results. However, delayed reconstruction of acetabular fractures remains a controversial subject. There is, to date, little published data reported for reconstruction of acetabular fractures on a delayed basis. Letournel and Judet divided surgical repair into three time periods: (*i*) injury to 21 days, (*ii*) 21 to 120 days, and (*iii*) beyond 120 days (9). Problems encountered after 21 days postinjury include changes in the soft tissue envelope, increased scar formation, resorption of fracture lines, and early callus, which ultimately hamper delayed reconstructive efforts.

Johnson et al. examined a cohort of 207 acetabular fractures, with follow-up available for 188 repaired on a delayed basis (between 21 and 120 days postinjury) (3). This series included the results of Letournel. The Kocher–Langenbeck approach was used in 105 fractures, the extended iliofemoral in 57 fractures, and the ilioinguinal in 26 fractures (Fig. 1A–I). Five fractures required both Kocher–Langenbeck and

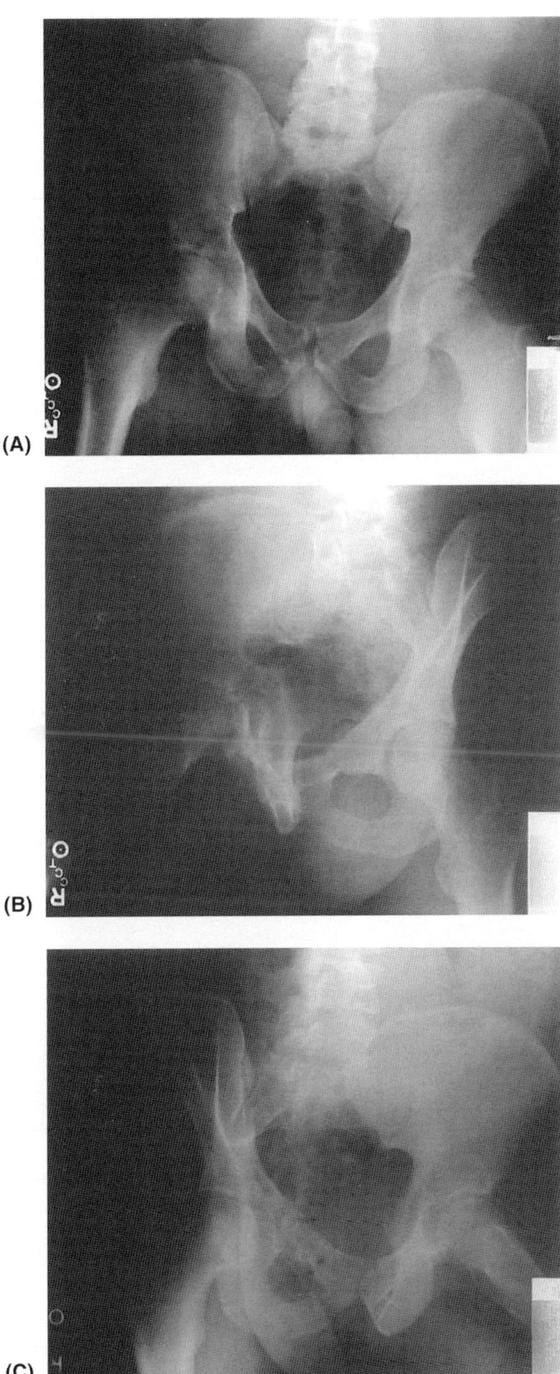

Figure 1A–H This is a case example of delayed open reduction internal fixation. (Case contributed by Phil Kregor, MD.) (**A**) Anteroposterior (AP) pelvis demonstrating initial injury view. (**B**) Iliac oblique view with displacement of posterior column acetabular fracture shown. (**C**) Illustrates obturator oblique view of posterior column acetabular fracture (*Continued*).

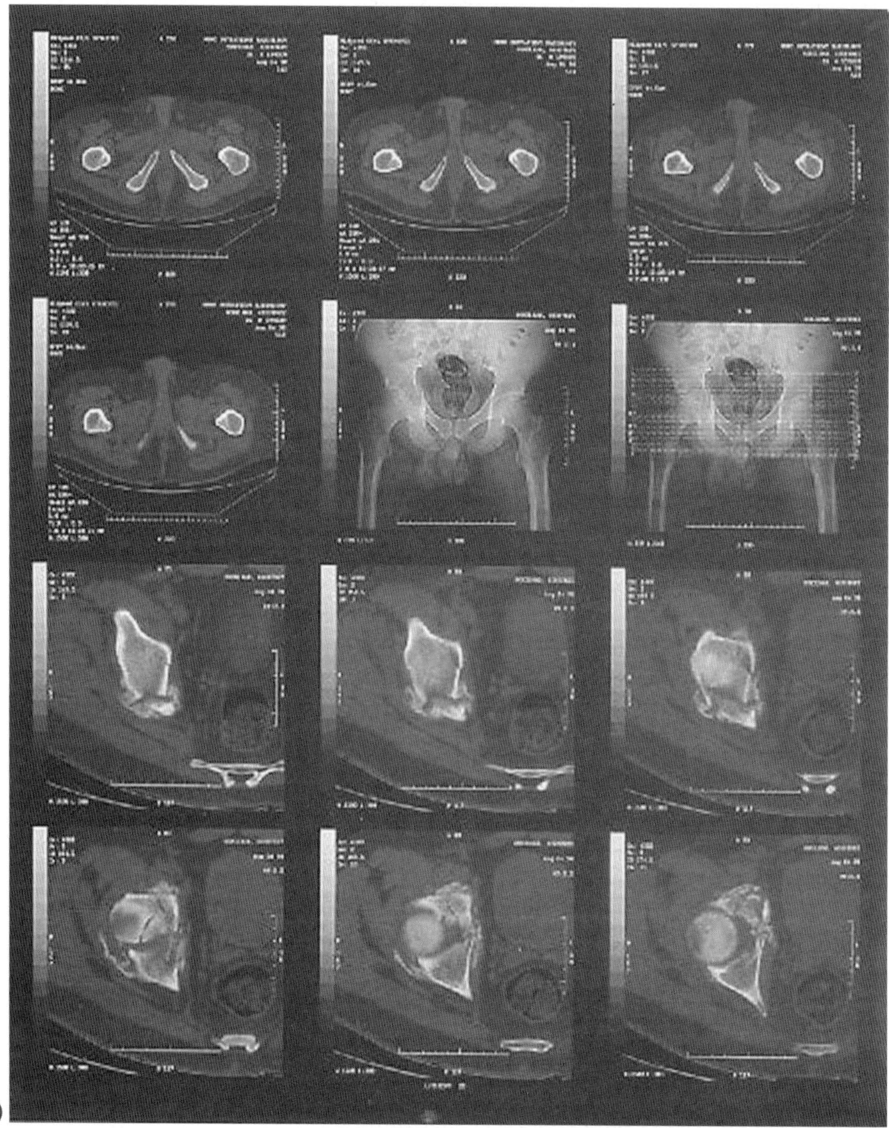

(D)

Figure 1A–H (*Continued*) (**D**) Illustrates preoperative computed tomography of displaced posterior column fracture (*Continued*).

ilioinguinal approaches. The average operation time was four hours, which ranged from two to nine hours. Overall they reported an overall good/excellent result in 65% of patients, fair result in 9%, and a poor result in 26%. Simple column fractures had the best overall results with good/excellent results in 89% and 100% of posterior and anterior column fractures, respectively. Isolated wall fractures fared less well with good/excellent results in about 60% for both. The isolated posterior wall fracture, the associated transverse plus posterior wall fracture, and T-type fractures did the worst overall with good/excellent results in 51%, 59%, and 61%, respectively (3).

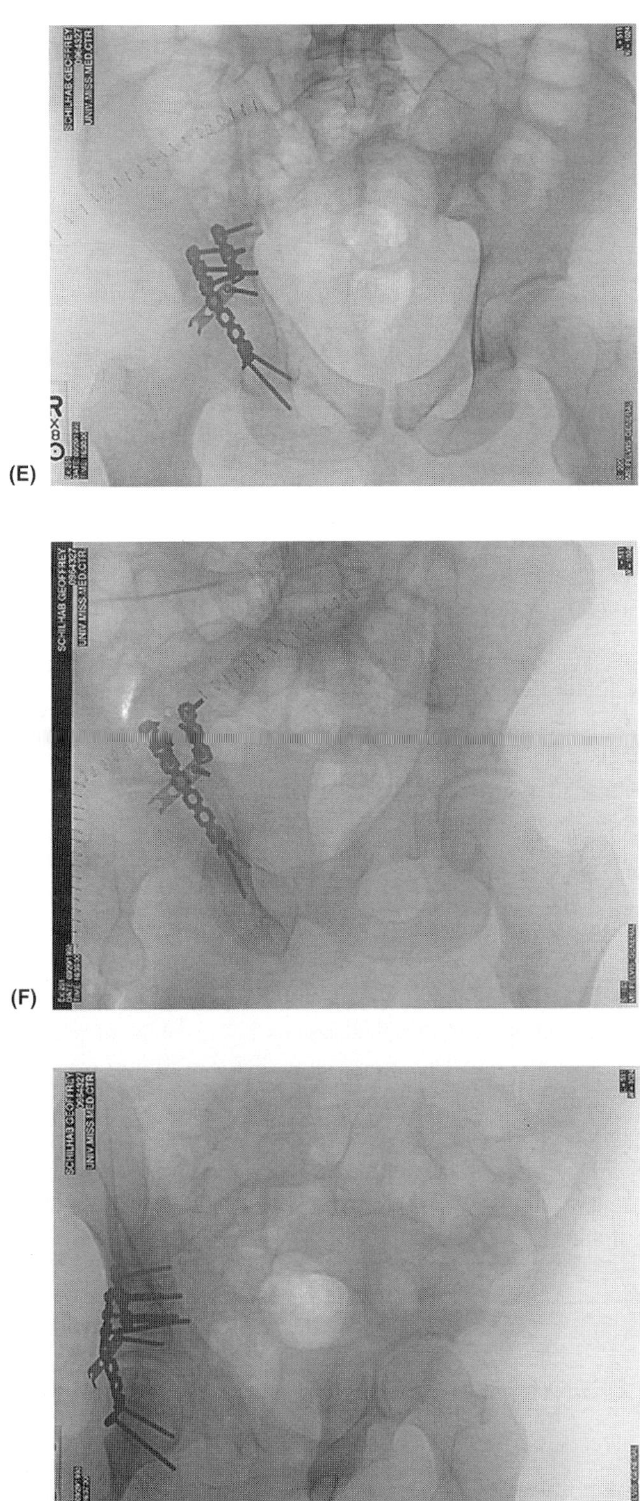

Figure 1A–H (*Continued*) (**E–G**) Illustrate the initial postoperative AP, iliac oblique, obturator oblique radiographs (*Continued*).

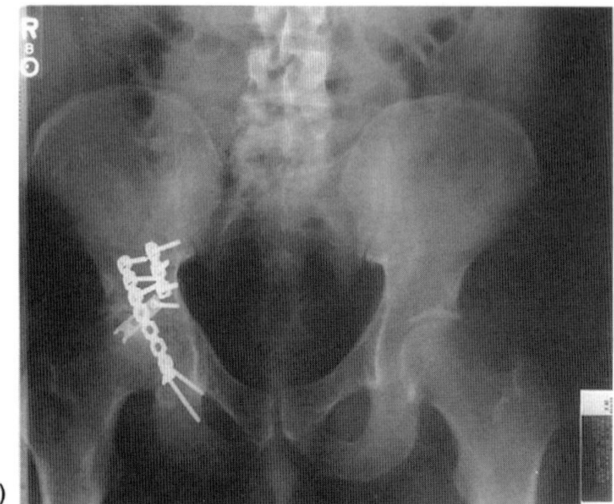

Figure 1A–H (*Continued*) (**H**) Follow-up radiograph taken at eight months postinjury. Note that despite revision fixation and anatomic reduction, there is early loss of joint space heralding post traumatic arthritis. Yet with a better base or foundation of bone, hip arthroplasty is still possible and has a better chance of success.

RESULTS OF REVISION ORIF OF ACETABULAR FRACTURES

Surgical revision of malreduced acetabular fractures is an area with little data focusing on outcomes. Mayo et al. published a series of 64 patients treated within 12 weeks of the index procedure for either surgical malreduction or loss of reduction (2). The authors used the Kocher–Langenbeck for revision of 30 fractures, an extensile lateral approach for 22 fractures (extended iliofemoral 15, triradiate 7), the ilioinguinal approach for eight fractures, and both Kocher–Langenbeck and ilioinguinal for four fractures. Articular reduction following revision was able to be restored to <2 mm displacement in only 56% of patients, 3 to 5 mm in 38%, and >5 mm in 6% of patients (Fig. 2). Overall results demonstrated good to excellent results in only 42% of patients overall at an average of four-year follow-up. The strongest predictor of failure was time from original repair to revision surgery. There were 13 of 23 patients (56%) with good/excellent results when surgery was performed within three weeks of the index procedure; 10 of 27 patients (37%) had a good/excellent result when revised between 3 and 12 weeks after initial repair; and the results worsened to 4 of 14 patients (29%) if revision was delayed for more than 12 weeks (Fig. 3). There were no significant differences between fracture patterns in this small group (2).

COMPLICATIONS WITH DELAYED OR REVISION SURGICAL TREATMENT

The most common serious complications following operative treatment of an acetabulum fracture include operative wound infection, iatrogenic nerve palsy, periarticular ectopic bone formation, and thromboembolic complications. Post trauma arthritis is the most common sequelae that can occur (Fig. 4) (1–3).

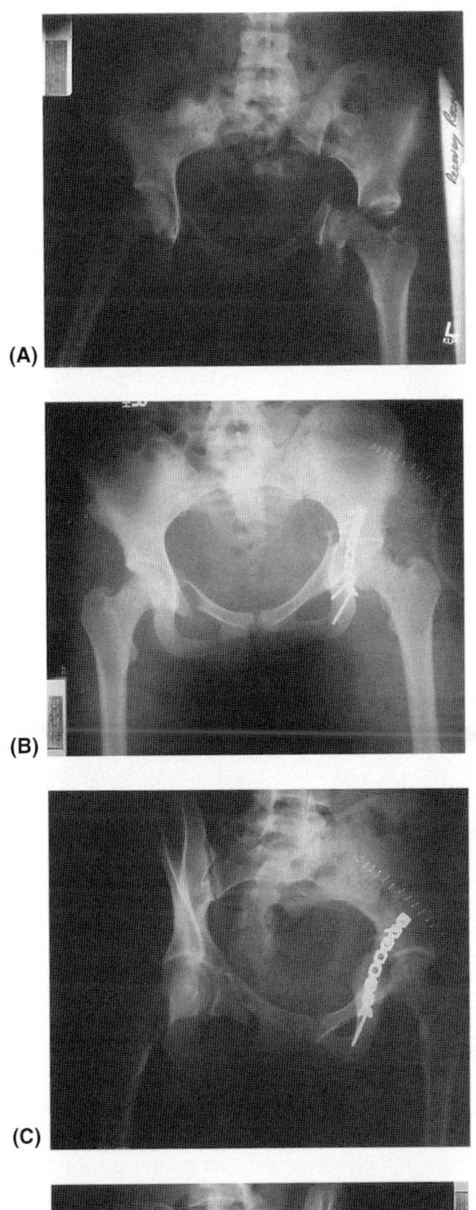

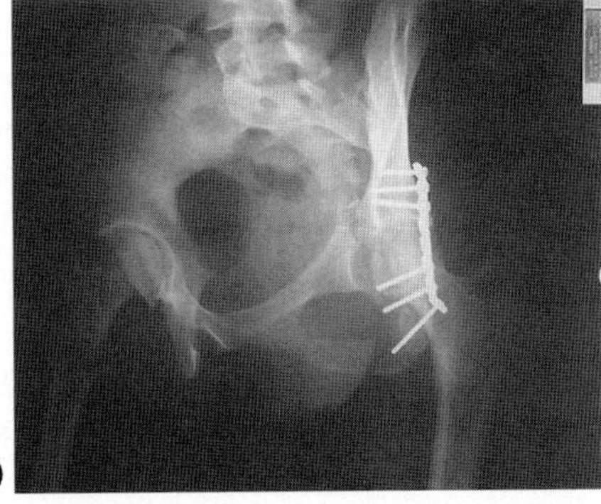

Figure 2A–H Revision reconstruction of acetabular fracture. (Case contributed by Phil Kregor, MD.) (**A**) A displaced transverse plus posterior wall acetabular fracture with associated ipsilateral sacroiliac joint injury. (**B–D**) Postoperative anteroposterior (AP), iliac oblique, obturator oblique radiographs of the acetabular fracture operated through a Kocher-Langenbach approach (*Continued*).

(E)
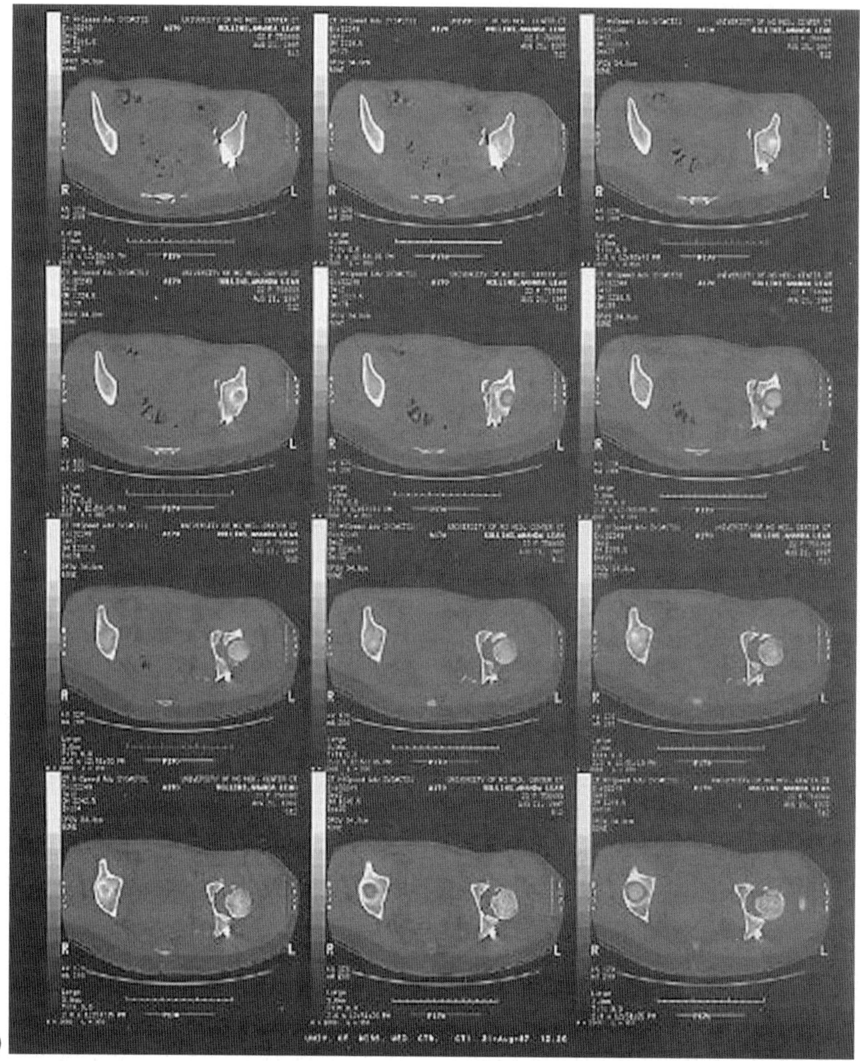

Figure 2A–H (*Continued*) (**E**) Postoperative computed tomography with illustration of malreduction (*Continued*).

If the patient's general condition is good, and no associated injuries are present, the risk of infection should not be higher than for other types of hip surgery. Unfortunately, most patients with acetabulum fractures have associated injuries. These can include injuries of the abdominal or pelvic viscera or of the extremities. A bladder rupture or a bowel, rectal, or vaginal injury can increase the chance of operative wound infection and can influence the indications for operation (2,3). Open fractures of the ipsilateral lower extremity can also increase the risks for wound infection in the acetabulum fracture. Revision open reduction should not be performed until the original surgical wound is dry and free of signs of infection (4).

Wound infection does remain a danger, however, even without associated injuries. Infection occurred in 8 of 207 delayed acetabular repairs and 3 of 64 revision fixations

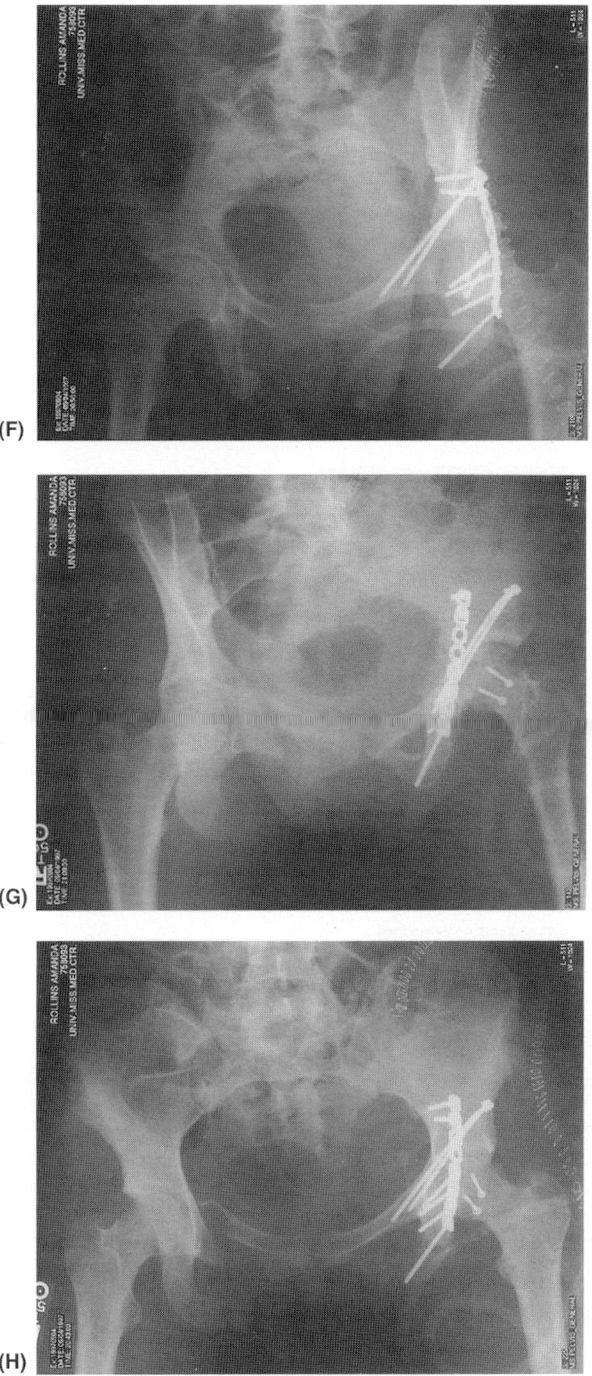

Figure 2A–H (*Continued*) (**F**) The patient underwent revision open reduction internal fixation through an extended iliofemoral approach at 24 days post the original surgery. The obturator oblique radiograph is shown in this view. (**G**) Iliac oblique view film. (**H**) AP radiograph status postrevision open reduction.

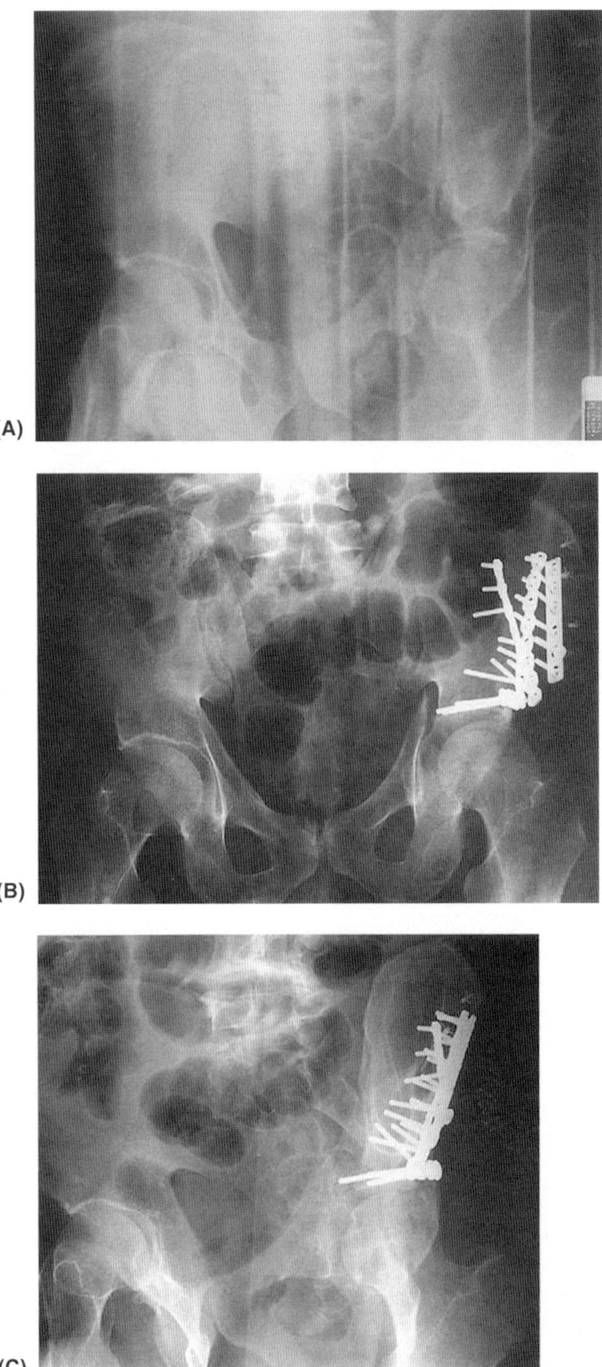

Figure 3A–F Case of a revision open reduction internal fixation of an acetabular fracture. (**A**) Initial anterioposterior (AP) radiograph demonstrating displaced both column acetabular fractures. (**B**) Postoperative fixation. The patient was operated through a Smith-Petersen approach with detachment of all of his abductors from the iliac wing. (**C**) Iliac oblique view of initial fixation demonstrating residual articular displacement (*Continued*).

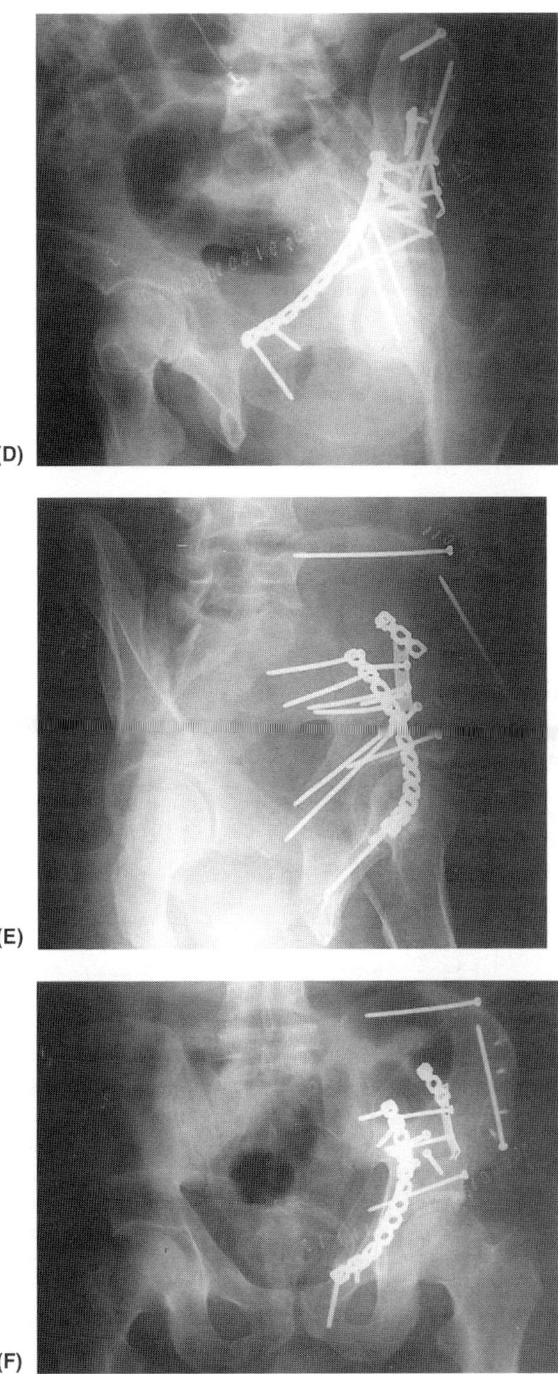

Figure 3A–F (*Continued*) (**D** and **E**) AP, obturator oblique, and iliac oblique views following revision open reduction internal fixation through ilioinguinal approach. This revision open reduction was performed at two weeks following the original surgical intervention. (**F**) Follow-up AP radiograph at eight months post-revision surgery. The patient fortunately had regained near normal abductor function postoperatively.

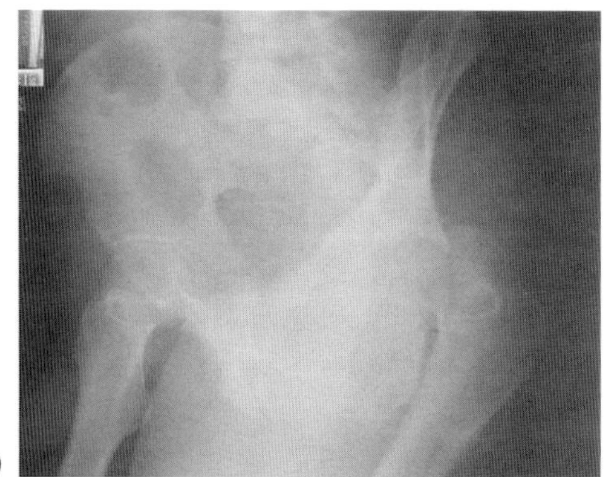

(A)

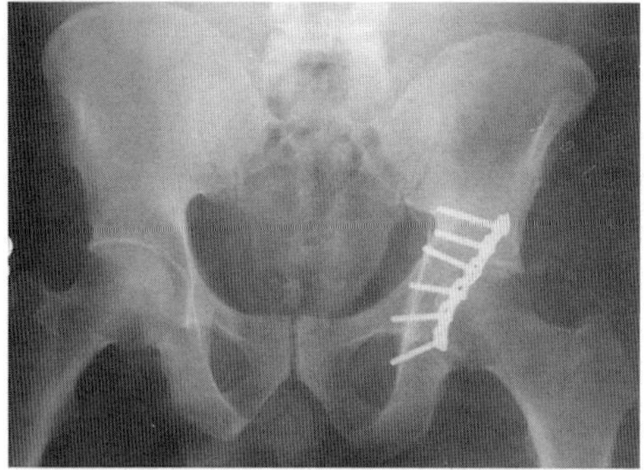

(B)

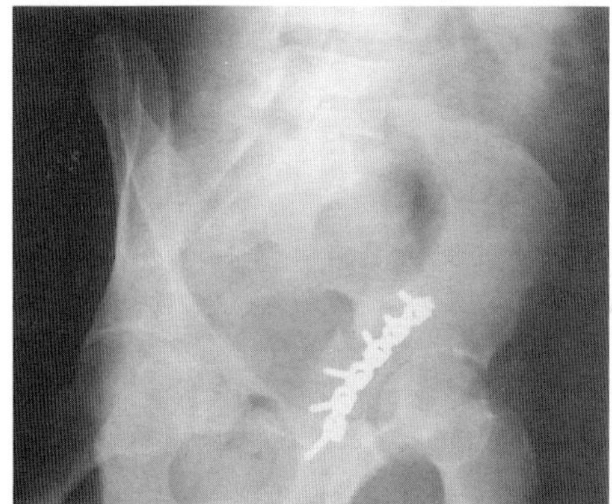

(C)

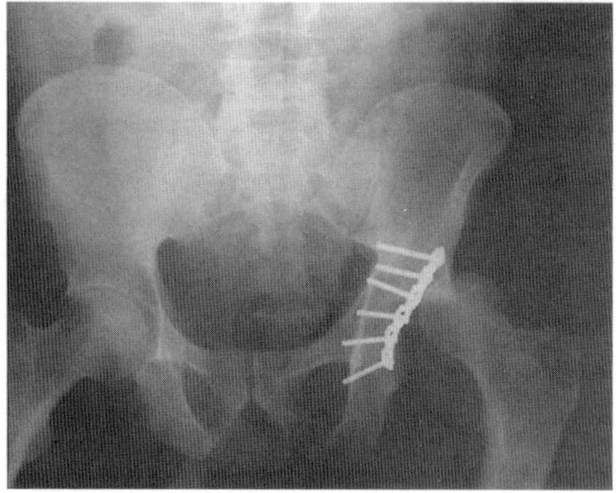

(D)

Figure 4A–H A failed posterior wall reconstruction. (**A**) Obturator oblique radiograph of initial injury at presentation. The patient has a transverse plus posterior wall acetabular fracture with the major displacement in the transverse component in the posterior column. Instability of the hip is noted in these radiographs. (**B**) Demonstrates anterio-posterior (AP) radiograph following open reduction internal fixation. Careful examination of the radiograph illustrates that a substantial portion of the posterior wall is missing following open reduction internal fixation. This portion of the ilioischial line is also displaced. (**C**) Illustrates an iliac oblique view following initial open reduction internal fixation. The posterior column is seen to be malreduced on this view. (**D**) Demonstrates instability of the hip with frank dislocation following open reduction internal fixation (*Continued*).

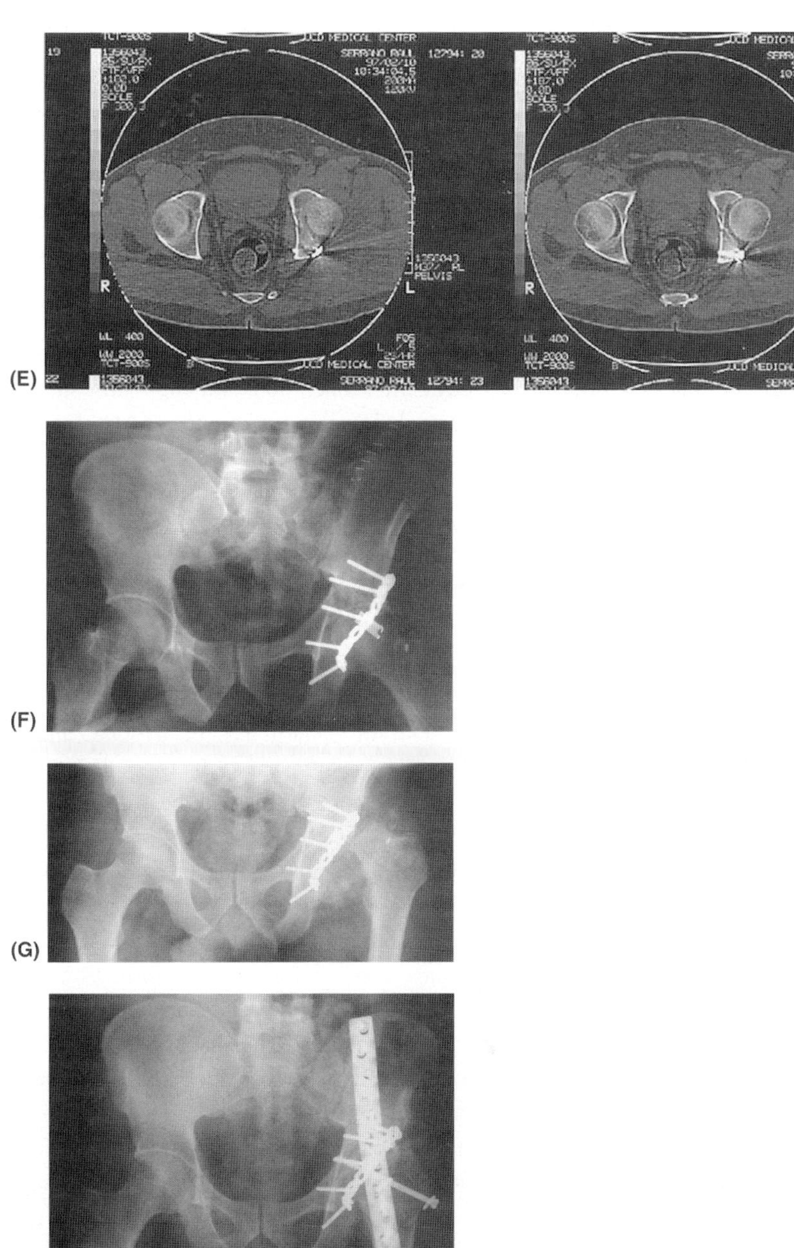

Figure 4A–H (*Continued*) (**E**) Postoperative computed tomography scan illustrating that the majority of the posterior wall is missing, having been excised in the original open reduction internal fixation. (**F**) Attempt at reconstruction with an iliac crest bone graft is performed. (**G**) Demonstrates subsequent failure with erosion of the femoral head secondary to intra-articular wear and displacement of the femoral shaft. (**H**) Reveals salvage of this case with a hip arthrodesis. With improvements in modern arthroplasty implants and results, hip fusion may be well accepted by patients and should be considered as a viable alternative.

(2,3). There is an increased risk of postoperative hematoma formation in the large wounds that are necessary for acetabulum surgery. Liberal use of suction drains should be employed (1). Hemostasis at the time of wound closure is always desirable. During the procedure, the large areas of exposed soft tissue should be kept moist and irrigated frequently with solution. It is often helpful to place moist sponges over exposed soft tissue to prevent desiccation. The surgeon should always strive to preserve soft tissue pedicles to all bone fragments to maintain vascularity of the bone (1–3). If a fragment is devascularized, it generally revascularizes rapidly as long as no infection develops. In the presence of infection, however, bacteria rapidly colonize an avascular fragment and it will usually need to be debrided and excised. Some bloody drainage can seep from the wound for the first one or two days after operation, although this should subside rapidly. It is not uncommon for a clear, yellow, serous drainage to be present for as long as 10 days after surgery without infection being present. If the wound has been benign for a number of days, however, and bloody or cloudy yellowish drainage then occurs, the patient should be returned to the operating room immediately for irrigation and debridement of the wound. If a wound hematoma is present, the amount of hematoma is usually much greater than initially suspected by inspecting the wound, and surgical drainage is indicated (1).

If infection is suspected, the surgeon should not wait for definitive results of wound culture but should proceed with reopening the wound on the clinical basis alone (1,10). If it is later found that no infection was present, little harm has been done, and a possible infection has been prevented. If an infection was present at the time of the earliest clinical suspicion, then the surgeon has acted properly by treating the infection expeditiously (10).

After evacuation of a wound hematoma, the wound is usually closed over suction drainage. In the case of debridement for infection, all implants that are stable and aid in the fixation are left in place. Avascular and infected bone fragments must be removed. If the diagnosis of infection is made early, before abscess formation, the wound can be closed over suction drainage tubes and appropriate antibiotic therapy instituted. Also, use of resorbable calcium sulfate mixtures that can be mixed with antibiotics and shaped into beads using molds can be used as local depots. These agents are useful when implants are left behind in an infected tissue bed and do not require removal as do traditional bone cement antibiotic depot methods. If the infection is extra-articular, it can probably be controlled successfully and the functional result will not be impaired. In the case of an intra-articular infection, however, the cartilage of the joint is almost invariably destroyed and hip function is significantly impaired (1–3,9).

Iatrogenic nerve palsy is caused almost exclusively by vigorous or prolonged retraction of the sciatic nerve. Sciatic nerve palsy occurred in 25 of 207 delayed fixations of acetabular fractures and 2 of 64 revision fixations, substantially more than in acute injuries (1–3). This occurs primarily with the Kocher–Langenbeck approach, and mainly involves the peroneal branch of the sciatic nerve. There is also a small chance of a stretch injury to the sciatic nerve with the extended iliofemoral approach, and a slight possibility of injuring the femoral nerve by stretch injury during the ilioinguinal approach, but this is unusual (1–3).

The surgeon must constantly monitor the force and duration of pull that the surgical assistants place on the sciatic nerve. It is helpful to keep the patient's knee flexed at least 60°, and the hip extended whenever the Kocher–Langenbeck or extended iliofemoral approach is used (1). Neurologic monitoring with somatosensory evoked potentials and/or electromyography has been reported by several authors (11,12). This technique is not available in every center. If a nerve palsy develops, it is best treated with an ankle-foot orthosis. There is some chance for recovery of the sciatic nerve for up to three years following injury. Iatrogenic nerve palsies are often a form of axonotmesis. The superior gluteal nerve can also be injured at the time of injury or at the time of surgical repair. Electromyography can be helpful in determining reinnervation of affected muscle groups. Tendon transfer procedures to correct a footdrop should not be performed during the initial three years.

Ectopic bone formation occurs almost exclusively with the lateral exposure of the innominate bone (1–3,7). The incidence of significant ectopic bone formation is highest with the extended iliofemoral approach, followed by the Kocher–Langenbeck approach; it is almost nonexistent with the ilioinguinal approach (1). Three of 207 fractures developed Brooker grade III or IV ectopic bone following delayed fixation of acetabular fractures [all occurred with the extended iliofemoral approach (EIF) approach] (3). Three of 64 fractures developed Brooker grade III or IV ectopic bone following revision fixation (2). Part of the prevention of ectopic bone formation should be directed toward choosing the ilioinguinal approach, whenever possible, and limiting muscle trauma during surgery by careful soft tissue handling. Indomethacin given in a dose of 25 mg tid perioperatively, and for several months following surgery, has been reported to be helpful in decreasing the incidence and extent of ectopic bone formation (13). A single dose of low dose (e.g., 500 Gray) radiation therapy is also very effective for prevention of hetertopic bone and may avoid the gastrointestinal side effects of indomethacin. The combination of indomethacin and postoperative radiation has been reported to be very effective at preventing nearly all heterotopic ossification (13). The surgical field should be debrided, devitalized tissue following completion of internal fixation of the acetabular fracture. Ectopic bone formation is influenced by the surgical approach, and probably also by the initial muscle trauma suffered by the patient. The combination of the two creates an inflammatory response that triggers the formation of bone.

Avascular necrosis of the femoral head occurred in 26 of 188 fractures with delayed reduction and fixation (3). Significant vascular injury occurred in 2 of 64 patients with revision fixation, both through the ilioinguinal approach (2).

There is significant potential for deep venous thrombosis and pulmonary embolism with fractures of the acetabulum (1,10). A 33% incidence of preoperative proximal deep venous thrombosis (DVT) detected with magnetic resonance imaging (MRI) venography has been reported (14). We normally use pneumatic compression boots on both lower extremities from the time of admission until the patient is fully ambulatory. In older patients and high-risk patients, partial anticoagulation is begun with heparin postoperatively (15). The patient is discharged to home with warfarin anticoagulation until they are ambulating actively, typically for three to four weeks following surgery (15). The level of anticoagulation with warfarin is maintained at about 1.5 times the normal international normalized ratio (INR) of 2 to 3. As warfarin management may be difficult and require frequent hematologic monitoring, as well as potentially complicating any emergent surgical procedure, the recent utilization of low molecular weight heparins has mostly supplanted oral coumadin use. The injections are well tolerated and side effects are minimal. Furthermore, if emergent procedures are required, their short half life avoids the issues found with warfarin. The duration of anticoagulation is not well elucidated but most commonly done for somewhere between 4 to 12 weeks and highly dependent on regional and individual preference. Although the potential for thromboembolic complications is always present, the surgeon must be cautious about too much anticoagulation because a large wound hematoma can have a devastating effect on the patient if a deep infection to the hip results.

ACKNOWLEDGMENT

The author thanks Phil Kregor, MD, for case contribution and editorial assistance.

REFERENCES

1. Letournel E, ed. Fractures of the Acetabulum, 2nd ed. New York: Springer-Verlag, 1993.
2. Mayo, KA, Letournel E, Matta JM, Mast JW, Johnson EE, Martimbeau CL. Surgical revision of malreduced acetabular fractures. Clin Orthop 1994; 305:47–52.
3. Johnson EE, Matta JM, Mast JW, Letournel E. Delayed reconstruction of acetabular fractures 21–120 days following injury. Clin Orthop 1994; 305:20–31.
4. Mears DC, Rubash H. Pelvic and Acetabular Fractures. Thorofare, New Jersey: Slack, February 1986.
5. Olson SA, Matta JM. The CT subchondral arc: a preliminary report of a new method to assess acetabular articular continuity following fracture. J Orthop Trauma 1993; 7(5): 402–413.
6. Fassler PR, Swiontkowski MF, Kilroy AW, Routt MR Jr. Injury of the sciatic nerve associated with acetabular fracture. J Bone Joint Surg 1993; 75A:1157–1166.
7. Ghalambor N, Matta JM, Bernstein L. Heterotopic ossification following operative treatment of acetabular fracture: an analysis of risk factors. Clin Orthop 1994; 305:96–106.
8. Tile M (ed.), Olson SA. Management of Acetabular Fractures. In: Fractures of the Pelvis, 3rd ed. Lippincott-Raven Publishers, 2003.
9. Matta JM. Fractures of the acetabulum: reduction accuracy and clinical results of fractures operated within three weeks of injury. J Bone Joint Surg 1996; 78A:1632–1645.
10. Olson SA, Matta JM. Surgical treatment of acetabular fractures. Skeletal Trauma, 2nd ed. Philadelphia: W.B. Saunders, 1997.
11. Helfet DL, Schmeling GJ. Somatosensory evoked potential monitoring in the surgical treatment of acute, displaced acetabular fractures. Results of a prospective study. Clin Orthop 1994; 301:213–220.
12. Vrahas M, Gordon RG, Mears DC, Krieger D, Sclabassi RJ. Intraoperative somatosensory evoked potential monitoring of pelvic and acetabular fractures. J Orthop Trauma 1992; 6:50–58.
13. Moed BR, Letournel E. Low-dose irradiation and indomethacin prevent heterotopic ossification after acetabular fracture surgery. J Bone Joint Surg 1994; 76B:895–900.

14. Montgomery KD, Potter HG, Helfet DL. Magnetic resonance venography to evaluate the deep venous system of the pelvis in patients who have an acetabular fracture. J Bone Joint Surg 1995; 77A:1639–1649.
15. Fishmann AJ, Greeno RA, Brooks LR, Matta JM. Prevention of deep vein thrombosis and pulmonary embolism in acetabular and pelvic fracture surgery. Clin Orthop 1994; 305: 133–138.

15
Management of Perioperative Complications

Kyle J. Jeray
Department of Orthopaedic Surgery, Greenville Hospital System, Greenville, South Carolina, U.S.A.

Enes M. Kanlic, Miguel Pirela-Cruz, and Hector O. Pacheco
Department of Orthopaedic Surgery and Rehabilitation, Texas Tech University Health Sciences Center, El Paso, Texas, U.S.A.

POSTOPERATIVE MANAGEMENT OF PELVIC AND ACETABULAR FRACTURES

Complications are part of fracture care. The complications may differ as to whether or not surgical treatment is involved. Complications may be early or late, iatrogenic or related directly to the injury, and may vary depending on age and sex. Regardless, our goal as physicians is to recognize, prevent, and at times treat the complications of pelvic and acetabular surgery. This chapter covers most of the complications related to the treatment of pelvic and acetabular fractures.

Thromboembolism

The exact incidence of DVT and pulmonary embolism (PE) associated with fractures of the pelvis and acetabulum is unknown. The incidence varies from 5% to as high as 61% (2–10). Equally as variable is the use of screening methods and prophylaxis in patients with these injuries. Letournel, in his series of 569 acetabular fractures treated operatively within 21 days of injury, had a 6% incidence of DVT or PE (2). Seven incidents occurred prior to any prophylaxis; however, 22 occurred after using routine prophylaxis. When no prophylaxis is used in trauma patients, a documented 58% incidence of DVT was detected by impedance plethysmography and venography in a prospective study (6). Further, a documented 61% incidence of DVT was identified following patients with pelvic fractures in the same population who had received no prophylaxis (6). Surprisingly, only 1.5% of the patients in this study with DVT had clinical characteristics suggestive of thrombosis prior to the diagnosis on venography (6). In patients using some form of prophylaxis for DVT, the incidence is reported as low as 2% to as high as 33% (11,12). The goal of DVT prophylaxis is to prevent long-term morbidity associated with DVT and ultimately the potential mortality associated with PE. By prevention of DVT, the hope is to decrease the incidence of PE. DVT of the lower extremities is believed to be the source of emboli in 75% to 95% of the cases (13,14). However, PE is often reported in patients without a documented lower extremity DVT. The source of the emboli may be from the veins in the pelvis (11). With trauma to the pelvis or acetabulum, such emboli in the veins of the pelvis are more likely, but identification is difficult. Conventional screening methods cannot reliably identify thrombi proximal to the inguinal ligament. Ultrasonography, arguably the current, most commonly used screening test for DVT, has been shown to have a poor positive predictive value for screening, especially more proximally, and is operator dependent (15,16). The current "gold standard," ascending venography, does not visualize the internal iliac or deep femoral venous system adequately (12,17–19). To visualize the veins proximal to the inguinal ligament, cannulation of the femoral system can be done, but requires an additional invasive procedure, and is not suited for routine screening (17,20). More recently, in patients with pelvic and acetabular fractures, magnetic resonance venography (MRV) and contrast-enhanced computed tomography have been studied with variable results (12,20,21). At this point, neither technique has received nationwide acceptance for routine screening.

Currently, the natural history of pelvic vein thrombosis is not known, but evidence suggests that more proximal clots are more likely to embolize (13,22,23). Pulmonary embolism is a potentially lethal complication in patients with pelvic and acetabular fractures, and has been reported as the most common fatal complication after operation or trauma to the lower extremities (24,25). The incidence of PE in these patients is reported to be between 0.5% and 10%, and fatal PE to be between 0.1% and 5% (2,3,5,26). Clearly, with the varying results related to DVT screening and prophylaxis, and the potential for PE, virtually all orthopedic surgeons agree that preoperative and postoperative prophylaxis is necessary (1). However, no consensus exists as to the most effective protocol for DVT prophylaxis in patients with pelvic and acetabular fractures. Current chemical prophylactic methods include aspirin, LMWH, low-dose heparin, adjusted-dose heparin, Dextran 40, and warfarin. All have studies to support and dispute their relative effectiveness, most of which are from the total joint arthroplasty literature. With the use of chemical prophylaxis, the risk of bleeding and associated complications is present (25,27–30). They include, but are not limited to, wound hematoma, wound dehiscence, infection, peripheral nerve palsy, internal bleeding, disseminated intravascular coagulopathy, heparin-induced thrombocytopenia, warfarin-induced skin necrosis, stroke, and death (31–33). With preoperative use of chemical agents, the patients should be monitored for a drop in their hemoglobin and platelet count.

While warfarin has been the mainstay of anti-coagulation therapy, it requires weekly monitoring and venipunture. Also, the practitioner or mid-level provider will need to monitor levels and make appropriate adjustments. With operative indications extending into more elderly patients, who frequently take multiple medications, there is a significant risk of medication interactions as well. All of these issues have paved the way for newer low molecular weight heparin (LMWH) agents that are easier to manage and with less adverse effects. These agents are usually injected subcutaneously once or twice daily and require less frequent hematologic surveillance. Also, due to their half life, they can be discontinued in the event that some emergent surgical procedure is needed. While they were initially associated with significant expense, the competitive market place has reduced their costs, and there are now a plethora of agents from which to choose. There are even newer oral agents under development that could make their use even easier. There are existing studies, mostly from the arthroplasty literature, that document their efficacy and use, but they have also been shown to be effective in the trauma population (11,19,26).

Mechanical devices for prophylaxis include thigh-calf low-pressure sequential-compression devices and calf-foot and foot high-pressure pulsatile-compression devices. These devices have support of effectiveness against DVT and PE in total arthroplasty patients but less literature support in trauma patients (5,10,34). The mechanical devices work by improving venous blood flow and by stimulating endogenous fibrinolytic activity (35). The devices carry no bleeding risk but can cause skin ulcerations and often patient compliance with its use in the hospital is poor. Often the mechanical devices are used in conjunction with chemical prophylaxis, but their combined efficacy is not additive. Another major concern is whether or not the compression devices are effective at inhibiting proximal thrombi as seen in the pelvic and acetabular population (36). Published DVT and PE rates in this population using only mechanical devices, with a similar reported incidence of DVT as other prophylactic methods (37).

Another alternative for prophylaxis is vena cava filters. Filters are placed in the inferior vena cava and act as a trap for thrombi, preventing the thrombus from entering the pulmonary vasculature, thereby preventing a PE. They do not however prevent DVTs. Filters are recommended in patients with a contraindication to chemical anticoagulation (e.g., head injury, patients managed nonoperatively for splenic or liver laceration) or in patients with pelvic or acetabular fractures that warrant surgical management and are considered high risk for a thromboembolic event (4,24). Risk factors include age over 60, hypercoagulable state, delay in surgery beyond 10 days, hormonal factors (oral contraceptives, postpartum), malignancy, obesity, and prior history of DVT or PE (24). Patients that are screened preoperatively, by whatever method the surgeon selects, and are positive, are considered for vena cana filter. The use of filters is not without complications. Patients may develop complete caval occlusion. The secondary phlegmasia cerulean dolens syndrome can be severe and represents both a life and limb threat (38). To avoid possible occlusion, anticoagulant prophylaxis after filter insertion has been recommended once safe for the patient. However, this is not universally agreed upon, and others do not use anticoagulant prophylaxis after filter placement (39). Additional complications include insertion problems, misplacement with potential for injury to renal vessels, perforation, and migration (39–41). As well there is uncertainty as to the long-term consequences of filter placement, especially in younger patients.

The protocol outlined above under postoperative care is one algorithm for DVT prevention. Many alternative protocols exist. A similar protocol was studied in the literature with excellent results, but no preoperative heparin was administered. Noninvasive screening with duplex ultrasound was performed preoperatively in patients transferred from an outside institution with a greater than 24-hour delay. If positive, a vena cava filter was placed preoperatively. Low-dose heparin was started postoperatively and continued for four to five days. Once the drains were removed, warfarin was started concurrently and continued for 12 weeks. If negative, mechanical devices were used preoperatively and continued throughout the hospital course. Warfarin was started once the drains were removed and continued for 3 weeks. The incidence of DVT was 3%, the incidence of PE was 1%, and no fatal PEs occurred following this protocol (10). With no clearly proven "best" screening technique for DVT and, no clearly proven "best" prophylactic method for DVT, any recommendation is just that. Although there is agreement for prophylaxis, the wide variation in type of prophylaxis and in the rationale for use suggests that controversy will continue, and a standard of care has yet to be defined.

Vascular Complications in Pelvic and Acetabular Fractures

Vascular complications, aside from DVT, are rare in both pelvic and acetabular surgery. Femoral artery thrombosis, femoral artery laceration, and femoral vein laceration have been described with ilioinguinal approaches with a reported incidence of 0.8% to 2% (2,3,42,43). This may occur from intraoperative traction, direct injury due to the vessels' proximity with the surgical approach, and extrinsic compression of the femoral artery by prominent screws placed in the anterior column (44). Equally in jeopardy of injury is the lymphatic system when using the ilioinguinal approach. Damage to the lymphatic system medial to the vessels can result in chronic lymphedema of the lower extremities (26). The incidence of this complication is unknown, but thought to be rare.

With the anterior approach to the pubic symphysis, whether for pelvic or acetabular surgery, there is a risk of significant bleeding from the vessels overlying the superior ramus. Although not a typically reported complication of pelvic and acetabular surgery in the literature, these anastomotic vessels between the external iliac or inferior epigastric systems and the obturator system can result in significant blood loss during surgery (45). This anastomotic connection has been described as the "corona mortis," and may be present in as low as 10% of the cases to as high as 84% of the cases (2,46–48). This connection may be arterial or venous, and the average distance from the symphysis to the anastomotic vessels averages 6.2 cm, ranging from 3 to 9 cm (48). With the knowledge of this anatomic variation, the surgeon can be prepared and look for, identify, and ligate the vessels to prevent significant intraoperative bleeding, avoiding a serious potential complication.

Iatrogenic injury to the superior gluteal vessels can occur during acetabular exposures utilizing a variety of posterior approaches because of the proximity of the vessels exiting superiorly from the greater sciatic notch. Injury can result in significant blood loss and gluteal muscle necrosis (2,3,49). Other than significant intraoperative bleeding, the clinical significance related to this iatrogenic injury and possible muscle necrosis is still in question (50).

The inciting traumatic event that causes a pelvic or acetabular fracture may also cause injury to the surrounding vessels. Injury to femoral, iliac, and hypogastric vessels can occur via direct injury or from laceration of the vessels from bony fragments usually of the anterior column (51,52). These traumatic vascular injuries associated with acetabular fractures are very rare and consist primarily of case reports in the literature (51,53–56). Because they can occur in patients presenting with an acetabular fracture and hemodynamic instability, this should be considered if other major sources of bleeding have been ruled out.

The association of vascular injury with pelvic fractures is much more common and well documented in the literature, with more severe fracture patterns associated with a higher prevalence of vessel injury (2,3,57–64). These vascular complications occur as a result of acute laceration, an intimal tear leading to vessel thrombosis, late formation of a pseudoaneurysm, or most commonly rupture from displacement of the pelvis (51,54,65–68). Although the treatment algorithms and diagnostic tools will be dealt with in other chapters, the vessel injuries warrant mention. Major arterial injury has been associated with only 20% of pelvic hemorrhage related deaths, the remainder of the bleeding sources result from either venous injury or fracture sites (69). Arterial injury was noted, in decreasing order of frequency, from the superior gluteal, the internal pudendal, the obturator, and the lateral sacral artery (63). The internal pudendal artery is the most commonly found site for active bleeding (63).

Soft Tissue Complications and Infection

Infection

Acetabular fracture surgery initially had high infection rates. Letournel, in his early series, reported a 30% incidence of surgical wound infection (70–72). With the use of prophylactic antibiotics and improved soft tissue management, the surgical infection rates have fallen dramatically to 2% to 5% in most large series (2,3,10,43,73–77). However, obese patients, patients with ipsilateral open fractures, patients with visceral injuries, patients with nutritional compromise, patients with some degree of immunocompromise, patients with local soft tissue injury, and patients with associated urologic and gastrointestinal injuries are at increased risk for infection, but how much is not known.

Infection rates associated with pelvic fractures are much less defined, with incidences varying from 0% to greater than 50% if associated with an open pelvic fracture (78,79). The same risk factors above for acetabular fractures apply to pelvic fractures. In particular, many of the pelvic ring disruptions are associated with lower urologic injury and rectal injury. These combined injuries require a planned surgical approach with the trauma surgeon to help avoid complications. This includes the orthopedic surgeon's presence at the time of laparotomy to help select appropriate sites for colostomies, if indicated, and to determine if or where a suprapubic catheter should be placed. With open pelvic fractures, the mortality rate is usually reported as opposed to the infection rates. However, if the patients survive the initial resuscitation, the mortality is usually related to infection. Through use of an early diverting colostomy, aggressive soft tissue debridement, and early stabilization, survival rates have been reported as high as 95% (80). With urologic injuries associated with pelvic or acetabular fractures, most of the literature supports urethral drainage as opposed to suprapubic catheters to avoid possible contamination of the surgical site through anterior approaches (81). However, with the use of antibiotics and local care of the cystostomy tube site, a small study used anterior approaches to treat anterior ring fractures without infection (7).

Soft Tissue Complications

Recognition and treatment of local soft tissue injury associated with pelvic and acetabular fractures is as equally important in preventing infection. This includes lacerations, abrasions, and closed degloving injuries. Pelvic fractures, with lacerations or abrasions located over the surgical site, should be managed as open fractures with early intervention for fracture fixation. In the case of an acetabular fracture where one can wait days before fixation, waiting for re-epithelialization of the abrasion or laceration prior to surgery may lower the risk for infection (82). Closed degloving injuries may often go unrecognized until surgery and potentially increase the infection rate once the incision is made. In the mid-19th century, Morel–Lavallee described this closed degloving lesion as a traumatic detachment of skin from the subjacent layers. Further studies more fully defined the degloving as a detachment of skin and subcutaneous tissue from the underlying fascia, with resultant disruption of segmental perforating blood and lymphatic vessels, caused by a violent, direct, and tangentially applied force to the superficial integument over unyielding aponeurotic fascia (83). This separation of layers and injury to the vessels creates a potential space allowing for hematoma or lymphocele to develop, further jeopardizing the vascular supply to the contused skin. The skin is then dependent on the randomly oriented dermal plexus for viability. If the injury occurs with direct force to the skin, the skin is at high risk for sloughing. Although the Morel–LaVallee lesion is not always associated with underlying fractures, if it is and potentially communicates with the surgical incision, proper treatment of the lesion is important for prevention of infection. Several studies noted both superficial and deep bone infections when operating through these lesions (83). With aspiration of the hematoma, positive cultures have been reported from 19% to 46% (84). Treatment is controversial. Recommendations include aggressive repeated surgical debridement with open packing followed by fixation either at the initial debridement or in a delayed fashion (84). More recent papers advocate early percutaneous surgical drainage with percutaneous debridement using a plastic brush and irrigation and suction drainage, followed by delayed surgery if open procedures are to be done, thus hopefully preserving the skin over the fractured areas (84).

With open approaches to posterior ring fixation of pelvic fractures, there has been a traditionally high infection rate reported—up to 27%—depending on the timing of surgery (78,79,85). This led to the use of indirect reduction techniques and percutaneous posterior ring fixation, which has dramatically dropped the infection rate to as low as 0%. However, there are some pelvic fractures that are not able to be reduced in an indirect fashion and require open reduction and internal fixation. With newer techniques and careful evaluation of the soft tissues, the infection rate for open posterior approaches to the pelvis has been reported at 3.9% in a large multicenter trial (85).

Pin Tract Infections

Pin tract infections are the most common complication after pelvic external fixation and frequently indicate pin loosening (86). Pin tract infections in the pelvis are treated with oral antibiotics like any other pin tract infection. Examination for pin loosening and skin necrosis is carried out at each visit. Loose pins should be removed and, depending on the construct of the fixation, pins added if necessary for stability. Skin problems can be addressed with relaxing incisions under local anesthetic if pressure necrosis is present. If osteomyelitis is present at the pin tract, intravenous antibiotics and surgical debridement may be indicated.

Pin care is most effective when the skin is stabilized by a minimally compressive dressing. There is no benefit to chemical treatments with peroxide or mechanical probing with cotton swabs. In fact, it has been shown that daily and weekly pin care fare better than more aggressive treatments. The pin sites of an external fixator, which are placed in the emergency department or intensive care unit, should be treated by orthopedic personel and routine nursing. Pin care in such areas should be avoided due to the known risks of nosocomial infections. The pins can be wrapped with gauze and changed periodically. Showers and cleansing with soap and water followed by a pin cleaning with an alcohol wipe may be the easiest and most effective technique. If there are signs of purulence or exudate, a short (7–10 day) course of oral antibiotics can be considered but should only be administered in full doses. Underdosing (e.g., cephalexin 500 mg BID) is not only ineffective but may breed resistant organisms.

Genitourinary Complications

Bladder rupture associated with pelvic fractures has a reported incidence as high as 20% (87–89). The majority of the time the bladder rupture will present with gross hematuria. Rupture of the bladder may be retroperitoneal (85%), intraperitoneal, or, infrequently, both (90). An intraperitoneal rupture commonly occurs at the dome of the bladder, when the patient has a full bladder, and is treated by primary repair. Retroperitoneal ruptures commonly occur on the anterolateral wall. Once identified by retrograde urethrogram or cystogram, primary repair is recommended to avoid the placement of a suprapubic catheter if anterior open reduction and internal fixation is carried out to treat the fractures.

Injury to the ureter has been reported only once in a pelvic fracture and rarely with isolated acetabular fractures (91). Once identified on CT, urologic consult and surgical repair is warranted.

Bladder entrapment during internal fixation of a pelvic or acetabular fracture has been reported only three times (92–94). The bladder entrapments were thought to be caused by either bony fragments penetrating the bladder during reduction and fixation or herniation of the filled bladder into the iliopubic fracture segment. Patients present with hematuria after fixation. The diagnosis is made using cystogram followed by CT. Surgical repair is required.

Female Genitourinary Complications

In the female population, traumatic injuries of the urethra are rare. This, at least in part, has been attributed to the relatively mobile and short course of the urethral channel behind the pubis. The incidence has varied from 1% to 6% (95,96). Because of the low incidence and rarity of blood at the meatus, this injury can be missed initially (96,97). If presenting with an associated bladder rupture and pelvic hematoma, the injury to the urethra may not be obvious. Once identified, the treatment remains controversial. The choices include immediate repair with realignment of the separated urethral ends indirectly over a catheter, with or without suprapubic catheter drainage, thus avoiding tissue dissection in the traumatized area, versus initial urinary diversion with delayed surgical reconstruction. As expected with injury to the female urethra, resulting incontinence is not uncommon and may necessitate additional surgery.

Vaginal lacerations may also accompany injury to the urethra. Vaginal lacerations occur in about 4% of pelvic fractures (98). Most present with bleeding, but at times with vaginal wall spasms bleeding may not be obvious, and if missed can lead to life-threatening sepsis. Detection, irrigation, debridement, and surgical repair of the injury are recommended (98).

With associated soft tissue injury accompanying pelvic and acetabular fractures, late genitourinary sequelae are common, but have been poorly documented in the literature. The largest study consisting of a retrospective review and questionnaire found that physiologic problems with arousal or orgasm were rare in females. However, female patients with pelvic fractures had a significantly higher rate of urinary complaints (21% vs. 7%), a significantly higher rate of gynecologic pain (19.6% vs. 9.5%), and a significant increase in the rate of postinjury cesarean section than the general female population (99).

Male Genitourinary Complications

Unlike female patients, males are more likely to have significant urologic injury related to pelvic and acetabular fractures, with incidences as high as 21%, the majority of these injuries to the urethra (as high as 16%). The urethra's longer length makes it more likely to be injured. Most commonly the injury occurs as an avulsion of the membranous urethra from the bulbar urethra rather than a shearing through the membranous urethra. Some degree of urethral sphincter function is preserved in a significant percentage of patients (100). With partial preservation of the urethral sphincter, incontinence is not a frequent sequelae in males with a urethral injury. Although an abundance of literature is available evaluating treatment options, the choice remains controversial. Recent studies favor early primary repair or endoscopic realignment to avoid suprapubic drainage if anterior open reduction and internal fixation is necessary for the treatment of the fractures. However, others still favor suprapubic drainage and delayed repair. The sexual and physiologic functions of the genitourinary system seem unchanged regardless of the urologic treatment.

Most of the injuries to the genitourinary system occur with anterior pelvic fractures and occasionally acetabular fractures. However, posterior ring fractures, which damage the lower sacral nerves, can result in sexual dysfunction, and should be discussed with the patient early if suspected. Recent work using the Brief Male Sexual Function Inventory (BMSFI) found that pelvic fractures of all types had a significantly profound negative effect on the sexual function of male patients, persisting for at least two years and possibly longer (101). Erectile dysfunction after blunt trauma and pelvic fracture has been documented to be between 20% and 80% (102).

Nerve Injury

Nerve Injury—Acetabular Fractures

Nerve injuries associated with acetabular fractures are iatrogenic or result from the initial injury. In either case, the sciatic nerve is by far the most commonly reported nerve injury and the peroneal division is more commonly involved than the tibial division (103–105). Proposed theories for why the peroneal division is more commonly injured include: (*i*) the anatomic relationship between the two divisions and the piriformis muscle; (*ii*) the peroneal division is tethered at the fibular neck and the sciatic notch, whereas the tibial division is tethered only at the sciatic notch; (*iii*) the funiculi of the peroneal division are fewer, larger, and less protected by connective tissue (106,107). Sciatic nerve palsy has an estimated prevalence ranging from less than 1% to as high as 35% (77,108,109). And iatrogenic sciatic nerve palsy has been reported between approximately 1% to 18% (2,43,64,77,110–115). The majority of the preoperative injuries to the sciatic nerve are associated with dislocation of the hip, resulting in direct trauma and compression of the nerve (116,117). Additionally, the nerve may become entrapped in the fracture, compressed by the fracture, or be lacerated or impaled by a bony fracture fragment (104,111,116,118). Late palsies of the sciatic nerve have been reported to occur from scar formation and massive heterotopic ossification (119–122). A thorough preoperative examination and documentation of the findings is critical. The examination should include individual muscle testing and sensory function by light touch and pin prick in all the dermatomes of the lower extremity. Although infrequently reported, femoral and obtorator nerve injuries can occur and will be missed unless looked for on preoperative examination. This would include muscle testing of the adductors, quadriceps femoris, and hip flexors. Weakness in the distribution of the injured nerve is the most common finding on examination, but patients may have paresthesias and subtle sensory loss depending on the nerve involved. A prompt reduction of the hip to relieve the pressure is important. If the reduction attempt is unsuccessful or the situation does not permit an attempt at reduction, an effort to reduce the tension on the sciatic nerve by placing the hip in extension and flexing the knee should be done. If the nerve was working prior to the reduction and subsequently is not, surgical exploration acutely is recommended for fear of entrapment of the nerve (123).

Although little can be done when patients present with a nerve injury, every effort should be made to minimize or prevent iatrogenic sciatic nerve injury. Letournel reported an initial incidence of 18% sciatic nerve injury associated with the Kocher–Langenbeck approach. However, with experience, careful attention to leg positioning (keeping the hip extended and knee flexed), retractor placement, and direct visualization of the nerve, he subsequently reported an incidence of 6.5% (124). Additionally, careful use of traction, limiting its use to short time intervals of 8 to 10 min, helps avoid iatrogenic injury. Even with great surgical care, iatrogenic nerve injuries still occur and may result in permanent disability in up to 24% of these patients (2,124). In an effort to decrease the incidence of iatrogenic nerve injury during acetabular fracture fixation, intraoperative nerve monitoring has been used; however, its use still remains controversial (1). Intraoperative nerve monitoring using somatosensory evoked potentials (SSEPs) has been supported by several studies (64,110,112,114). However, others have reported iantrogeic nerve injury despite negative intraoperative monitoring (64). SSEP monitoring does not provide information on the motor conduction pathways nor does it allow for real-time or instantaneous monitoring. In an attempt to offset these limitations, electromyography (EMG) has been used by itself or in combination with SSEP to improve on the success of monitoring during surgery (113,125). Despite the addition of EMG, the success of monitoring is still in question, with a recent study showing a higher rate of iatrogenic nerve injury in their monitored patients (125). Further studies report a 3% or lower rate of iatrogenic nerve injury in unmonitored patients (72,77,123). Monitoring adds time and expense, requiring an experienced staff and expensive equipment, making its use less attractive.

Most of the iatrogenic sciatic nerve injuries have been reported to occur when the Kocher–Langenbeck approach or the extended iliofemoral approach is used. Interestingly, two papers found that the majority of the iatrogenic injuries to the sciatic nerve occurred through the ilioinguinal approach (110,125). This was attributed to indirect reduction maneuvers of the posterior column through the sciatic notch combined with the leg slightly flexed at the hip and only minimally flexed at the knee, placing the nerve in greater tension. It has also been suggested that patients with preoperative nerve injury are at risk for iatrogenic injury but a recent study questions this finding (125,126). Still, if one considers that there may be a "sub-clinical" injury to the nerve, as has been described with plexopathies of pelvic fractures, and as are commonly seen during surgery in the form of physical nerve damage, it would not be implausible that such a damaged nerve represents a nerve "at risk." Also, accepting that a clinical motor grading exam is rather crude and does not necessarily reflect objective nerve injury, a nerve that is damaged but clinically functional may be at risk during the slightest and appropriately performed retraction maneuvers during surgery. In such cases, the patient with a weak or seemingly normal physical exam can awaken with a complete palsy. While considered "iatrogenic," the actual cause may be a sequelae of the injury, and an objective description of any damage to the nerve or sheath may not only alert the surgeon of such a possibility but will be supportive explanation to avoid any misunderstandings about the nature of post operative problems. In such cases, if appropriate and gentle retraction was utilized with findings of nerve injury, the cause of nerve palsy ought not be placed on the surgeon and should be considered a sequelae of the injury itlelf. Ultimately, each patient should have a thorough examination pre- and postoperatively, and great care should be taken in surgery regardless of the approach to minimize iatrogenic sciatic nerve injury.

The recovery of acute traumatic and iatrogenic nerve injuries in acetabular fractures vary widely, with functional return reported in 30% to 84% of the patients, occurring as early as six weeks or as late as three years (57,104,105,111,116–118, 127,128). The prognosis for recovery from sciatic nerve palsies is related to the severity of the initial deficit, with the tibial division having a better recovery than the peroneal (26,111). In cases of late developing palsies, with resection of the scar or heterotopic bone, the functional recovery is excellent (119,122).

Unlike injuries to the sciatic nerve or lumbar plexus, femoral nerve injuries are much less common and rarely reported. The prevalence of iatrogenic injury to the femoral nerve has been reported to range from 0.2% to 0.4% (72,129). As well, the prevalence of traumatic femoral nerve palsy is equally low. The injury to the femoral nerve is thought to be low because of its anatomic location, essentially protected between the iliac and psoas muscles as it exits the pelvis deep to the inguinal ligament. Femoral nerve palsy associated with iliac hematomas has been well described (130). However, in the reported cases of nerve palsy associated with acetabular fractures, none have been attributed to a hematoma. Traumatic causes include complete laceration of the nerve trapped in the fracture site, while other etiologies can only be speculated (108,131). The cause of iatrogenic femoral nerve palsies is likewise uncertain. Possible causes include excessive intraoperative traction during the ilioinguinal approach as described by Letournel in his reported two cases of femoral nerve palsy (2). Direct compression with the patient in the prone position may result in femoral nerve palsy (129). Regardless of the etiology, unless lacerated, the return of function is excellent in the described cases. Motor return has been 100%, with return occurring as early as four weeks to as late as 52 weeks (129). Sensory return has been reported in all cases, but remained incomplete in most, though not debilitating. Although a rare occurrence, a thorough examination of the quadriceps muscle function and femoral nerve sensation, both pre- and postoperatively, is the key to identification of this complication.

Iatrogenic injury to the lateral femoral cutaneous nerve can occur with placement of an anterior external fixator on the pelvis. In 10% of the patients, the lateral femoral cutaneous nerve was found to course over the iliac wing, making it vulnerable to injury during pin placement (132). It may also occur with anterior approaches to the acetabulum or to the sacroiliac joint. With these approaches, the lateral femoral cutaneous nerve may be injured as high as 30% to 40% of the time (86). Injury to the nerve results in decreased sensation or loss of sensation over the anterolateral thigh and a potentially painful neuroma. If injured, sharp debridement and soft tissue coverage of the proximal nerve end may decrease neuroma formation, reducing the need for further surgery later. Although no functional impairment results, the patient should be informed prior to surgery of the potential for decreased sensation.

Pelvic Nerve Injuries

The incidence of neurologic injuries associated with pelvic fractures is unknown. The literature has reported an incidence as low as 0.7% to as high as almost 60% when unstable vertical shear fractures of the pelvis or medial sacral fractures are examined (133–137). Many of these studies are retrospective, making the accuracy of the initial and follow-up examinations subject to error.

Neurologic injury is a major part of the disability associated with pelvic fractures and is increasing with the increase in high-energy accidents in which polytraumatized patients are surviving, in part because of improvement in safety of vehicles and improvement in resuscitation and fixation techniques for the pelvis (138,139).

As expected, most neurologic injuries are related to disruption of the posterior ring of the pelvis with a few notable exceptions discussed later (140). Lateral compression injuries tend to compress the sacral nerves or have bony fragments encroach on the exiting nerves in the foraminal canal, whereas vertically unstable injuries and, to a lesser extent, unstable anterior posterior compression injuries are more likely to stretch or avulse the nerve roots (141). Yet, the extent of the displacement of the fracture has not been shown to correlate with the resulting neurologic injury (142). The location of the injury, whether the sacrum or the sacroiliac joint, has not revealed any difference in incidence of nerve injury. The location of the fracture in the sacrum as classified by Denis showed an increased incidence: zone 1 (fracture lateral to the foramen), which was 5.9% and more likely to involve the L5 nerve to zone 2 (through the foramen), which was 28.4% and involved the L5, S1, and S2 ventral roots to zone 3 (fractures medial to the foramen), which was 56.8% and involved, nearly 80% of the time, bladder, bowel, and/or sexual function (143). However, a later study showed no difference in incidence of nerve injury with sacral fracture location (144). The location of the fracture does help to predict the potential nerve or nerves injured and corresponding clinical findings. The lumbosacral trunk and the superior gluteal nerve are the most frequent sites of injury. The lumbosacral trunk located anterior to the lateral sacral ala and sacroiliac joint is commonly injured with external rotation and posterosuperior displacement of the hemipelvis. The superior gluteal nerve is most vulnerable to injury after comminuted fractures of the sacroiliac joint (142). The obturator nerve injury occurs infrequently, but can occur with a posterior ring disruption more so than with a fracture involving the obturator foramen. Sacral nerves S2, S3, and S4 require only unilateral preservation to maintain bowel, bladder, and usually sexual function, although this often is multifactorial (145). For this reason pelvic ring fractures are less likely to see loss of bowel and bladder function. Transverse fractures of the sacrum carry a higher incidence of bowel and bladder dysfunction, but they are rarely seen with a pelvic ring fractures, and are more appropriately considered spinal injuries (142–144).

A thorough examination and continued repeat examinations are critical to identify the neurologic injuries especially in the multiply injured patient. With a pelvic injury, special attention to bowel and bladder function, sphincter tone, and peroneal sensation will help avoid missing a nerve injury or having a delay in the diagnosis of nerve injury.

Recovery of neurologic injuries varies widely in the literature. Partial recovery has been reported as high as 100%, complete recovery as high as 68%, but no sign of recovery has also been reported in all the nerve-injured patients (134,136,140, 146–148). The time interval to recovery varies from early signs of return in two to three months to some continued return at three to four years (142). Currently there is no way to guarantee improvement in recovery. Exploration and decompression may be of benefit in compression injuries, but, with the majority of the lesions from traction or avulsion, decompression is unlikely to help unless a CT scan can clearly document bony impingement. However, early stabilization of the pelvis and restoration of the anatomy of the pelvis may remove tension and aid in decompression of the nerves, enhancing the chance for recovery.

Heterotopic Ossification

Heterotopic ossification (HO) is a common complication following acetabular surgery and can jeopardize the functional outcome of patients. Overall, rates of HO have been reported to vary from 45% to 100%, with the rate of severe HO between 14% and 50% when no prophylaxis is used (2,3,57,62,149,150–152). When nonoperative treatment is selected, HO is rare (50). A direct relationship between the severity of HO and loss of function has been demonstrated, thus making prophylaxis routine for most surgeons (151). Significant reported potential risk factors for HO development include head injury, type and severity of the fracture, time delay to surgery, trochanteric osteotomy, and associated injuries to the abdomen and chest (50,153–155). The most commonly reported and convincing risk factor for HO is the surgical approach, with the extended iliofemoral and the Kocher–Langenbeck approaches having the highest rate of HO and the ilioinguinal approach the lowest (50,63,152,154). The major difference in approaches involves the stripping of the gluteal muscles off the external iliac fossa. Unless the ilioinguinal approach is extended onto the external fossa, no HO prophylaxis is recommended (2,3,43,62). Unfortunately, without a clear understanding of the etiology of HO, multiple methods of prophylaxis currently are in use, all with literature to support and refute their effectiveness.

Heterotopic bone experimentally occurs with soft tissue trauma, with transplantation of cells which form bone, and with undifferentiated mesenchymal cells that are exposed to bone growth factors (156). These theories support the idea that, with tissue injury and/or dissection, the process of HO is more likely to occur, especially in situations that displace bony fragments into the surrounding soft tissue. The process of HO formation is thought to begin within 16 hours of the injury/surgery and is maximal at 36 to 48 hours (50,152,157,158). Therefore, whatever treatment selected, the optimal time for initiation of preventative treatment is within the first 48 hours following the surgery.

Heterotopic ossification is usually evident on radiographs by six weeks and has shown little likelihood of progression after three months (57,63). Once identified on radiographs, the classification of HO has been described by Brooker, which is based on a single AP pelvic radiograph. Although commonly used, the classification system has been modified by Moed, and most published articles refer to the modified Brooker classification system. The modified system uses two additional radiographic views to identify the extent of HO formation (159). The views are the iliac oblique and obturator oblique (Judet views) views of the acetabulum. The modified system allows for better correlation with hip motion (159). Ultimately, HO formation is only important if it affects the range of motion of the hip, and as the grade of HO increases the range of motion diminishes, thus the importance for prevention rather than treatment after formation (50,62,63,149,154,159–162).

Various prophylactic treatments have been attempted in the past, much of which was based on the literature for HO prevention in total hip arthroplasty. In the 1970s, ethyl hydroxydiphosphonate was thought to prevent osteoid mineralization, but not osteoid production (163,164). Unfortunately, diphosphonates only delayed the mineralization of osteoids, rather than preventing HO. In subsequent experimental animal studies and in patients after surgery about the hip, diphosphonates have been shown to be ineffective (165,166).

Indomethacin, a nonsteroidal antiinflammatory drug (NSAID), has been shown to diminish the incidence of HO after pelvic surgery (2,57,62,63). The pathway for indomethacin's use in HO prevention is felt to be related to its ability to affect the inflammatory process by acting through an inhibitory action on prostaglandin synthesis (167). Therefore, early administration of the medication for prophylaxis, usually within the first 24 to 48 hours of surgery, is important. Current recommended prophylactic dose is 25 mg three times a day, administered orally or by rectal suppository, beginning on the first postoperative day and continuing for three to six weeks (26). Specific to acetabular surgery, the incidence of HO with indomethacin prophylaxis is 5% to 47% with significant ectopic bone formation in up to 22% of the patients (57,62,63,155). The benefits of indomethacin include both cost and ease of administration. However, a randomized, prospective study in 1997, using three-dimensional CT reconstruction to assess the HO, determined that indomethacin was not effective as a prophylactic agent, raising again the question of its use. Patient compliance can be an issue, with a reported noncompliance rate as high as 33% (168). Furthermore, although rarely reported in most studies, indomethacin can have serious complications, including gastric ulcerations, decreased platelet function, renal toxicity, impaired fracture healing, and increased risk of long bone nonunion (162,169–171).

Radiation has been proven effective in reducing the severity and overall incidence of HO after acetabular surgery (50,57,62,149,151). Irradiation acts by altering DNA transcription. This affects rapidly dividing cells and prevents osteoblastic precursor cells from multiplying and forming active osteoblasts (149,172). Several studies noted that the timing of the radiation may effect the success, and therefore recommend the radiation be given within 48 to 72 hours of the surgery, if not preoperatively (50,149,155). Following the fourth postoperative day, the success of HO prevention fell from 98% to 33% in one study (155). Treatment recommendations vary from as little as 500 to 1000 cGy in a one time single low-dose to 1000 to 1200 cGy given in five or six divided doses daily over five to six days. A major benefit of the radiation is that prophylactic treatment is administered while still in the hospital, eliminating compliance issues. However, radiation therapy is not always available and may be costly at some institutions, but considering the complexity of such cases, and the trend for such patients to be transferred to tertiary institutions or trauma centers, as well as the increasing level of oncologic services at such centers, obtaining radiation therapy is not very difficult. It would not be justified to transfer a multiply injured patient in the rare case that it is not available; other methods should be employed. Radiation therapy has major risks, including induction of malignancy, genetic alterations of offspring, and sterility. However, these risks are dose-related, and none have been shown to occur with the recommended single low-dose treatment, although its long-term effects have not been determined (50,62,149,156,160,173).

A more aggressive prophylactic treatment for HO includes a combination therapy, of both indomethacin and radiation (160). This has reported results as good as the best individual treatments, but carries the risks of both treatments.

Another recommendation for prevention of HO is resection of the necrotic muscle at the time of surgery, specifically resection of the damaged/necrotic gluteus minimus and medius muscles. One study reports a decrease in the incidence of significant HO with resection of the necrotic muscle and no adjuvant treatment (156). The obvious advantages include no compliance issues and no complications related to radiation or NSAIDs; however, most surgeons already remove necrotic muscle, bringing into question the ultimate success of this treatment alone.

Even with prophylactic treatment, HO does occur and in some instances can become disabling for the patient by limiting hip motion. Surgical excision should only be considered if hip motion is limited and even then must be decided upon on a case-by-case basis. Verification that the ossification process has subsided is important since resection in the active phase can result in an even more significant recurrence. Monitoring blood alkaline phosphatase and bone scan activity for stabilization are two accepted methods for determing the appropriate timing of resection, should it be contemplated. If resection is planned, a preoperative CT is helpful for preoperative planning. Resection of the bone is usually done through the original approach used for fracture fixation. Care must be taken when resecting bone because the sciatic and superior gluteal nerves can be entrapped in the bone or surrounding scar tissue. If done carefully, excision of the HO can result in an improved range of motion in the hip. After excision, HO prophylaxis is recommended using NSAIDs, or a combination of both.

Osteonecrosis

Osteonecrosis is a complication associated with acetabular fractures. The incidence has generally ranged from 3% to 9%, and is most commonly associated with posterior hip dislocations and ipsilateral femoral neck fractures (26,72,76). The incidence increases to 13% when only posterior fracture dislocations are examined (174). Most of the cases of avascular necrosis (AVN) are identified by two years postinjury with changes sometimes noted as early as three weeks (18). With early AVN, there often arises the question of early post-traumatic chondrolysis and wear of the head secondary to an imperfect reduction. It is very difficult to make a distinction in many cases. Nonetheless, these patients tend to have poor results. Avascular necrosis of the acetabulum can also occur. It is usually of the posterior wall, which often is devoid of soft tissue, but AVN of the anterior column has also been described. Both can lead to early cartilage loss and a painful hip. Currently, the feeling is that the damage is done with the injury and our current treatments may not affect the outcome of the AVN. However, controversy exists regarding early hip reduction as a potential method of reducing AVN and does have support in the literature. As well, with acetabular surgery care should be taken to preserve the femoral head blood supply by avoiding dissection through the quadratus femoris muscle, and limiting devascularization of the fracture fragments to prevent AVN.

Intra-articular Hardware

Intra-articular hardware has been reported in up to 4% of operatively treated acetabular fractures (43,175). With a better understanding of the anatomy and improvements in intraoperative orthogonal fluoroscopy assessing the quality of the reduction and the position of the hardware, this complication is now seldom reported. With the intraoperative use of fluoroscopy, if any screw can be visualized out of the acetabulum, in any one view, the hardware is truly out of the joint (176). In obese patients, in which fluoroscopic visualization is poor, auscultation intraoperatively with an esophageal stethoscope along the quadrilateral surface and the lateral ilium may help to detect intra-articular hardware (177). If there remains a question of screw positioning, post-operative radiographs and/or a CT scan may be needed to conclusively determine the position of the hardware.

RARE AND UNUSUAL COMPLICATIONS

Entrapment of bowels within pelvic fractures has been reported in at least 20 cases in the literature (178). Of these cases, five resulted in eventual death from sepsis. The typical presentation is that of an ileus, not an unusual finding in trauma patients. This often leads to a delay in the diagnosis. Therefore, in patients with an unknown source of fevers or a persistent ileus, a CT with enteric contrast is recommended to fully evaluate such patients. Another possible indicator of bowel entrapment is a disruption of the iliacus muscle. With disruption of the muscle the peritoneal contents can communicate with the fracture and become entrapped or punctured. When the general surgeon addresses the bowels either with resection and primary anastomosis or diverting colostomy, consideration should be given to repair of the fracture and if possible the iliacus muscle, if a defect exists.

Perineal soft tissue and urogenital injuries are associated with pelvic and acetabular fractures. Most often these injuries are a result of the energy transferred to the bone and soft tissue. However, with the use of skeletal traction against a perineal post for assistance with surgical treatment, further injury to the perineum can occur. Utilizing traction in femoral shaft fractures, pudendal nerve palsy and wound slough have been well described (179–182). Recently a similar injury has been reported after treatment of a pelvic fracture and bilateral acetabular fractures. Perineal wound sloughs have multifactorial causes, including the initial injury and the pressure applied during surgery. By increasing the size of the perineal post, limiting the force of traction used, limiting the time of traction, appropriately padding the perineal post, and intermittently releasing traction, complications to the perineal area can be minimized, short of not using traction altogether.

Spontaneous urinary voiding of a screw after operative fixation of the pelvis has been reported. The patient presented, seven years after plate and screw fixation of the pubic symphysis, with dysuria, hematuria, and spontaneous urethral voiding of a screw. Further work-up revealed that a loose screw eroded through the anterior bladder wall and amazingly was eventually voided (183). In patients with retained pelvic hardware and urinary symptoms, this may represent a very rare cause of their symptoms.

REFERENCES

1. Morgan SJ, Jeray KJ, Phieffer LS, et al. Attitudes of orthopaedic trauma surgeons regarding current controversies in the management of pelvic and acetabular fractures. J Orthop Trauma 2001; 15(7):526–532.
2. Letournel E, Judet R. Fractures of the Acetabulum. 2nd ed. Berlin: Springer-Verlag, 1993.
3. Matta JM. Operative treatment of acetabular fractures through the ilioinguinal approach: a 10-year perspective. Clin Orthop 1994; 305:10–19.
4. Collins DN, Barnes CL, McCowan TC, et al. Vena caval filter use in orthopaedic trauma patients with recognized preoperative venous thromboembolic disease. J Orthop Trauma 1992; 6(2):135–138.
5. Fisher CG, Blachut PA, Salvain AJ, Meek RN, O'Brien PJ. Effectiveness of pneumatic leg compression devices for the prevention of thromboembolic disease in the orthopaedic trauma patients: a prospective, randomized study of compression alone versus no prophylaxis. J Orthop Trauma 1995; 9(1):1–7.
6. Geerts WH, Code KI, Jay RM, Chen E, Szalai JP. A prospective study of venous thromboembolism after major trauma. N Engl J Med 1994; 331(24):1601–1606.
7. Matta JM. Indications for anterior fixation of pelvic fractures. Clin Orthop 1996; 329:88–96.
8. National Institute of Health Consensus Development. Prevention of venous thrombosis and pulmonary embolism. JAMA 1986; 256(6):744–749.
9. White RH, Goulet JA, Bray TJ, et al. Deep-vein thrombosis after fracture of the pelvis: assessment with serial duplex-ultrasound screening. J Bone Joint Surg 1990; 72A(4):495–500.
10. Fishmann AJ, Greeno RA, Brooks LR, Matta JM. Prevention of deep vein thrombosis and pulmonary embolism in acetabular and pelvic fracture surgery. Clin Orthop 1994; 305:133–137.
11. Knudson MM, Morabito DM, Paiement GD, Shackleford S. Use of low molecular weight heparin in preventing thromboembolism in trauma patients. J Trauma 1996; 41(3): 446–459.
12. Montgomery KD, Potter HG, Helftet DL. Magnetic resonance venography to evaluate the deep venous system of the pelvis in patients who have an acetabular fracture. J Bone Joint Surg 1995; 77A(11):1639–1649.
13. Moser KM. Pulmonary embolism. Am Rev Respir Dis 1997; 115(5):829–852.
14. Ramsa LE. Impact of venography on the diagnosis and management of deep vein thrombosis. Br Med J (Clin Res Ed) 1983; 286(6366):698–699.
15. Burns GA, Cohn SM, Frumento RJ, Degutis LC, Hammers L. Prospective ultrasound evaluation of venous thrombosis in high-risk trauma patients. J Trauma 1993; 35(3): 405–408.
16. Davidson BL, Elliot CG, Lensing AW. Low accuracy of color Doppler ultrasound in the detection of proximal leg vein thrombosis in asymptomatic high-risk patient. The RD Heparin Arthroplasty Group. Ann Intern Med 1992; 117(9):735–738.
17. Bettmann MA, Robbins AM, Braun SD, et al. Contrast venography of the leg: diagnostic efficacy, tolerance, and complication rates with ionic and nonionic contrast media. Radiology 1987; 165(1):113–116.
18. Carpenter JP, Holland GA, Baum RA, et al. Magnetic resonance venography for the detection of deep venous thrombosis: comparison with contrast venography and duplex Doppler ultrasonography. J Vasc Surg 1993; 18(5):734–741.
19. Geerts WHJ, Jay R, Code KR. Thromboprophylaxis after major trauma—a doubler blind RCT complaining LDH and the LMWH enoxaparin. Thrombo Haemost 1995; 73:284.

20. Stover MD, Morgan SJ, Bosse MJ, et al. Prospective comparison of contrast-enhanced computed tomography versus magnetic resonance venography in the detection of occult deep pelvic vein thrombosis in patients with pelvic and acetabular fractures. J Orthop Trauma 2002; 16(9):613–621.
21. Montgomery KD, Potter HG, Helfet DL. The detection and management of proximal deep venous thrombosis in patients with acute acetabular fractures: a follow-up report. J Orthop Trauma 1997; 11(5):330–336.
22. Kakkar VV, Howe CT, Flanc C, Clarke MB. Natural history of postoperative deep-vein thrombosis. Lancet 1969; 2(7614):230–232.
23. Moser KM, LeMoine JR. Is embolic risk conditioned by location of deep venous thrombosis? Ann Intern Med 1981; 94:439–444.
24. Webb LX, Rush PT, Fuller SB, Meredith JW. Greenfield filter prophylaxis of pulmonary embolism in patients undergoing surgery for acetabular fracture. J Orthop Trauma 1992; 6(2):139–145.
25. Salzman EW, Harris WH. Prevention of venous thromboembolism in orthopaedic patients. J Bone Joint Surg 1976; 58A(7):903–913.
26. Sims SH. Acetabular fractures: postoperative management and complications. In: Levine AM, ed. Orthopaedic Knowledge Update, Trauma. Am Acad Orthopaed Surg 1996; 273–280.
27. Gillman AG, Rall TW, Nies AS, Taylor P. Goodman and Gilman's The Pharmacologic Basis of Therapeutics, 8th ed. New York: Pergamon Press, 1990:1320–1321.
28. Glenny RW. Pulmonary embolism: complications of therapy. South Med J 1987; 80(10):1266–1276.
29. Poller L. Oral anticoagulants reassessed. Br Med J 1982; 284(6327):1425–1426.
30. Proter JM, Edwards JM, Taylor Jr LM. Drugs in vascular surgery. In: Moore WS, ed. Vascular Surgery: A Comprehensive Review. Orlando: Grune & Stratton, 1986.
31. Hacker LA. Antithrombotic therapy. In: Bennett JC, Plum F, eds. Cecil Textbook of Medicine, 20th ed. Philadelphia: WB Saunders, 1996:115–122.
32. Handin RI. Oncology and hematology. In: Braunwald E, Fauci AS, Kasper DL, Hauser SL, Longo DL, Jameson JL, eds. Harrison's Principles of Internal Medicine. New York: McGraw-Hill, 2001.
33. Woolson ST, Harris WH. Greenfield vena caval filter for management of selected cases of venous thromboembolic disease following hip surgery. A report of five cases. Clin Orthop 1986; 204:201–206.
34. Elliott CG, Dudney TM, Egger M, et al. Calf-thigh sequential pneumatic compression compared with plantar venous pneumatic compression to prevent deep-vein thrombosis after non-lower extremity trauma. J Trauma 1999; 47(1):25–32.
35. Comerota AJ, Chouhan VM, Harada RN, et al. The firbrinolytic effects of intermittent pneumatic complression: mechanism of enhanced fibrinolysis. Ann Surg 1997; 226(3):306–313.
36. Montrey JS, Kistner RL, Kong AY, et al. Thromboembolism following hip fracture. J Trauma 1985; 25(6):534–537.
37. Stannard JP, Riley RS, McClenney MD, et al. Mechanical prophylaxis against deep-vein thrombosis after pelvic and acetabular fractures. J Bone Joint Surg 2001; 83A(7):1047–1051.
38. Schwartz SI, Shires GT, Spencer FC, Storer EH. Principles of Surgery, 3rd ed. New York: McGraw-Hill, 1979.
39. Greenfield LJ, Peyton R, Crute S, Barnes R. Greenfield vena caval filter experience. Late results in 156 patients. Arch Surg 1981; 116(11):1451–1456.

40. Greenfield LJ, McCurdy JR, Brown PP, Elkins RC. A new intracaval filter permitting continued flow and resolution of emboli. Surgery 1973; 7(4):599–606.
41. Stewart JR, Peyton JW, Crute SL, Greenfield LJ. Clinical results of suprarenal placement of the Greenfield vena cava filter. Surgery 1982; 92(1):1–4.
42. Probe R, Reeve R, Lindsey RW. Femoral artery thrombosis after open reduction of an acetabular fracture. Clin Orthop 1992; 283:258–260.
43. Mayo KA. Open reduction and internal fixation of fractures of the acetabulum: results in 163 fractures. Clin Orthop 1994; 305:31–37.
44. Johnson EE, Eckardt JJ, Letournel E. Extrinsic femoral artery occlusion following internal fixation of an acetabular fracture: a case report. Clin Orthop 1987; 217:209–213.
45. Teague DC, Graney DO, Routt ML. Retropubic vascular hazards of the ilioinguinal exposure: a cadaveric and clinical study. Final Program, Orthopaedic Trauma Association, 1994.
46. Braithwaite JL. Variations in origin of the parietal branches of the internal iliac artery. Am J Anat 1952; 86:423–430.
47. Fernandez LA. Hemorragia de la “corona mortis.” Pren Med Argent 1968; 55:382–385.
48. Tornetta P, Hochwalkd N, Levine R. Corona mortis: incidence and location. Clin Orthop 1996; 329:97–101.
49. Juliano PJ, Bosse MJ, Edwards KJ. The superior gluteal artery in complex acetabular procedures: a cadaveric angiographic study. J bone Joint Surg 1994; 76A:244–248.
50. Anglen JO, Moore KD. Prevention of heterotopic bone formation after acetabular fracture fixation by single dose radiation therapy: a preliminary report. J Orthop Trauma 1996; 10(4):258–263.
51. Frank JL, Reimer BL, Raves JJ. Traumatic iliofemoral arterial injury. An association with high anterior acetabular fractures. J Vasc Surg 1989; 10(2):198.
52. Yosowitz P, Hobson II RW, Rich NM. Iliac vein laceration caused by blunt trauma to the pelvis. Am J Surg 1972; 124:91–93.
53. Chen AL, Wolinsky PR, Tejwani NC. Hypogastric artery disruption associated with acetabular fracture. J Bone Joint Surg 2003; 85A(2):333–338.
54. Hammami NM. An aneurysm of the superior gluteal artery presenting as buttoch pain 6 months after a missed fracture of the acetabulum. Br J Surg 1981; 68:442–444.
55. Cheng SL, Rosati C, Waddell JP. Fatal hemorrhage caused by vascular injury associated with an acetabular fracture. J Trauma 1995; 38:208–209.
56. Wolinsky PR, Johnson KD. Delayed catastrophic rupture of the external iliac artery after an acetabular fracture. A case report. J Bone JointSurg Am 1995; 77:1241–1244.
57. McLaren AC. Prophylaxis with indomethacin for heterotopic bone after open reduction of fractures of the acetabulum. J Bone Joint Surg 1990; 72A:245–247.
58. Reinert CM, Bosse MJ, Poka A, et al. A modified extensile approach for the treatment of complex or malunited acetabular fractures. J Bone Joint Surg 1988; 70A(3):329–337.
59. McMurtry RY, Walton D, Dickinson D, Kellam J, Tile M. Pelvic disruption in the polytraumatized patient: a management protocol. Clin Orthop 1980; 151:22–30.
60. Moreno C, Moore EE, Rosenberger A, Cleveland HC. Hemorrhage associated with major pelvic fracture: a mulitspecialty challenge. J Trauma 1986; 26:987–994.
61. Rothenberger DA, Fischer RP, Strate RG, Velasco R, Perry JF Jr. The mortality associated with pelvic fractures. Surgery 1978; 84:356–361.
62. Johnson EE, Kay RM, Dorey FJ. Heterotopic ossification prophylaxis following operative treatment of acetabular fracture. Clin Orthop 1994; 305:88–95.
63. Moed BR, Maxey JW. The effect of indomethacin on heterotopic ossification following acetabular fracture surgery. J Orthop Trauma 1993; 7(1):33–38.

64. Calder HB, Mast J, Johnstone C. Intraoperative evoked potentials monitoring in acetabular surgery. Clin Orthop 1994; 305:160–167.
65. Belley G, Gallix BP, Derossis AM, Mulder DS, Brown RA. Profound hypotension in blunt trauma associated with superior gluteal artery rupture without pelvic fracture. J Trauma 1997; 43:703–705.
66. Birchard JD, Pichora DR, Brown PM. External iliac artery and lumbosacral plexus injury secondary to an open book fracture of the pelvis: report of a case. J Trauma 1990; 30:906–908.
67. Brown JJ, Greene FL, McMillin RD. Vascular injuries associated with pelvic fractures. Am Surg 1984; 50:150–154.
68. Smith K, Ben-Menachem Y, Duke JH Jr, Hill GL. The superior gluteal artery: an artery at risk in blunt pelvic trauma. J Trauma 1969; 9:126–134.
69. Bosse MJ, Poka A, Reinert CM, et al. Preoperative angiographic assessment of the superior gluteal artery in acetabular fractures requiring extensile surgical exposures. J Orthop Trauma 1988; 2:303–307.
70. Judet R, Judet J, Letournel E. Fractures of the acetabulum: classification and surgical approaches for open reduction. J Bone Joint Surg 1964; 46A:1615.
71. Matta JM. Operative indications and choice of surgical approach for fractures of the acetabulum. Tech Orthop 1986, 1:13.
72. Matta JM. Fractures of the acetabulum: accuracy of reduction and clinical results in patients managed operatively within three weeks after the injury. J Bone Joint Surg 1996: 78A:1632–1645.
73. Letournel E. The treatment of acetabular fractures through the ilioinguinal approach. Clin Orthop 1993, 292:62–76.
74. Mears DC, Rubash HE. Extensile exposure of the pelvis. Contemp Orthop 1983; 6:21–32.
75. Matta JM, Merritt PO. Displaced acetabular fractures. Clin Orthop 1988; 230:83–97.
76. Matta JM, Anderson LM, Epstein HC, Hendricks P. Fractures of the acetabulum: a retrospective analysis. Clin Orthop 1986; 205:230–240.
77. Matta JM, Mehne DK, Roffi R. Fractures of the acetabulum: early results of a prospective study. Clin Orthop 1986; 205:241–250.
78. Kellam JF, McMurtry RY, Paley D, Tile M. The unstable pelvic fracture: operative treatment. Orthop Clin North Am 2987; 18:25–41.
79. Goldstein A, Phillips T, Sclanfani SJ, et al. Early open reduction and internal fixation of the disrupted pelvic ring. J Trauma 1986; 26:325–333.
80. Richardson JD, Harty J, Amin M, Flint AM. Open pelvic fractures. J Trauma 1982; 22: 533–538.
81. Routt ML Jr, Simonian PT, Ballmer F. A rational approach to pelvic trauma: resuscitation and early definitive stabilization. Clin Orthop 1995; 318:61–74.
82. Jeray KJ, Banks DM, Phieffer LS, et al. Evaluation of standard surgical preparation performed on superficial dermal abrasions. J Orthop Trauma 2000; 14(3):206–211.
83. Mir y Mir L, Novell AM. Repair of necrotic cutaneous lesions secondary to tangential trauma over detachable zones. Plast Reconst Surg 1950; 6:264–274.
84. Hak DJ, Olson SA, Matta JM. Diagnosis and management of closed internal degloving injuries associated with pelvic and acetabular fractures: the Morel–Lavallee lesion. J Trauma 1997; 42(6):1046–1051.
85. Stover MD, Sims SH, Templeman DC, Merkle P, Matta JM. Is the posterior approach to pelvic ring injuries associated with a high rate of soft tissue complications? Vancouver, British Columbia: 14th Annual Orthopaedic Trauma Assocation Meeting, Oct 8–10, 1998. Paper number 1:39–41.
86. Wiss DA. Master Techniques in Orthopaedic Surgery: Fractures. Philadelphia: Lippincott-Raven, 1998.

87. Fallon B, Wendt JC, Hawtrey CE. Urological injury and assessment in patients with fractured pelvis. J Urol 1984; 131(4):712–714.
88. Iverson HG, Jessing P. Urinary tract lesions associated with fractures of the pelvis. Acta Chir Scand 1973; 139:201–207.
89. Palmer JK, Benson GS, Corriere JN Jr. Diagnosis and initial management of urologic injuries associated with 200 consecutive pelvic fractures. J Urol 1983; 130(4):712–714.
90. Campbell JE. Urinary tract trauma. J Can Assoc Radiol 1983; 34(3):237–248.
91. Bick C, Oesterwitz H, Ziegler PF. Traumatic injuries of the lower ureter associated with pelvic fractures. Eur Urol 1984; 10(2):143–144.
92. Salomé F, Cazaux P, Setton D, Bothorel P, Colombeau P. Bladder entrapment during internal fixation of a pelvic fracture. J Urol 1999; 161(1):213–214.
93. Wright DG, Taitsman L, Laughlin RT. Pelvic and bladder trauma: a case report and subject review. J Orthop Trauma 1996; 10(5):351–354.
94. Kumar R, Schaff DC, Ostrowski ES. Entrapped urinary bladder: complication of pelvic trauma. Urology 1980; 16:82–83.
95. Orkin LA. Trauma to the bladder, ureter and kidney. In: Sciarra JJ, ed. Gynecology and Obstetrics, Vol. 1. Philadelphia: Lippincott, 1991:1.
96. Podesta ML, Jordan GH. Pelvic fracture urethral injuries in girls. J Urol 2001; 165:1660–1665.
97. Casselmann RC, Schillinger JF. Fractured pelvis with avulsion of the female urethra. J Urol 1977; 117:385–386.
98. Niemi TA, Norton LW. Vaginal injuries in patients with pelvic fractures. J Trauma 1985; 25(6):547–551.
99. Copeland LW, Bosse MJ, McCarthy ML, et al. Effect of trauma and pelvic fracture on female genitourinary, sexual, and reproductive function. J Orthop Trauma 1997; 11(2):73–81.
100. Andrich DE, Mundy AR. The nature of urethral injury in cases of pelvic fracture urethral trauma. J Urol 2001; 165(5):1492–1495.
101. Ozumba D, Starr AJ, Beneditti G, et al. Male sexual function after pelvic fracture. San Diego, CA: 17th Annual Meeting of the Orthopaedic Trauma Association, Oct 18–20, 2001, Poster No. 83.
102. Munarriz MR, Yan QR, Nehra A, Udelson D, Goldstein I. Blunt trauma: the pathophysiology of hemodynamic injury leading to erectile dysfunction. J Urol 1995; 153:1831–1840.
103. Epstein HC. Posterior fracture-dislocations fo the hip: long-term follow-up. J Bone joint Surg 1974; 56A:1103–1127.
104. Stewart MJ, Milford LW. Fracture-dislocation of the hip: an end-result study. J Bone Joint Surg 1954; 36A:315–342.
105. Stewart MJ, McCarroll HR Jr, Mulhollan JS. Fracture-dislocation of the hip. Acta Orthop Scand 1975; 46:507–525.
106. Gregory CF. Early complications of dislocation and fracture dislocations of the hip joint. Instr Course Lect 1973; 22:105–114.
107. Sunderland S. Nerve and Nerve Injuries, 2nd ed. Edinburgh: Churchill-Livingstone, 1978.
108. Hardy SL. Femoral nerve plasy associated with an associated posterior wall transverse acetabular fracture. J Orthop Trauma 1997; 11:40–42.
109. Helfet DL, Schmeling GJ. Somatosensory evoked potential monitoring in the surgical treatment of acute, displaced, acetabular fractures. Results of a prospective study. Clin Orthop 1994; 301:213–220.
110. Baumgaertner MR, Wegner D, Brooke J. SSEP monitoring during pelvic and acetabular fracture surgery. J Orthop Trauma 1994; 8(2):127–133.
111. Fassler PR, Swiontkowski MF, Kilroy AW, Routt ML Jr. Injury to the sciatic nerve associated with acetabular fracture. J Bone Joint Surg 1993; 75(A):1157–1166.

112. Helfet DL, Hissa EA, Sergay S, Mast JW. Somatosensory evoked potential monitoring in the surgical management of acute acetabular fractures. J Orthop Trauma 1991; 5(2):161–166.
113. Helfet DL, Anand N, Malkani ALL, et al. Intraoperative monitoring of motor pathways during operative fixation of acute acetabular fractures. J Orthop Trauma 1997; 11(1):2–6.
114. Middlebrooks ES, Sims SH, Kellam JF, Bosse MJ. Incidence of sciatic nerve injury in operatively treated acetabular fractures without somatosensory evoked potentials monitoring. J Orthop Trauma 1997; 11(5):327–329.
115. Vrahas M, Gordon RG, Mears DC, Krieger D, Sclabassi RJ. Intraoperative somatosensory evoked potentials monitoring of pelvic and acetabular fractures. J Orthop Trauma 1992; 6:50–58.
116. Epstein HC. Traumatic dislocations of the hip. Clin Orthop 1973; 92:116–142.
117. Nerubay J, Glancz G, Katznelson A. Fractures of the acetabulum. J Trauma 1973; 13:1050–1062.
118. Armstrong JR. Traumatic dislocation of the hip joint: review of one hundred and one dislocations. J Bone Joint Surg 1948; 30B:430–445.
119. Derian PS, Bibighaus AJ. Sciatic nerve entrapment by ectopic bone after posterior fracture-dislocation of the hip. South Med J 1974; 67:209–210.
120. Hart VL. Fracture dislocation of the hip. J Bone Joint Surg 1942; 24A:458–460.
121. Haw DWM. Complication following fracture dislocation of the hip. Br Med J 1965; 1:1111–1112.
122. Kleiman SG, Stevens J, Kolb L, Pankovic A. Late sciatic-nerve palsy following posterior fracture-dislocation of the hip: a case report. J Bone joint Surg 1971; 53A: 781–782.
123. Russell GV Jr, Nork SE, Routt MLC Jr. Perioperative complications associated with operative treatment of acetabular fractures. J Trauma 2001; 51(6):1098–1103.
124. Letournel E, Acetabulum fractures: classification and management. Clin Orthop 1980; 151:81–106.
125. Haidukewych GJ, Scaduto J, Herscovici D, Sanders RW, DiPasquale T. Iatrogenic nerve injury in acetabular fracture surgery: a comparison of monitored and unmonitored procedures. J Orthop Trauma 2002; 16(5):297–301.
126. Moed BR, Maxey JW, Minister GJ. Intraoperative somatosensory evoked potential monitoring of the sciatic nerve: an animal model. J Orthop Trauma 1992; 6:59–65.
127. Epstein HC, Wiss DA, Cozen L. Posterior fracture dislocation of the hip with fractures of the femoral head. Clin Orthop 1985; 201:9–17.
128. Baumgaertner MR, Wegner D, Booke J. SSEP monitoring during pelvic and acetabular fracture surgery. J Orthop Trauma 1994; 8(2):127–133.
129. Gruson KI, Moed BR. Injury of the femoral nerve associated with acetabular fracture. J Bone Joint Surg 2003; 85A(3):428–431.
130. Nobel W, Marks SC Jr, Kubik S. The anatomical basis for femoral nerve palsy following iliacus hematoma. J Neurosurg 1980; 51:531–534.
131. Barrington RL. Haemorrhagic femoral neuropathy. Injury 1982; 14:170–173.
132. Ghent WR. Further studies on meralgia paresthetica. Can Med Associ J 1961; 6:871–875.
133. Connolly JF. Closed treatment of pelvic and lower extremity fractures. Clin Orthop 1989; 240:115–128.
134. Patterson FP, Morton KS. Neurological complications of fractures and dislocations of the pelvis. J Trauma 1972; 12(12):1013–1023.
135. Henderson RC. The long-term results of non-operatively treated major pelvic disruptions. J Orthop Trauma 1989; 3(1):41–47.
136. Huittinen VM, Slatis P. Nerve injury in double vertical pelvic fractures. Acta Chir Scand 1972; 138(6):571–575.

137. Huittinen VM, Slatis P. Fractures of the pelvis: trauma mechanism, types of injury and principles of treatment. Acta Chir Scand 1972; 138(6):563–569.
138. Asprinio DE, Helfet DL, Tile M. Complications. In: Tile M, ed. Fractures of the Pelvis and Acetabulum, 2nd ed. Baltimore: Williams and Wilkins, 1995:224–245.
139. Burgess AR, Tile M. Fractures of the pelvis. In: Rockwood CA, Green DP, Bucholz RW, eds. Fractures in Adults, Vol. 2, 2nd ed. Philadelphia: JB Lippincott, 1991: 1399–1442.
140. Majeed SA. Neurologic deficits in major pelvic injuries. Clin Orthop 1992, 282:222–228.
141. Huittinen VM. Lumbosacral nerve injury in fracture of the pelvis: a postmortem radiographic and patho-anatomical study. Acta Chir Scand 1972; 429(suppl):3–43.
142. Reilly MC, Zinar DM, Matta JM. Neurologic injuries in pelvic ring fractures. Clin Orthop 1996; 329:28–36.
143. Denis F, Davis S, Comfort T. Sacral fractures: an important problem. Retrospective analysis of 236 cases. Clin Orthop 1988; 227:67–81.
144. Gibbons KJ, Soloniuk DS, Razack N. Neurological injury and patterns of sacral fractures. J Neurosurg 1990; 72(6):889–893.
145. Gunterberg B. Effects of major resection of the sacrum. Clinical studies on urogenital and anorectal function and a biomechanical study on pelvic strength. Acta Orthop Scand 1976; 162(suppl):1–38.
146. Semba R, Yasukawa K, Gustilo R. Critical analysis of results of 53 Malgaigne fractures of the pelvis. J Trauma 1983; 23(6):535–537.
147. Sidhu JS, Dhillon MK. Lumbosacral plexus avulsion with pelvic fractures. Injury 1991; 22:156–158.
148. Helfet D, Koval K, Hissa EA, et al. Intraoperative somatosensory evolked potential monitoring during acute pelvic fracture surgery. J Orthop Trauma 1995; 9(1):28–34.
149. Bosse MJ, Poka A, Reinert CM, Ellwanger R, Slawson R, McDevitt ER. Heterotopic ossification as a complication of acetabular fracture: prophylaxis with low-dose irradiation. J Bone Joint Surg 1988; 70A(8):1231–1237.
150. Matta JM, Siebenrock KA. Does indomethacin reduce heterotopic bone formation after operations for acetabular fractures? A prospective randomised study. J Bone Joint Surg 1997; 79B(6):959–963.
151. Slawson RG, Poka A, Bathon H, et al. The role of postoperative radiation in the prevention of heterotopic ossification in patients with post-traumatic acetabular fracture. Int J Radiat Oncol Biol Phys 1989; 17(3):669–672.
152. Wright R, Barrett K, Christie MJ, Johnson KD. Acetabular fractures: long-term follow-up of open reduction and internal fixation. J Orthop Trauma 1994; 8(5):397–403.
153. Kaempffe FA, Bone LB, Border JR. Open reduction and internal fixation of acetabular fractures: heterotopic ossification and other complications of treatment. J Orthop Trauma 1991; 5(4):439–445.
154. Webb LX, Bosse MJ, Mayo KA, et al. Results in patients with craniocerebral trauma and an operatively managed acetabular fracture. J Orthop Trauma 1990; 4(4):376–382.
155. Daum WJ, Scarborough MT, Gordon W Jr, Uchida T. Heterotopic ossification and other perioperative complications of acetabular fractures. J Orthop Trauma 1992; 6(4):427–432.
156. Rath EMS, Russell GV Jr, Washington WJ, Routt MLC Jr. Gluteus minimus necrotic muscle debridement diminishes heterotopic ossification after acetabular fixation. Injury 2002; 33(9):751–756.
157. Ayers DC, Pelligrini VD Jr, Evarts CM. Prevention of heterotopic ossification in high-risk patients by radiation therapy. Clin Orthop 1991; 263:87–93.
158. Sawyer JR, Myers MA, Rosier RN, Puzas JE. Heterotopic ossification: clinical and cellular aspects. Calcif Tissue Int 1991; 49(3):208–215.

159. Moed BR, Smith ST. Three-view radiographic assessment of heterotopic ossification after acetabular fracture surgery. J Orthop Trauma 1996; 10(2):93–98.
160. Moed BR, Letournel E. Low-dose irradiation and indomethacin prevent heterotopic ossification after acetabular fracture surgery. J Bone Joint Surg 1994; 76B(6):895–900.
161. Routt Jr ML, Swiontkowski MF. Operative treatment of complex acetabular fractures. Combined anterior and posterior exposures during the same procedure. J Bone Joint Surg 1990; 72A(6):897–904.
162. Burd TA, Lowry KJ, Anglen JO. Indomethacin compared with localized irradiation for the prevention of heterotopic ossification following surgical treatment of acetabular fractures. J Bone Joint Surg 2001; 83A(12):1783–1788.
163. Plasmans C, Kuypers W, Sloof TJ. The effect of of ethane-1-hydroxy-1, 1-diphosphonic acid (EHDP) on matrix induced ectopic bone formation. Clin Orthop 1978; 132:223–243.
164. Russell RGG, Smith R. Disphosphonates: experimental and clinical aspects. J Bone Joint Surg 1973; 55B:66–86.
165. Ahrengart L, Lindgren U, Reinhold FP. Comparative study of the effects of radiation, indomethacin, prednisolone, and ethane-1-hydroxy-1, 1-disphosphonate (EHDP) in the prevention of ectopic bone formation. Clin Orthop 1988; 229:265–273.
166. Thomas BJ, Amstutz HC. Results of the administration of diphosphonate for the prevention of heterotopic ossification after total hip arthroplasty. J Bone Joint Surg 1985; 67A:400–403.
167. Vane JR. Inhibition of prostaglandin synthesis as a mechanism of action for aspirin-like drugs. Nature New Biol 1971; 231:232–235.
168. Cella JP, Salvati EA, Sculco TP. Indomethacin for the prevention of heterotopic ossification following total hip arthroplasty. Effectiveness, contraindications and adverse effects. J Arthroplast 1988; 3:229–234.
169. Altman RD, Latta LL, Keer R, et al. Effect of nonsteroidal antiinflammatory drugs on fracture healing: a laboratory study in rats. J Orthop Trauma 1995; 9(5):392–400.
170. Bhalla AK, Simon LS. A clinical evaluation of the antiarthritic agents. Compr Ther 1984; 10(8):40–50.
171. Burd TA, Hughes MS, Anglen JO. Heterotopic ossification prophylaxis with Indomethacin increases the risk of long bone nonunion. Toronto, Ontario: 18th Annual Meeting Orthopaedic Trauma Association, Oct 11–13, 2002, Paper # 20.
172. Pittenger DE. Heterotopic ossification. Orthop Rev 1991; 20:33–39.
173. Kim JH, Chu FC, Woodard HQ, et al. Radiation-induced soft-tissue and bone sarcoma. Radiology 1978; 129:501–508.
174. Alonso JE, Volgas DA, Giorano V, Stannard JP. A review of the treatment of hip dislocations associated with acetabular fractures. Clin Orthop 2000; 377:32–43.
175. Ruesch PD, Holdener H, Ciaramitaro M, Mast JW. A prospective study of surgically treated acetabular fractures. Clin Orthop 1994; 305:38–46.
176. Norris BL, Hahn DH, Bosse MJ, Kellam JF, Sims SH. Intraoperative fluoroscopy to evaluate fracture reduction and hardware placement during acetabular surgery. J Orthop Trauma 1999; 13(6):414–417.
177. Anglen JO, DiPasquale T. The reliability of detecting screw penetration of the acetabulum by intraoperative auscultation. J Orthop Trauma 1994; 8:404–408.
178. Stubbart JR, Merkley M. Bowel entrapment within pelvic fractures: a case report and review of the literature. J Orthop Trauma 1999; 13(2):145–150.
179. Hammit MD, Cole PA, Kregor PJ. Massive perineal wound slough after treatment of complex pelvic and acetabular fractures using a traction table. J Orthop Trauma 2002; 16(8):601–605.

180. Kellam JF, Browner BD. Fractures of the pelvic ring. In: Browner BD, Jupiter JB, Levine AM, Trafton PG, eds. Skeletal Trauma, 2nd ed. Philadelphia, PA: Saunders, 1998: 1120–1174.
181. Chan PTK, Schondorf R, Brock GB. Erectile dysfunction induced by orthopaedic trauma managed with a fracture table: a case report and review of the literature. J Trauma 1999; 47(1):183–185.
182. Lyon T, Koval KJ, Kummer F, Zuckerman JD. Pudendal nerve palsy induced by fracture table. Orthop Rev 1993; 22(5):521–525.
183. Fridman M, Glass AM, Noronha JAP, Carvalhal EF, Martini RK. Spontaneous urinary voiding of a metallic implant after operative fixation of the pubic symphysis. J Bone Joint Surg 2003; 85A:1129–1132.

16
Psychosocial Sequelae of Pelvic Injury

Allison E. Williams and Wade R. Smith
Department of Orthopaedics, Denver Health Medical Center, University of Colorado School of Medicine, Denver, Colorado, U.S.A.

INTRODUCTION

Although pelvic fractures represent a small percentage of all fractures, they are a significant health problem in the United States. It is estimated that 61,000 people in the United States suffer a pelvic injury each year, and that the incidence of severe pelvic injury is increasing (1–3). For multiple reasons, pelvic fractures are associated with significant physical and psychological morbidity. Among these are mechanism of injury, severity of injury, and unique anatomical and physiological aspects of the pelvic region. Pelvic injuries typically result from high-energy, blunt force trauma, with motor vehicle collisions (MVCs) being the major cause of pelvic fractures in younger persons and falls in the elderly population. Pelvic fractures are often accompanied by other injuries. These associated injuries usually occur in areas surrounding the pelvis and the lower extremities such as the genitourinary organs, liver, spleen, lumbosacral plexus, iliac vessels, femur, and tibia. Given the vital functions located in the pelvic region, pelvic injury not only restricts mobility, but may also interfere with highly personal activities such as elimination and sexual relations. These interacting factors make pelvic fracture a condition that is ripe for psychosocial problems, including psychological disorders, genitourinary and sexual dysfunction, and alterations in social identity. While improvements in critical care have decreased mortality and physical morbidity, the psychosocial sequelae of pelvic fractures have not been adequately explored.

PSYCHOLOGICAL DISORDERS FOLLOWING TRAUMA

Presently, few studies have specifically evaluated the psychological impact of pelvic fractures in an adult population. However, studies have indicated that psychological distress following pelvic fracture is a significant issue in the pediatric population (4,5). Subasi et al. (4) examined 58 children who experienced unstable pelvic fractures and assessed urologic outcomes as well as psychiatric data. To assess psychiatric status, both the parents and children were interviewed by a psychiatric specialist. Fifty-six percent (31) of the children were found to have a psychiatric disorder, five of whom had two diagnoses and three of whom had three diagnoses. The diagnoses included dysthymic disorder, social phobia, post-traumatic stress disorder (PTSD), major depression, and specific phobia. The prevalence of psychiatric disorders was significantly higher than the normal population. Similar results were found in 49 children who sustained a posterior urethral rupture secondary to pelvic fracture. Twenty-one (42.9%) of the children developed a psychiatric disorder, including dysthymic disorder, social phobia, PTSD, separation anxiety, major depression, and generalized anxiety disorder. The development of a psychiatric disorder was significantly associated with number of urologic procedures, long-term complications, and total number of hospitalizations consequent to the injury.

While there are physical characteristics of the pelvis unique to children, and developmental differences that distinguish pediatric and adult mental health, current literature indicates that adults are also at risk for developing a psychological disorder following a pelvic fracture. Over the past decade, psychological sequelae have become recognized as potential consequences of injury that can have a deleterious effect on patient outcomes. In particular, a large number of studies have demonstrated psychological problems related to MVCs, which likely capture people who have had pelvic fractures. The most extensively examined psychological disorders are PTSD and depression.

Post-traumatic Stress Disorder

PTSD is an anxiety disorder that follows exposure to an event that is perceived as life threatening or has the potential to cause a serious injury (6). PTSD is characterized by a constellation of symptoms that fall into three domains: intrusion, avoidance, and arousal. The intrusion domain includes symptoms such as recurrent flashbacks and frightening dreams in which the person relives the experience. The avoidance domain consists of symptoms that function to isolate the person from memories of the trauma and significant others. The arousal domain includes symptoms such as insomnia, irritability, and hypervigilance. Persons with PTSD may experience symptoms in one or all of these domains. Symptoms that have persisted for less than three months are considered acute, and symptoms that have persisted for more than three months are considered chronic. In some cases, symptoms may develop more than six months following exposure to a traumatic event. This is referred to as delayed onset PTSD.

PTSD following an injury has been recognized as a significant source of morbidity. Multiple prospective studies have demonstrated that a significant percentage of people develop symptoms of PTSD following general traumatic injury (7–9). However, in the orthopedic trauma population, the incidence of PTSD appears to be even higher than it is in the general trauma population. One multisite study indicated that more than half of the patients with traumatic orthopedic injuries (51% of 580 patients) developed PTSD (10).

Significantly, studies examining patient outcomes demonstrate that PTSD is among the most predictive variables of functional outcome following injury. In a retrospective study examining persons with moderate traumatic injury, PTSD was found to contribute more to perceived general health than injury severity or the degree of physical functioning (7). A prospective study examining posttraumatic stress, problem drinking, and functional outcome after injury also found that, one year after injury, PTSD was the strongest predictor of an adverse outcome (9). Another prospective study demonstrated that the most predictive variable for health, work satisfaction, and general functional outcomes was mental health as measured by the SF-36 mental health subscale. While this subscale is inclusive of PTSD, it also suggests that other psychological symptoms and conditions may explain variation in patient outcomes. Michaels et al. (8) identified major depression as one of those conditions.

Depression

Few studies have examined depression following traumatic injury, however, there is evidence that depression is a problem that affects many injured patients. Estimates of depression following injury range from 14.2% to 42% (8,11,12). Significantly, Michaels et al. (7,8) found that the prevalence of depression increased with time from 18.6% at baseline to 40% at six months and 42% one year postinjury. In contrast, the prevalence of PTSD within this sample decreased from 41.3% to 38% at six months and one year, respectively. Baseline PTSD was not measured. Studies have also indicated that a large percentage of persons with PTSD following injury have comorbid depression. In one study, 59% of persons with PTSD also had major depression four months postinjury (12). Importantly, persons with cooccurring PTSD and major depression report more symptoms, greater distress from their symptoms, and are judged to have poorer functioning than persons who have PTSD or major depression alone (12).

ETIOLOGY OF POST-TRAUMATIC PSYCHOLOGICAL SEQUELAE

There is no single conceptual framework that explains the etiology of psychological sequelae following trauma. Although most people who are exposed to a traumatic event experience psychological symptoms, there is limited information concerning what distinguishes persons who will develop chronic psychological problems from those whose psychological symptoms will resolve independently (13). Among the potential predictors of PTSD that researchers have identified are personal characteristics and injury circumstances.

Personal Characteristics

Personal characteristics that have been examined include body awareness, pre-existing psychological conditions, history of trauma, and physiological response patterns.

Additionally, there is evidence that there may be a genetic predisposition not only toward the development of post-traumatic psychological sequelae, but also to exposure to traumatic events (14–16). Some studies have indicated that persons who are overly focused on internal sensations are more likely to experience physical discomfort as well as cognitive and psychological symptoms (17). The researchers imply that, for these persons, the perception is incongruent with the actual condition and may amplify it. Consequently, it may be that persons who are more focused on internal sensations are more likely to develop—or perceive—physical and psychological discomfort following an injury.

There is also evidence that a history of trauma may predispose a person to PTSD following a traumatic injury. In particular, retrospective studies have shown that persons who are exposed repeatedly to prolonged traumatic events are more likely to develop PTSD than persons who experience an isolated trauma. Additionally, these studies have indicated that exposure to trauma frequently exacerbates pre-existing psychological conditions (18–20).

Yehuda et al. (13), however, challenged the results of these studies. Their review of the literature indicated that while retrospective studies show clear relationships between psychological variables and the development of PTSD, these findings are not confirmed in prospective studies. Indeed, in one prospective study (21), no significant relationships were found between gender, age, past psychiatric history, prior trauma, injury severity, pain severity, and the subsequent development of PTSD. Instead, the literature indicates that the most predictive indicators of the development of PTSD following trauma are not psychological characteristics but biological responses. Yehuda et al. (13) stated that, in the aggregate, studies suggest that people who develop PTSD have aberrant physiological responses to stress. For example, victims of trauma who subsequently develop PTSD have lower cortisol levels when they are in the emergency department (ED) than those who do not develop PTSD. Additionally, persons who went on to develop PTSD had a higher mean heart rate in the ED and at the one-week follow-up visit than those who did not.

Yehuda et al. (13) speculate that PTSD emerges as a result of "disruptions in the normal cascade of the fear response and its resolution" (p. 11). In addition, they propose that the disruption can lead not only to PTSD, but also to other psychological disturbances such as depression.

Further support for a relationship between biological factors and posttraumatic psychological conditions is demonstrated in a study examining differences in inflammatory markers between healthy persons and patients diagnosed with PTSD (22). Plasma levels of pro- and anti-inflammatory markers were measured and the groups were compared. The proinflammatory markers included C-reactive protein (CRP), interleukin (IL)-1β, IL-6, and tumor necrosis factor (TNF)-α. Antiinflammatory markers measured included IL-4 and IL-10. For the PTSD group, the inflammatory markers were also analyzed in relation to symptom clusters. The study findings indicated that patients with PTSD had significantly higher levels of proinflammatory circulating interleukin IL-1β and TNF-α and significantly lower levels of antiinflammatory circulating IL-4. Additionally, TNF-α was found to have a significant positive relationship with severity of PTSD as well as the individual symptom clusters avoidance, hyperarousal, and re-experiencing. IL-1β had a significant, positive correlation with avoidance symptoms.

Although lack of premorbid data prohibit establishing a causal relationship, the study does indicate that patients with PTSD may be more likely to experience a proinflammatory state that could have a negative effect on overall health. Significantly, the relationship between proinflammatory markers and symptom clusters suggest that prior to meeting the criteria for a PTSD diagnosis, persons may exhibit a proinflammatory response following trauma.

A biological relationship between depression and trauma has also been indicated. A recent study suggests that IL-6 is a component in the pathogenesis of stress-induced depression (23). This study compared behavioral responses to basal, stressful, and learned helpless conditions in IL-6 knockout versus wild-type male mice. No behavioral differences were found between groups during the basal activity, during which the mice were observed during regular open field activity. However, differences were found in the stress-inducing and learned helplessness activities.

To induce stress the mice were place in a dark-light box. As mice prefer dark sheltered spaces, it was presumed that the light would present an anxiety-inducing situation, which would encourage the mice to move to the dark area. In this test, the knockout mice displayed increased anxiety and spent less time in the brightly illuminated area. A learned helplessness model was used to assess depression-like behavior. The model evaluated the coping capabilities of mice by subjecting them to a series of unpredictable and uncontrollable foot shocks. Knockout mice exhibited less depression-like behavior as demonstrated by significantly fewer escape latencies and escape failures. To measure despair, the mice participated in a forced swim test and were subjected to a tail suspension test. For both of these tests, the knockout mice demonstrated significantly less time immobile. Hedonic alterations were also assessed. The reinforcing properties of glucose were evaluated to determine if there was a difference in sensitivity to rewards between knockout IL-6 mice and wild-type mice. The findings indicated that IL-6 knockout mice were significantly more sensitive to glucose reinforcement than the wild-type mice. Upon necropsy, alteration in IL-6 levels in the brain was measured, and the wild-type mice were compared to sham-treated mice. The wild-type mice exhibited significantly higher levels of IL-6 in the hippocampus than the sham group. The study suggests that the production of IL-6 is associated with the development and/or maintenance of depression and despair.

Injury Characteristics

Injury characteristics have also been examined in the literature. A somewhat unexpected, but consistent finding is that the development of PTSD cannot be predicted according to the severity of injury (9,13,18,20). People who experience minor physical injuries appear to be as vulnerable to psychological sequelae as those who suffer severe physical injuries. Two factors relating to the event have been explored to explain this finding. The first is the person's perception of the traumatic event. Those who perceive the event as a threat to their life are more likely to develop PTSD than those who do not, regardless of the actual outcome of the event. The second is peritraumatic dissociation. People who experience an alteration in awareness around the time of the accident—for example, alterations in perceptions of time, feeling as if they are separated from their body—are more likely to develop symptoms of PTSD than persons who do not experience peritraumatic dissociation (24). Of interest, this study also found that people with a history of major depression were more vulnerable to peritraumatic dissociation. Thus, it appears that a person's psychological history is related to the evolution of post-traumatic psychological sequelae, suggesting that there is a complex interaction between psychology and physiology that influences a person's psychological response to trauma.

Clearly, the etiology of PTSD as well as other post-traumatic psychological sequelae remains unknown. Nonetheless, it is evident that there is a high incidence of psychological sequelae that results from trauma.

SEXUAL FUNCTIONING

Pelvic fractures have also been shown to affect genitourinary and sexual functioning in both males and females. These effects have been found to be both physiological and psychological in nature. All studies have reported that pelvic fractures create a risk for genitourinary and sexual dysfunction, and that multifactorial, genitourinary, and sexual dysfunction have been shown to have a profound impact on a person's life.

In males, sexual function following pelvic fracture has been studied in relation to sexual drive and erectile function. Sexual drive focuses on overall satisfaction with sexual life as well as whether the man finds his sexual functioning personally problematic. Erectile function includes the quality, or firmness, of an erection, and the ability to attain an erection, maintain an erection, and ejaculate.

Several studies have focused on erectile function following a pelvic fracture. A detailed description of all of these investigations is beyond the scope of this chapter; however, a review article summarizing articles concerning erectile dysfunction after pelvic fracture estimated postinjury male sexual dysfunction to be as high as 30% (25). This percentage was even higher in males who incurred a concomitant urethral injury. Harwood et al. (25) state that studies as a whole have indicated that for these males the incidence of erectile dysfunction (ED) following pelvic injury was 42%.

Harwood et al. (25) describe the pathogenesis of ED as a combination of neurogenic, vascular, corporal, and psychogenic injury. Thus, ED is a complex condition that likely involves multiple systems. What remains to be determined is whether these injuries contributing to ED result from the initial insult, treatment, or both. Fracture management, pelvic arteriography and embolization, and timing of urological interventions have all been indicated as having the potential to prevent or create further physical injury that may result in ED. Additionally, the patient's psychological experience of invasive procedures and prolonged hospitalization may mitigate or exacerbate psychological responses. It is remarkable that sexual dysfunction in persons with PTSD has been reported as high as 80%. Given the high percentage of persons reporting PTSD following trauma, this prevalence underscores the need for providers to address the patients' psychological needs.

While most studies of ED have used physiological evaluations, such as electromyography (EMG), pharmacologic testing, and penile angiography, a notable exception is a study that evaluated male sexual function after bilateral internal iliac artery embolization (BIIAE) for pelvic fracture (26). Ramirez et al. (26) conducted a telephone survey using a questionnaire consisting of 24 items that assessed medical history, urinary function, and male sexual function. Three groups were surveyed: those who had a pelvic fracture and received BIIAE (group 1), those who had a pelvic fracture and did not receive BIIAE (group 2), and a healthy control group (group 3). There were 16 subjects in each group. Items assessing male sexual function included subjective rankings of sexual drive, erection firmness, ejaculatory function, and overall sex life. Additionally, subjects were queried regarding how personally problematic they found their sex life.

No differences for any of these items were found between the fracture groups. However, both group 1 and group 2 reported significantly lower scores for erectile function, sexual drive, and overall satisfaction with sexual life than the health control group. Furthermore, sexual function was perceived as personally more problematic in a higher proportion of both fracture groups than it was by the healthy controls. Subjects in the fracture groups also gave lower scores for ejaculatory function. Overall, the incidence of ED in the fractures groups was 19% while no healthy controls reported ED. While the intent of the article was to demonstrate the safety of BIIAE, the study provided a unique window into male's perception of sexual functioning. These results indicate that pelvic fracture has a negative impact on physical and psychological aspects of male sexuality.

Ramirez et al. (26) also assessed urinary function. Items on the questionnaire queried participants regarding difficulty voiding and urinary continence. No differences for either of these items were found among the groups. However, studies have indicated that a significant number of men do experience urinary problems following pelvic fracture. Men who have suffered damage to the urethra are especially vulnerable (27,28).

Sexual and genitourinary functions following pelvic injury has not been as extensively studied in females as it has in males. However, studies suggest that pelvic injury does affect female sexuality and genitourinary function. A study of 223 women with pelvis fractures only ($n = 84$), a pelvis fracture and lower extremity fracture ($n = 39$), and a lower extremity fracture only ($n = 110$) indicated that pelvic fracture is significantly associated with negative changes in sexual functioning (29). In telephone surveys conducted by trained female interviewers, the patients were administered the SF-36, supplemented with questions concerning sexual functioning. Overall, women in all groups reported some effect of the injury on their sexuality. Forty-five percent reported feeling less attractive, 19% reported less frequent sexual activity, 39% experienced less sexual pleasure, and 24% reported dyspareunia and hip and lower back pain during intercourse. Women with a pelvic fracture, however, suffered more negative changes, which although not statistically significant, were likely clinically significant to them. Furthermore, severity of the pelvic injury was found to be significantly associated with dyspareunia, feeling less attractive, and experiencing less sexual pleasure. Interestingly, associated injuries, including facial, genitourinary, and abdominal injuries, were not associated with sexual function.

Another study examining the effect of trauma and pelvic fracture on female genitourinary, sexual, and reproductive function produced similar findings (30). This study also compared women with pelvic fractures (group 1, $N = 123$) to those with a lower extremity fracture (group 2, $N = 110$), and was composed of the same subjects in the study cited above. An outcomes questionnaire covering the following domains was administered over the telephone by professional female interviewers: demographics, urinary and gastrointestinal symptoms, reproduction, and sexual function.

With respect to sexual function, a small percentage reported problems with physiologic arousal. Seven percent of women in the pelvic fracture group and 12% of women in the lower extremity group indicated that they had problems reaching orgasm. In addition, only a small percentage of women indicated a higher threshold to orgasm (5% in group 1 vs. 7% in group 2), decreased intensity of orgasm (3% in group 1 vs. 4% in group 2), and decreased ability to lubricate (3% in group 1 vs. 6% in group 2). However, a larger percentage of women in both groups reported new onset of pain during sex following their injury (group 1, 31% and group 2, 24%). Coital musculoskeletal pain was similar between the groups, but gynecological pain during intercourse was significantly more in group 1 (19%) than group 2 (9.5%) ($p = 0.045$). For subjects in group 1, fracture displacement contributed to reports of musculoskeletal and gynecologic pain during intercourse. Significantly more subjects with fractures displaced $\geq$5 mm at follow-up reported musculoskeletal and gynecologic pain during intercourse than those with fractures displaced <5 mm (43% and 25%, respectively, $p = 0.04$). It is notable that the majority of women in group 1 (76%) and group 2 (87%) reported that they received no instructions or information from their health care providers regarding the resumption of sexual activity.

The study also revealed that subjects in group 1 were significantly more likely to have urinary complaints than those in group 2 (21% vs. 7%, $p = 0.003$), and the majority had more than one complaint. Among the urinary complaints were cystitis, nocturia, stress incontinence, frequency, incontinence, and retention. The most frequent complaints indicated by group 1 were stress incontinence (13%) and frequency of urination (13%), both of which were significantly higher than group 2 ($p = 0.007$ and $p = 0.02$, respectively). There was also a significantly higher incidence of nocturia in group 1 than in group 2 ($p = 0.04$). Urinary complaints, similar to sexual dysfunction, were also significantly associated with fracture displacement. Group 1 subjects with initial and residual fracture displacement $\geq$5 mm were significantly more likely to report urinary tract complaints than subjects with fracture displacement <5mm ($p = 0.02$ and $p = 0.018$, respectively).

Findings concerning the impact of trauma and pelvic fracture on reproduction were inconclusive. No significant differences were found between the groups for miscarriage rates, and 6% of both groups reported infertility after the injury. A significant difference was found in the number of Cesarean sections performed for group 1 subjects before and after the injury ($p < 0.001$). However, it is not clear whether this was due to the pelvic fracture or other factors concerning parturition such as a prior Cesarean section. It is probable that reproductive function is of concern to young women who have experienced a pelvic injury and further research needs to be conducted to understand if and how pelvic fracture affects reproduction.

SOCIAL ROLE

The physical and psychological consequences of pelvic fracture have an impact on aspects of social functioning, including work status, interpersonal relationships, and life choices. Pelvic injuries frequently result in chronic pain and physical disability, which prevent a person from returning to his or her former employment. People who are able to return to employment may not be able to perform as effectively as before, and are forced to reduce their work commitment or modify their activities. In one study examining outcomes of patients with pelvic ring fractures, 76% of patients returned to work full-time, and, of these, 62% were full time and 14% had job modifications (30). Nonetheless, for nearly one-fourth of these patients, employment, and, inevitably, financial status, were negatively affected by their pelvic fracture.

Interpersonal relationships are also affected by injury, particularly when a person has to assume a prolonged role of dependency. Persons who experience a pelvic fracture have limited mobility and must rely on others to assist with basic, personal activities, such as bathing, dressing, and elimination. Loss of independence can be a difficult adjustment and can put stress on relationships with significant others. Furthermore, if the person develops a psychological condition following a pelvic fracture, this can add additional stress to important relationships. While studies indicate that strong support networks can have a positive affect on functional outcome, significant psychological morbidity can create tension that undermines interpersonal relationships. Family members and friends are often unprepared to manage psychological symptoms and may respond to symptoms inappropriately. Additionally, if one develops sexual dysfunction following pelvic injury, this can create or exacerbate problems in their relationship with their partner. Interpersonal relationships can be challenging in the absence of injury, and response to a significant injury is likely related to preinjury characteristics of the relationship system.

Social aspects of pelvic injury are particularly important to consider in the pediatric population. Pediatric pelvic fractures often require prolonged hospitalizations, multiple surgeries, and cause gait and genitourinary dysfunction that may lead to acute or chronic psychological conditions (4,5). In turn, these conditions may stunt social development and inhibit optimal life functioning. Subasi et al. (4) reported that, for children in their study, education had been negatively affected by long hospital stays, surgeries, and follow-up visits. Significantly, children who experienced prolonged hospitalization exhibited connection disorders with family, friends, and health care personnel. Physical problems exacerbated social isolation as well. Children who had an abnormal gait, urinary incontinence, or an indwelling catheter tended to avoid social situations.

CONCLUSION

Psychosocial consequences of pelvic injury include, but are not limited to, psychological symptoms, genitourinary and sexual dysfunction, and alterations in social identity. Although the etiology of symptom development has yet to be determined, the literature indicates that these are common problems for which all patients who experience pelvic fracture are at risk. Establishing multidisciplinary care plans that attend to the psychosocial as well as the physiological needs of patients with pelvic fractures can help diminish psychosocial sequelae and improve patient outcomes.

REFERENCES

1. Gänsslen A, Pohlemann T, Paul CH, Lobenhoffer PH, Tscherre H. Epidemiology of pelvic ring injuries. Injury 1996; 27(suppl 1):13–20.
2. Prevalence and incidence statistics for pelvic fractures. Available: http://www.wrenaldiagnosis.com/p/pelvic_fracture/stats.htm (accessed March 16 2000).
3. Inaba K, Sharkey PW, Stephen DJ, Redelmeier DA, Brenneman FD. The increasing incidence of severe pelvic injury in motor vehicle collisions. Injury 2004; 35;759–765.
4. Subasi M, Arslan H, Necmioglu S, et al. Long-term outcomes of conservatively treated paediatric pelvic fractures. Injury 2004; 35:771–781.
5. Onen A, Subasi M, Arslan H, Ozen S, Basuguy E. Long-term urologic, orthopaedic, and psychological outcome of posterior urethral rupture in children. Pediatr Urol 2005; 66(1):174–179.
6. American Psychiatric Association. Diagnostic and Statistical Manual of Mental Disorders, 4th ed. Washington, D.C.: American Psychiatric Association, 1994.
7. Michaels A, Michaels C, Moon C, et al. Posttraumatic stress disorder after injury: impact on general health outcome and early risk assessment. J Trauma 1999; 47:460–466.
8. Michaels A, Michaels C, Smith J, et al. Outcome from injury: general health, work status, and satisfaction 12 months after trauma. J Trauma 2000; 48:841–848.
9. Zatzick D, Jurkovich G, Gentilillo L, Wisner D, Rivara F. Posttraumatic stress, problem drinking, and functional outcomes after injury. Arc Surg 2002; 184(2):200–205.
10. Starr A, Smith W, Frawley W, et al. Symptoms of post-traumatic stress disorder after orthopaedic trauma. J Bone Joint Surg Am 2003; 86A(6):1115–1121.
11. McCarthy M, MacKenzie E, Edwin D, et al. Psychological distress associated with severe lower-limb injury. J Bone Joint Surg Am 2003; 85A(9):1689–1697.
12. Shalev A, Freedman S, Peri T, et al. Prospective study of posttraumatic stress disorder and depression following trauma. Am J Psyc 1998; 155:630–637.
13. Yehuda R, MacFarlane A, Shalev A. Predicting the development of posttraumatic stress disorder from the acute response to a traumatic event. Biol Psyc 1998; 44(12):1305–1313.
14. Lawford BR, Young R, Noble EP, Kann B, Ritchie T. The D_2 dopamine receptor (DRD2) gene is associated with co-morbid depression, anxiety and social dysfunction in untreated veterans with post-traumatic stress disorder. Euro Psyc 2006; 21:180–185.
15. Lee HJ, Lee MS, Kang RH, et al. Influence of the serotonin transporter promoter gene polymorphism on susceptibility to posttraumatic stress disorder. Depress Anxiety 2005; 21:135–139.
16. Stein, MB, Jang KL, Taylor S, Vernon PA, Livesley WJ. Genetic and environmental influences on trauma exposure and posttraumatic stress disorder symptoms: a twin study. Am J Psyc 2002; 159(10):1675–1681.
17. Van der Werf S, van de Vree B, van der Meer J, Bleijenberg G. The relations among body consciousness, somatic symptom report, and information processing speed in chronic fatigue syndrome. Neuropsyc, Neuropsychat Behavl Neurol 2002; 15(1):2–9.
18. Joy D, Probert R, Bisson J, Shepherd J. Posttraumatic stress reactions after injury. J Trauma 2000; 48:490–494.
19. Ursano R, Fullerton C, Epstein R, et al. Acute and chronic posttraumatic stress disorder in motor vehicle accident victims. Am J Psyc 1999; 156(4):589–595.
20. Schnyder U, Morgeli H, Nigg C, et al. Early psychological reactions to life-threatening injuries. Critic Care Med 2000; 28(1):86–92.
21. McFarlane AC. The prevalence and longitudinal course of PTSD. Implications for the neurobiological models of PTSD. Ann NY Acad Sci 1997; 821:10–23.

22. Von Kanel R, Hepp U, Kraemer B, et al. Evidence for low-grade systemic proinflammatory activity in patients with posttraumatic stress disorder. J Psyc Res 2006, in press.
23. Chourbaji S, Urani A, Inta I, et al. IL-6 knockout mice exhibit resistance to stress-induced development of depression-like behaviors. Neurobiol Dis 2006; 23:587–594.
24. Fullerton C, Ursano R, Epstein R, et al. Peritraumatic dissociation following motor vehicle accidents: relationship to prior trauma and prior major depression. J Nerv and Ment Dis 2000; 188(5):267–272.
25. Harwood PJ, Grotz M, Eardley I, Giannoudis PV. Erectile dysfunction after fracture of the pelvis. J Bone Joint Surg 2005; 87B:281–290.
26. Ramirez JI, Velmahos GC, Best CR, Chan LS, Demetriades D. Male sexual function after bilateral internal iliac artery embolization for pelvic fracture. JT 2004; 56(4):734–741.
27. Brandes S, Borrelli J. Pelvic fracture and associated urologic injuries. World J Surg 2001; 25:1578–1587.
28. Asci R, Sarikay S, Buyukalpelli R, et al. Voiding and sexual dysfunctions after pelvic fracture urethral injuries treated with either initial cystostomy and delayed urethroplasty or immediate primary urethral realignment. Scan J Urol Nephrol 1999; 33:228–233.
29. McCarthy ML, MacKenzie EJ, Bosse MJ, et al. Functional status following orthopedic trauma in young women. J Trauma 1995; 39(5):828–837.
30. Copeland C, Bosse M, McCarthy M, et al. Effect of trauma and pelvic fracture on female genitourinary, sexual, and reproductive function. J Orthop Trauma 1997; 11(2):73–81.
31. Hakin RM, Gruen GS, Delitto A. Outcomes of patients with pelvic-ring fractures managed by open reduction internal fixation. Physical Therapy 1996; 75(3):286–295.
32. King JA, Abend S, Edwards E. Genetic predisposition and the development of posttraumatic stress disorder in an animal model. Biological Society 2001; 50:231–237.

Index

Italics indicate pages containing illustrations.

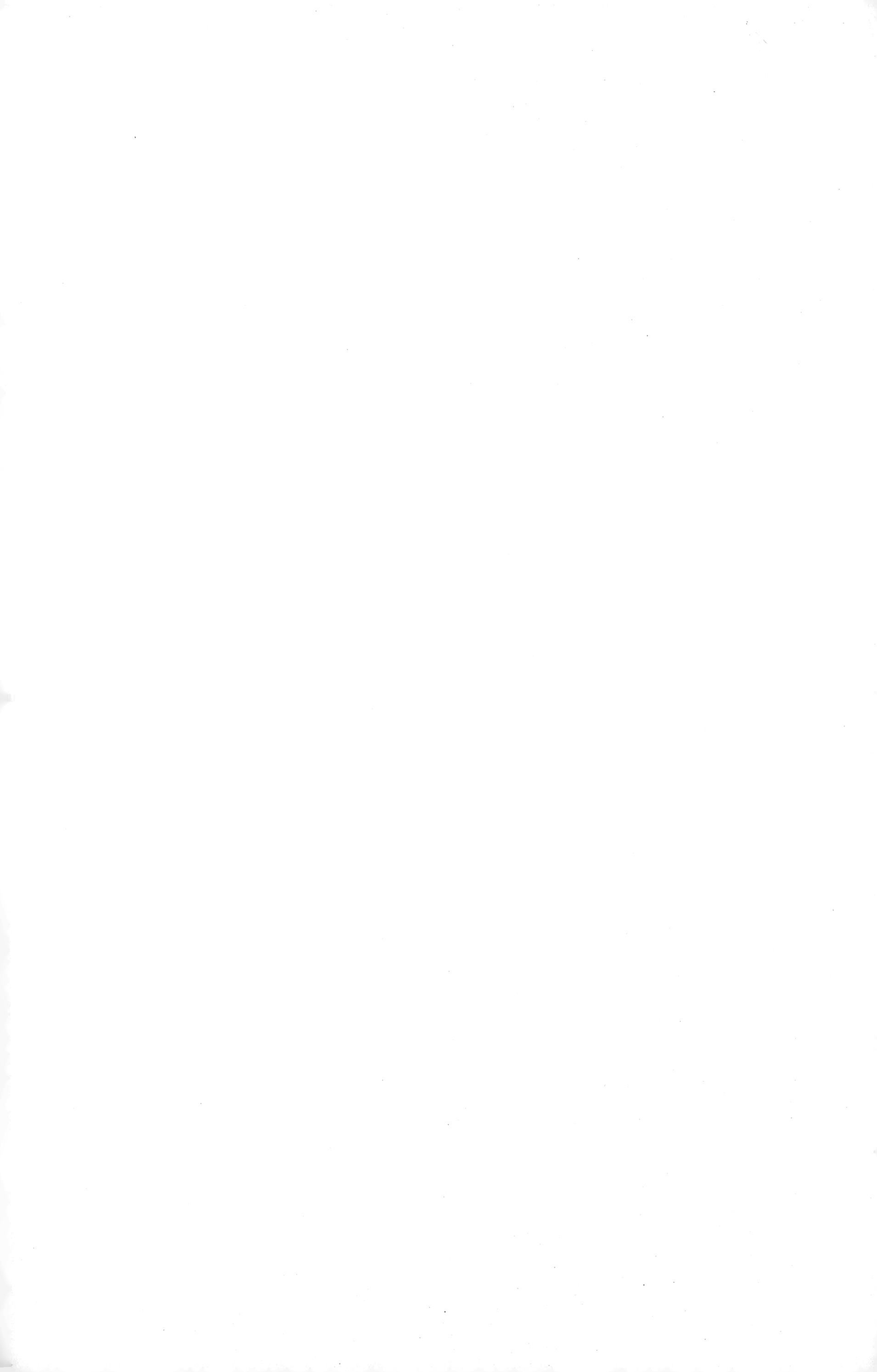